Gastrointestinal
Ultrasonography

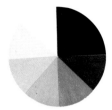

CLINICS IN DIAGNOSTIC ULTRASOUND
VOLUME 23

Volumes Already Published

Gastrointestinal Ultrasonography

Edited by

Alfred B. Kurtz, M.D.

Professor
Department of Radiology
Jefferson Medical College of
    Thomas Jefferson University
Associate Director
Division of Diagnostic Ultrasound
Department of Radiology
Thomas Jefferson University Hospital
Philadelphia, Pennsylvania

Barry B. Goldberg, M.D.

Professor
Department of Radiology
Jefferson Medical College of
    Thomas Jefferson University
Director
Division of Diagnostic Ultrasound
Department of Radiology
Thomas Jefferson University Hospital
Philadelphia, Pennsylvania

CHURCHILL LIVINGSTONE
NEW YORK, EDINBURGH, LONDON, MELBOURNE
1988

Library of Congress Cataloging-in-Publication Data

Gastrointestinal ultrasonography / edited by Alfred B. Kurtz, Barry B. Goldberg.
　　p. cm.—(Clinics in diagnostic ultrasound ; v. 23)
　Includes bibliographies and index.
　ISBN 0-443-08574-9
　1. Digestive organs—Diseases—Diagnosis.　2. Digestive organs—Ultrasonic imaging.　I. Kurtz, Alfred B.　II. Goldberg, Barry B., date– 　. III. Series.
　[DNLM: 　1. Gastrointestinal Diseases—diagnosis.
2. Gastrointestinal System—pathology.　3. Ultrasonic Diagnosis.
W1 CL831BC v. 23 / WI 141 G25795]
RC804.U4G37　1988
616.3'307543—dc19
DNLM/DLC
for Library of Congress　　　　　　　　　　　　　　　　88-10849
　　　　　　　　　　　　　　　　　　　　　　　　　　　CIP

© **Churchill Livingstone Inc. 1988**

Distributed in the United Kingdom by Churchill Livingstone, Robert Stevenson House, 1–3 Baxter's Place, Leith Walk, Edinburgh EH1 3AF, and by associated companies, branches, and representatives throughout the world.

Accurate indications, adverse reactions, and dosage schedules for drugs are provided in this book, but it is possible that they may change. The reader is urged to review the package information data of the manufacturers of the medications mentioned.

The Publishers have made every effort to trace the copyright holders for borrowed material. If they have inadvertently overlooked any, they will be pleased to make the necessary arrangements at the first opportunity.

Acquisitions Editor: *Linda Panzarella*
Copy Editor: *Kimberly Quinlan*
Production Designer: *Charlie Lebeda*
Production Supervisor: *Sharon Tuder*

Printed in the United States of America

First published in 1988

Contributors

Giovanna Casola, M.D.
Assistant Professor, Department of Radiology, University of California, San Diego, School of Medicine; Chief, Interventional Radiology and Abdominal CT, Veterans Administration Medical Center, La Jolla, California

Martin I. Cohen, M.D.
Fellow, Imaging and Interventional Radiology, Department of Radiology, University of California, San Diego School of Medicine, La Jolla, California; Fellow, UCDS Medical Center, San Diego, California

Paul A. Dubbins, F.R.C.R.
Consultant in Charge, Department of Diagnostic Ultrasound, Plymouth General Hospital, Freedom Fields, Plymouth, England

Barry B. Goldberg, M.D.
Professor, Department of Radiology, Jefferson Medical College of Thomas Jefferson University; Director, Division of Diagnostic Ultrasound, Department of Radiology, Thomas Jefferson University Hospital, Philadelphia, Pennsylvania

Michael C. Hill, M.B.
Professor, Department of Radiology, George Washington University; Tomography and Ultrasound Division, Department of Radiology, George Washington University Hospital, Washington, D.C.

Robert A. Kane, M.D.
Assistant Professor, Department of Radiology, Harvard Medical School; Director, Department of Diagnostic Ultrasound, New England Deaconess Hospital, Boston Massachusetts

Alfred B. Kurtz, M.D.
Professor, Department of Radiology, Jefferson Medical College of Thomas Jefferson University; Associate Director, Division of Diagnostic Ultrasound, Department of Radiology, Thomas Jefferson University Hospital, Philadelphia, Pennsylvania

Ian M. Lande, M.D., C.M., F.R.C.P.(C)
Assistant Professor, Department of Radiology, George Washington University; Senior Consultant, Magnetic Rosonance Imaging, Department of Radiology, George Washington University Hospital, Washington, D.C.

Laurence Needleman, M.D.
Assistant Professor, Department of Radiology, Thomas Jefferson Medical College; Attending Radiologist, Division of Diagnostic Ultrasound and Body CT, Thomas Jefferson University Hospital, Philadelphia, Pennsylvania

Kenneth J. W. Taylor, M.D.
Professor, Department of Diagnostic Imaging, Yale University School of Medicine, New Haven, Connecticut

Eric vanSonnenberg, M.D.
Associate Professor of Radiology and Medicine, Department of Radiology, University of California, San Diego, School of Medicine, La Jolla, California; Chief, Gastrointestinal and Interventional Radiology, UCSD Medical Center, San Diego, California

Contents

Preface

Since the publication of the first book in this series on gastrointestinal ultrasound over eight years ago, there has been a significant increase in knowledge both in terms of techniques and image quality. It is appropriate, therefore, to produce a second book in this area. Rather than attempt to duplicate the chapters in the previous book, we have used a more sophisticated approach. We have selected specific topics that would be of interest to those wanting to learn more about the gastrointestinal uses of ultrasound. All the major organ systems within the abdomen are discussed, including an in-depth review of its usefulness in the evaluation of the bowel. Techniques utilized for drainage and aspiration are also emphasized. Newer techniques, such as the use of Doppler in the evaluation of abnormalities within the abdomen, are also included. We have included general information along with the more specific information on some of the newer approaches in the ultrasonic examination of the gastrointestinal system. It is anticipated that this book will be useful to experienced physicians and sonographers not only as an update on the latest advances in gastrointestinal ultrasound, but also as a reference source. In addition, it should prove to be an excellent book for those just beginning to learn ultrasound.

Alfred B. Kurtz, M.D.
Barry B. Goldberg, M.D.

1 Focal Liver Lesions

IAN M. LANDE
MICHAEL C. HILL

EVALUATING THE FOCAL HEPATIC MASS

Diagnostic imagers have been confronted with the introduction of a variety of new imaging techniques that have had a dramatic impact on hepatic imaging. Despite these newer techniques, ultrasound, in large part because of its ease of use, low cost, and lack of ionizing radiation, continues to play a central role in hepatic imaging. In the hands of the experienced sonographer it is a sensitive and accurate modality for the identification, localization, and characterization of focal hepatic abnormalities.[1-4] At the same time ultrasound can also evaluate the retroperitoneum, porta hepatis, pancreas, kidneys, biliary tree, pleura, and major vascular structures of the upper abdomen.

In some institutions alternate imaging techniques such as computed tomography (CT) have replaced ultrasound as the primary screening modality for the assessment of focal hepatic lesions.[5] The rationale for this can be understood for patients that are obese, or critically ill, or for those patients that have abundant bowel gas, surgical wounds, sutures, or drainage tubes causing limited acoustic access. Images from real-time studies can be difficult for the non-radiologist to review for treatment planning. For the remaining patient population, however, issues of comparative costs and equipment availability must be considered in light of the perceived added benefits.

The ultimate choice among CT, ultrasound, scintigraphy, angiography, or magnetic resonance imaging (MRI) as the single best study for the evaluation of focal hepatic masses requires a knowledge of the natural history and pathophysiology of the disease under investigation, as well as a knowledge of the advantages and limitations of each imaging technique. There is no widely accepted protocol for assessing focal liver lesions, although many different algorithms have been suggested.[6-9] This chapter reviews the sonographic appearances of common focal liver lesions and evaluates the comparative role of ultrasound in light of newer competitive modalities.

LOCALIZATION OF RIGHT UPPER QUADRANT MASSES

The identification and exact localization of the right upper quadrant mass is a common diagnostic problem. The symptoms and signs may be obscured or nonspecific. Delineating the exact organ(s) involved, as well as delineating the localization of disease within involved organs, is of great importance for the treatment, surgical approach, and prognosis.

There have been recent improvements in oncologic hepatic surgery and improved survival rates with tumor debulking. Resection of primary and some metastatic liver tumors necessitate an understanding of segmental hepatic anatomy.[2, 10, 11] The liver is divided into two lobes, four segments, and eight subsegments based upon the segmental and lobar vascular and biliary anatomy.[11] Ultrasound readily identifies the hepatic venous structures that course between and fall into the boundaries of the various hepatic segments and lobes.[2] Tumor that is limited to a single hepatic lobe can theoretically be cured via lobectomy. Tumor that involves the right lobe of the liver as well as the medial segment of the left requires a trisegmentectomy. Tumor present in all hepatic segments is surgically incurable.

Ultrasound is of value in determining whether a right upper quadrant mass is intrahepatic vs. extrahepatic in origin. Sonographic features which suggest an intrahepatic location of a mass include external bulging of the liver capsule, posterior shift of the inferior vena cava, and displacement and distortion of intrahepatic portal and hepatic venous structures. Features suggesting an extrahepatic location include internal invagination of the liver capsule, discontinuity of the liver capsule, a triangular-shaped wedge of tissue formed between the mass and the liver, and anterior or medial shift of the inferior vena cava.[12, 13] Although these sonographic criteria are accurate for lesions less than 10 cm in diameter, there is diminished correlation in larger lesions.[12]

Sonography has advantages over CT for differentiating intrahepatic from extrahepatic lesions in that CT is limited to a standard transverse section and thus may pose some difficulty defining the interface between adjacent structures in the craniocaudad plane (Fig. 1.1). Ultrasound, which has limitless multiplanar possibilities, can more accurately delineate the tomographic orientation between contiguous viscera. Although current generation MRI provides images in multiple orthogonal plans, it has none of the "real-time" features of ultrasound. In addition, questions of availability, cost, imaging time, and image degradation from respiratory motion are factors which must be addressed.

HEPATIC PSEUDOLESIONS

Hepatic pseudolesions are frequently encountered and may be a source of diagnostic error for the inexperienced sonographer. Most of these lesions are the result of technical artifacts or anatomic variants. Most of these prob-

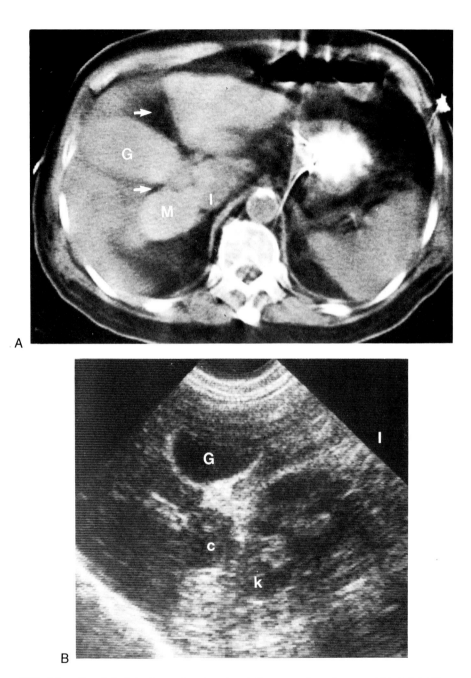

FIG. 1.1. Caudate lobe hypertrophy simulating an adrenal mass. (A) Axial CT scan at the level of the right adrenal gland reveals an apparent mass, *M* posterior and lateral to the inferior vena cava, *I*. The hepatic fissures (small arrows) are prominent, reflecting hepatic cirrhosis. *G* is the gallbladder. (B) Longitudinal oblique sonogram of the liver and upper pole of the right kidney. The caudate lobe, *c*, of the liver is prominent, extending into the hepatorenal space adjacent to the upper pole of the right kidney, *k*. The longitudinal orientation of the sonogram is accurate in identifying the craniocaudad interface between adjacent viscera.

lems can be overcome with a thorough knowledge of the anatomy, ultrasound physics, appropriate time gain compensation curves (TGC), and through the selection of transducers with the optimal frequency and focal length.

A number of pseudolesions have been described, not all of which can be listed here.[14–16] Those most frequently encountered include bowel gas and fluid-filled bowel loops which, if interposed between the anterior abdominal wall and the liver, may, in addition to obscuring visualization, generate beam transmission artifacts that may simulate focal or diffuse disease.[17] A prominent Riedel's lobe of the liver appearing as a right hepatic lobe mass can generally be recognized because of its isoechoic parenchymal pattern with that of the remainder of the normal liver and normal hepatic vascular anatomy. Accessory hepatic fissures found in up to 25 percent of patients result from diaphragmatic invaginations of peritoneal and extraperitoneal fat into the liver substance.[14] Accessory hepatic fissures may simulate focal echogenic lesions when obscured in part by shadowing from the lower ribs, or when viewed in cross section. If multiple they may be confused with macronodular cirrhosis. Pleural or pleural-based lung masses in the costophrenic sulci may mimic hepatic lesions particularly if they extend into one of these accessory fissures. Diagnostic errors can be avoided if the morphology and normal distribution of these fissures are understood.

Side lobe artifacts, which simulate focal hepatic disease, result from aberrant propagation of ultrasonic emissions at an angle to the main beam. These are particularly problematic adjacent to the periphery of a curved interface such as the diaphragm where these aberrant emissions are reflected to the center of the liver parenchyma.[14]

Other frequently encountered artifacts include acoustic shadowing related to vascular and biliary structures caused by fibrostroma within the portal triads, superimposition of the cardiac chambers on the lateral segment of the left lobe of the liver, and acoustic shadowing from fat or fibrous tissue within the ligamentum venosum that appear as a focal echogenic lesion, or that cause the caudate lobe of the liver to appear artifactially hypoechoic.[15] Hepatic pseudotumors have also been described in patients with cirrhosis and ascites. Foci of increased echogenicity caused by decreased attenuation from the underlying ascites in conjunction with a refractive artifact at the hepatic-ascites interface simulate lesions on the peripheral surface of the liver.[18] Air in the liver may be a cause of confusing artifacts. Whether in the biliary or portal venous system or within the liver parenchyma proper, the presence of gas is manifest as bright echoes with or without acoustic shadowing. Consequently, confluent air containing vascular or biliary structures in an anterior location may simulate an echogenic focal parenchymal process[19] (Fig. 1.2). Where confusion persists, comparative studies with plain radiographs or computed tomography will clarify the situation.

FATTY HEPATIC INFILTRATION

Although often considered a pseudolesion, fatty metamorphosis of the liver warrants separate consideration because it is the result of true morphologic change from increased deposition of triglyceride in hepatocytes. This can

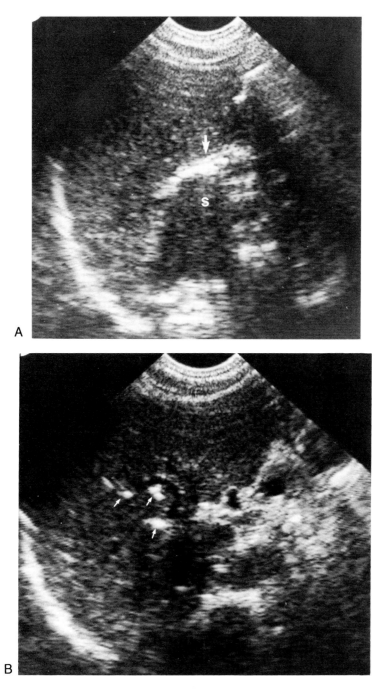

FIG. 1.2. Air in the biliary tree simulating a focal mass. (A) Longitudinal scan through the porta hepatis and right lobe of the liver demonstrating an echogenic band (white arrow) with distal shadowing, S, simulating a mass. (B) Transverse sonogram of the same region reveals multiple linear echogenic structures (small white arrows) converging towards the porta hepatis. This patient with status post choledochoenterostomy.

be associated with alcoholism, diabetes mellitus, obesity, nutritional deficiencies, steroids, pregnancy, hyperalimentation, hepatotoxic drugs, trauma, and hepatitis.[20, 21] Fatty metamorphosis appears as an area of increased echogenicity in contrast to the less echogenic normal liver parenchyma. Diagnostically, it is significant only in that it should not be confused with more ominous pathophysiologic processes. It may be difficult to decide which is the abnormal region, the hyperechoic or hypoechoic, as islands of normal parenchyma within a diffusely infiltrative fatty liver may be mistaken for hypoechoic focal neoplasms or abscesses (Fig. 1.3). The correct sonographic diagnosis depends on accurate TGC curve settings, so that normal areas of liver will not appear artifactly hypoechoic and thus simulate disease.[22]

Foci of fatty infiltration may appear as solitary echogenic masses simulating hemangiomas, hepatocellular carcinomas (HCC), hepatic adenomas (HA), focal nodular hyperplasia (FNH), and solitary metastases (Fig. 1.4).[23] Features that suggest focal fatty infiltration include a geographic process with sharp boundaries between normal and fatty liver with interdigitating angulated and geometric margins.[21] These angulated margins are not typically seen with primary liver tumors, metastatic disease, or with abscesses, all of which tend to be more rounded in configuration. Clinically, fatty changes can be seen as early as 3 weeks following an insult and may totally resolve as early

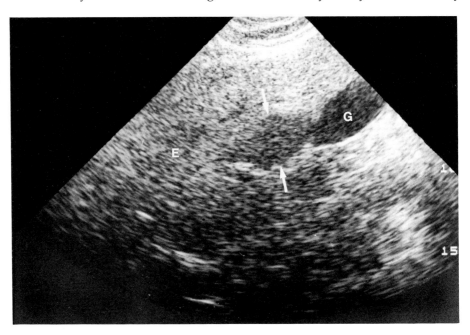

FIG. 1.3. Fatty metamorphosis of the liver with focal sparing simulating a focal hepatic lesion. Oblique sonogram of the liver and gallbladder, G reveals a focal area of hypoechogenicity (arrows). The liver texture is abnormally echogenic, E. Focal sparing of the liver may occur in any hepatic lobe, with an increased prevalence in the quadrate lobe.

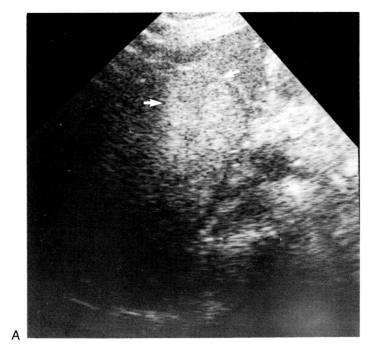

A

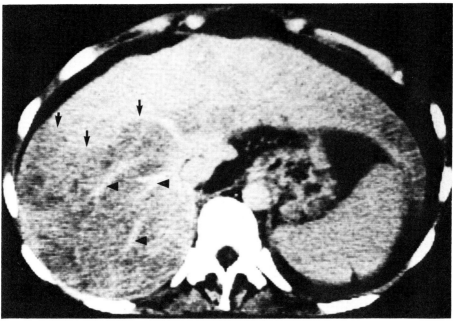

B

FIG. 1.4.   Focal fatty infiltration simulating an echogenic hepatic mass. (A) Transverse sonogram of the liver demonstrating a focal, slightly inhomogeneous echogenic mass (arrows). (B) Axial CT scan of the liver with intravenous contrast showing an inhomogeneous low density right lobe of the liver (black arrows). Note that the venous radicals (solid black arrow heads) are neither displaced nor effaced by the infiltrative fat.

as 6 days following appropriate therapy.[21, 24] This rapidly changing sonographic appearance can be a helpful clue to the correct diagnosis. Regrettably, fatty infiltration does not always have this classic appearance, and unusual manifestations that are nodular or multifocal, may be indistinguishable from metastatic disease.[25] In confusing cases, ^{133}Xe scintigraphy, Technetium-99m sulfur-colloid scintigraphy, or CT may be required for further clarification.[26, 27]

CYSTIC HEPATIC LESIONS

Ultrasound is accurate in the identification and differentiation of cystic from solid hepatic lesions and is generally considered superior to CT in determining the lesions internal morphologic characteristics.[1, 28] CT attenuation values alone are not reliable in differentiating truly benign cystic focal abnormalities from malignant cystic processes, as both may have similar attenuation coefficients.[29] Attenuation coefficients that are high may be found in benign hepatic cysts because of technical factors such as volume averaging or detector calibration drift. Recent hemorrhage, debris, or infection may also produce an increase in the density of a benign hepatic cyst. Provided that strict criteria are used, ultrasound is accurate in the evaluation of cystic structures.[1] Careful evaluation should include assessing for the presence or absence of internal echoes, septae, fluid levels, cyst wall smoothness or irregularity, and enhanced posterior sound transmission (Fig. 1.5). Changes in the sonographic pattern of contiguous liver parenchyma surrounding a cystic mass in the liver are usually indicative of an aggressive process. Ultrasound is helpful in visualizing mural nodules and internal septae, which on CT may be overlooked or appear as normal remaining hepatic parenchyma circumscribing the lesion.[29] Cystic lesions which are too small to characterize with certainty (i.e., < 2.0 cm) because of volume averaging may have indeterminate CT characteristics or can appear as solid masses. Ultrasound, despite the small size of the lesions, can accurately delineate the true cystic nature, due to their anechoic characteristics and presence of enhanced posterior sound transmission (Fig. 1.6).[28]

Most hepatic metastases appear sonographically as inhomogeneous solid masses with echo patterns distinct from normal liver and from simple cysts.[30] Rarely, metastatic lesions may appear primarily anechoic and thus be confused with simple cysts. In most cases there are sonographic clues such as a thick irregular wall, fluid interfaces, or echogenic mural nodules to aid in the differentiation.[1] Where confusion persists, differentiation of hypoechoic necrotic tumors from benign cysts or abscesses can be ascertained by percutaneous needle aspiration (Fig. 1.7).[30]

Simple hepatic cysts may be primary or secondary in etiology. Primary liver cysts result as a consequence of embryologic maldevelopment. They are uncommon and are unassociated with polycystic renal disease.[31] Acquired cysts are usually secondary to trauma, inflammation, or parasitic infestation. Usually asymptomatic, simple cysts may present with pain, right upper quadrant mass, hepatomegaly, or with symptoms secondary to superimposed

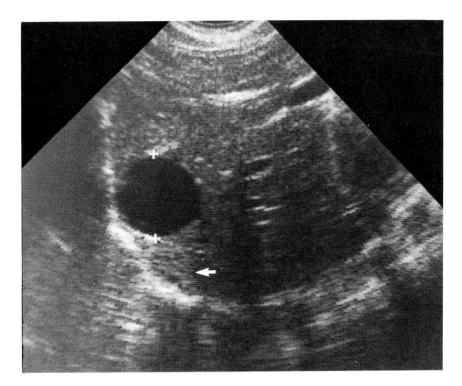

FIG. 1.5. Simple hepatic cyst. There is a well-defined lucent lesion (cursors) within the right lobe of the liver. Note the sharp margination, lack of internal echoes, and posterior sound transmission (solid white arrow).

complications from hemorrhage or infection.[30] Rarely, simple cysts may be confused with necrotic metastases, hematomas, hepatic cystadenocarcinomas, or with abscesses. In confusing or symptomatic cases, percutaneous ultrasound guided aspiration with cytologic analysis can be diagnostic and occasionally therapeutic.[30, 32]

While multiple cysts in the liver may occur as an isolated phenomenon, they are frequently observed in patients with underlying adult polycystic renal disease (Fig. 1.8). These cysts usually have smooth contours and are often concurrent with cysts in other abdominal viscera such as the kidneys and pancreas.

An intrahepatic gallbladder or a biliary cystadenoma may simulate a solitary intrahepatic cyst.[31, 33] Biliary cystadenomas may vary in size; some are as large as 30 cm in diameter. Sonographically they are quite distinctive, being cystic with multiple septations and papillary projections, not unlike those cystadenomas arising from the ovary or the pancreas (Fig. 1.9).[34, 35] Sonographic differentiation between the benign and malignant varieties is generally not possible.

Segmental nonobstructive dilatation of the bile ducts (Caroli's disease) is

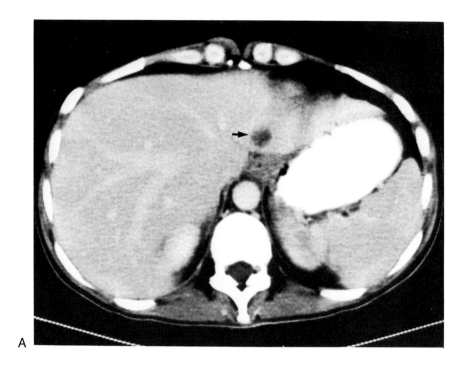

A

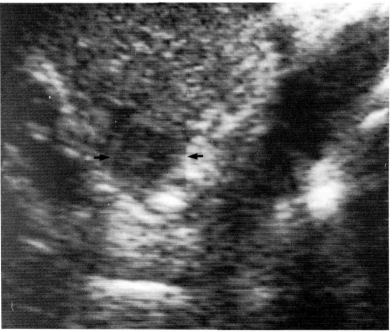

B

FIG. 1.6.   Small solid lesion appearing cystic on CT. (A) CT scan of the liver demon-strates a well-defined less than 2 cm hypodense cystic lesion (black arrow) in the lateral segment of the left lobe of the liver. (B) Magnified ultrasound of the same region demonstrating a solid mass (black arrows) with internal echoes. Biopsy proven metastatic clear cell carcinoma of the vagina.

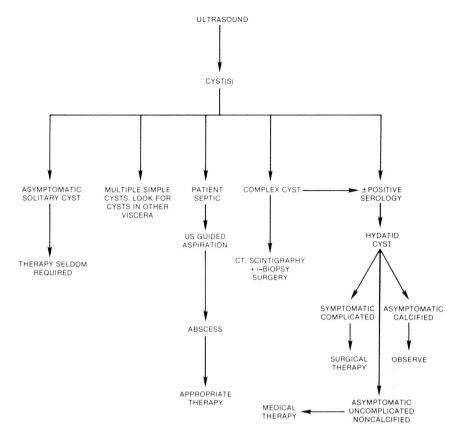

FIG. 1.7.   Management of cystic hepatic lesions.

associated with infantile polycystic kidney disease.[36, 37] Patients present with recurrent cholangitis and lithiasis in the dilated ducts. Caroli's disease may have a similar sonographic appearance to that of polycystic liver disease; the differentiation being that the former is comprised of sonolucent tubular structures communicating with each other and converging towards the porta hepatis.[38, 39] There is often accompanying intraductal echogenic calculi with acoustic shadowing.[38] Intraluminal biliary wall protrusions leading to partial or complete bridging of the ductal walls can, if visualized sonographically, be diagnostically helpful. Marshall has postulated that these protrusions are the result of arrested embryogenesis of the intrahepatic bile ducts.[36]

Choledochal cysts, which typically are solitary and involve the extrahepatic biliary tree, can on occasion be either multiple or intrahepatic in location.[40] When intrahepatic they can have a solid echogenic appearance and may appear solid on CT. This is thought to be the result of concentrated bile salts and old hemorrhagic contents. As a result, they may be inseparable from other solid appearing lesions in the liver. Tc-HIDA scans or percutane-

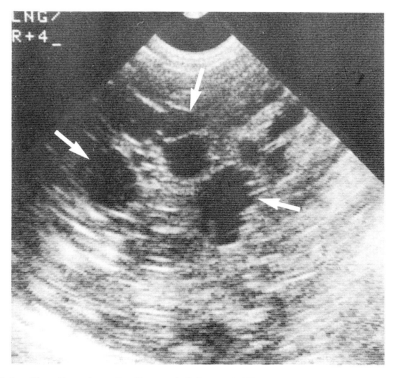

FIG. 1.8. Hepatic polycystic disease (adult type). There are multiple cysts (arrows) of variable size and shape identified throughout the liver. The underlying hepatic parenchymal architecture is markedly distorted. Cysts were also present in both kidneys (not shown).

ous transhepatic cholangiograms may aid in establishing the correct diagnosis.

METASTATIC LIVER DISEASE

Annual statistics show that nearly two million individuals in the United States are at risk of having liver metastases.[41] With recent refinement in surgical techniques, 5-year survival rates after resection of some types of liver metastases have been reported to be just under 30 percent. Five to ten percent of patients with metastatic disease may benefit from resection of liver metastases.[42, 43] Careful preoperative selection is needed to avoid unnecessary explorations that may reduce the quality of the short remaining life span of patients with unresectable tumors.

Patients may present with either solitary or multiple focal hepatic masses, or with diffuse distortion of the hepatic parenchymal architecture. Unless complicated by hemorrhage, infection, or necrosis, focal metastatic disease presents as one of three basic sonographic patterns. These include sonodense,

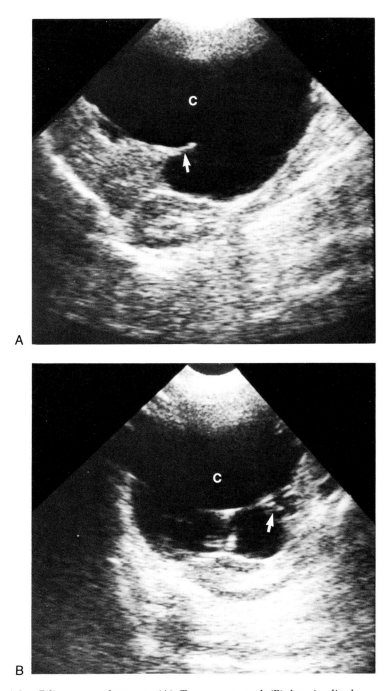

FIG. 1.9. Biliary cystadenoma. (A) Transverse and (B) longitudinal sonogram of the liver demonstrates a lobulated cyst, C, with multiple septa and mural nodules (arrow) typical of biliary cystadenomas. Sonographic differentiation of benign from malignant forms of the disease is not possible.

sonolucent, or a bull's eye appearance.[44] There is no consistent correlation between the primary tumor type and that of the varying echographic pattern. Colonic tumors tend to be the most frequent primary source which cause echogenic metastases (Fig. 1.10), however, no correlative histologic abnormality has been observed to account for this finding. An anechoic, thin, poorly defined halo is frequently seen surrounding solid liver metastases.[45] Marchal, et al, in histopathologic studies, claims that this is most often the result of peritumoral compression of normal hepatic parenchyma, and less often the result of tumoral infiltration into the surrounding hepatic parenchyma. Regardless of etiology, this finding is seldom present in slow growing lesions, and when present indicates an aggressive lesion.

Tumor necrosis, although a plausible explanation for the appearance of sonolucent focal lesions, is not consistently present at necropsy when this sonographic appearance is observed.[44] Marchal, et al, noticed a correlation between metastatic microangiopathic histology and the sonographic appearances of metastases. Lesions that were echogenic were found to contain

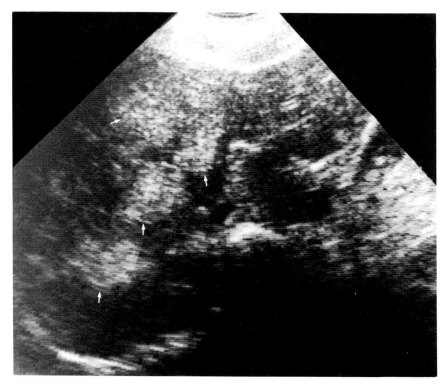

FIG. 1.10. Hyperechogenic colonic metastases. Transverse ultrasound of the liver reveals multiple rounded variably defined echogenic foci in the hepatic parenchyma (small arrows). Hyperechogenic metastases although frequently observed in colonic carcinoma, may be seen with other forms of metastatic disease.

multiple tortuous vessels of variable definition, frequently demonstrating dysplastic neovascularity. Complex lesions with central sonolucency revealed peripheral dysplastic tumor vessels with a progressive reduction to central avascularity, suggesting that tumor vascularity may be the main cause of the echogenic appearance of liver metastases, and that the echogenicity is related to the abundance of blood/solid tissue interfaces rather than to the walls of the tumor vessel themselves.[46] Necrosis, fibrosis, or fatty metamorphosis are often factors accounting for the variable echogenicity of liver metastases.

Bernardino, et al, found that ultrasound is valuable in assessing the therapeutic response to focal liver metastases and correlates well with other imaging techniques.[47] The sonographic appearances of these lesions undergoing treatment are extremely variable and alone are unreliable in determining the response to therapy (Fig. 1.11).[44, 47] In this setting ultrasound is primarily useful in determining a change in the overall liver size, detecting changes in the size of existing lesions, and for the detection of new lesions.

It is uncommon for hepatic lymphoma to present with focal liver masses. The sensitivity of detection of focal hepatic lymphomatous involvement is low, around 4.5 percent in advanced cases, down to 0.9 percent in early stages of the disease, for a total of 5.4 percent.[48, 49] At autopsy lymphomatous involvement of the liver is reported to be as high as 51 percent. The poor ultrasound detection rates relate to the diffuse rather than focal distribution of the disease.[48] Exceptions to this are in patients with acquired immune deficiency syndrome (AIDS), where Hodgkins or non-Hodgkins lymphomatous transformation in extranodal sites such as the liver, kidney, and spleen is frequent (Fig. 1.12). Twenty-five percent of patients with AIDS-related lymphoma will have solitary or multiple focal hepatic deposits.[50] The sonographic appearance of lymphomatous involvement of the liver is difficult to distinguish from other forms of metastases, primary hepatic carcinomas, or cirrhosis. The sonographic pattern of hepatic lymphoma varies from hypoechoic to target lesions to highly echogenic.[48] Hypoechoic and diffuse disease is seen in all types of lymphoma, while target and echogenic lesions are more prevalent in non-Hodgkin's lymphoma. AIDS-related lymphomas may appear markedly sonolucent with internal septations, appearing more as a fluid collection rather than as a solid lymphomatous deposit.

Hepatic leukemia is uncommon, but when it does occur it usually is in patients with acute myelogenous or lymphocytic leukemia, usually in the form of microscopic infiltration.[51] Hepatic sonography, although usually normal, on occasion may show nonspecific liver enlargement and disorganization of the normal hepatic echo pattern. Focal masses are unusual, but may occasionally be observed (Fig. 1.13).[52] Hepatic chloromas, although rare, are indistinguishable from other multiple hepatic metastases or abscesses.[51]

Studies have been performed comparing the relative diagnostic accuracy of ultrasound, scintigraphy, CT, arteriography, and MRI for the detection of focal metastatic disease.[53, 54, 55] Gunven, et al, noted that both CT and ultrasound were equally accurate in correctly localizing detectable lesions.

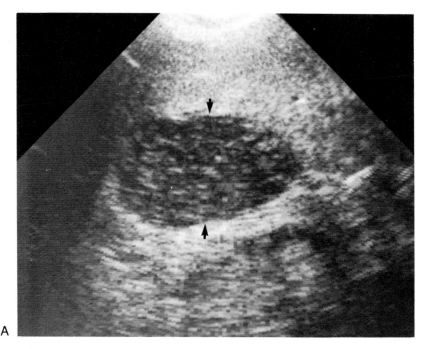

A

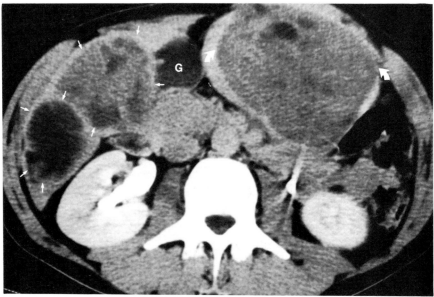

B

FIG. 1.11. Post therapeutic embolization necrosis of metastatic leiomyosarcoma of the liver. (A) There is a well defined hypoechoic lesion (black arrows) with medium level internal echoes. (B) Axial CT scan demonstrates multiple necrotic metastases in the right lobe of the liver (small arrows). To the left of the gallbladder, G, is a large inhomogeneous lesion (curved arrows) correlating to the lesion in Fig. A. (*Figure continues.*)

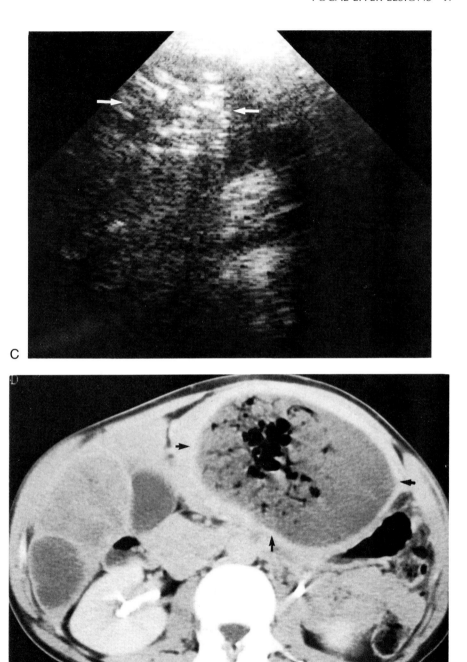

FIG. 1.11 (*Continued*).   (C) Sonogram and (D) axial CT scan of the same lesion identified in Fig. A, following therapeutic embolization. There are multiple bright internal reverberation echoes (white arrows) resulting from post-embolization air and necrosis.

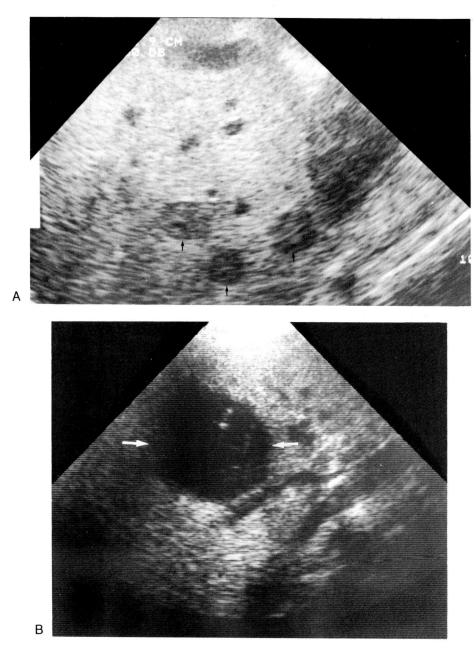

FIG. 1.12.   AIDS related lymphoma. (A) Oblique sonogram of the liver demonstrating multiple rounded lesions (small black arrows). This patient succumbed to disseminated AIDS related Burkitts lymphoma. (B) Sonogram of a solitary hepatic mass (arrow) in an AIDS patient. Note the hypoechoic cystic appearance of the mass. Biopsy proven non-Hodgkins lymphoma.

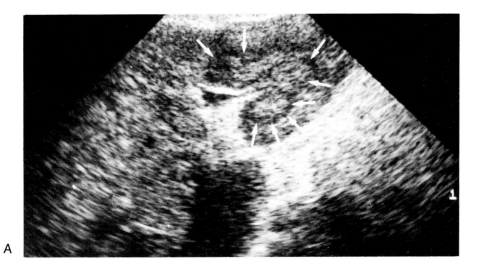

A

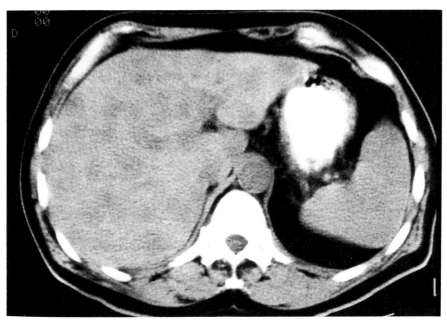

B

FIG. 1.13.   Focal leukemic deposits in the liver. Ultrasound (A) and CT (B) reveal multiple nodular lesion (small arrows) in all segments and lobes of the liver. Discrete leukemic lesions in the liver are unusual. The hypoechoic rings (white arrows) surrounding the lesions are frequently seen with metastatic disease. This finding usually suggests an aggressive process (See text).

CT was superior to ultrasound in detecting the numbers of metastases, particularly in lesions measuring less than 1 cm.[54] Alderson, et al, has shown that CT has a higher sensitivity than scintigraphy or ultrasound in the detection of metastatic colon or breast lesions in the liver. He also showed that

CT had the highest true positive ratio and that ultrasound had the lowest, while CT revealed more extrahepatic metastatic disease than did ultrasound.[55] Improved lesion detection with CT, either in combination with intra-arterial infusion of contrast and dynamic sequential imaging or following arterio-portography, has been observed.[56, 57] Ultrasound limitations are greatest in detecting lesions in the posterior segment of the right lobe of the liver and within regions of the liver that are located far away from the transducer, such as high up under the diaphragm.[54]

Angiography, although most helpful in evaluating the vascular architecture of metastatic implants, can be limited in detecting small metastatic foci that are avascular or superimposed over the spine. Comparatively, ultrasound is more accurate in the architectural evaluation of the portal and hepatic venous systems.[54]

Deciding which modality is the ideal screening technique in a given clinical setting is dependent upon many factors, including availability of equipment, cost, and the potential that additional imaging information will lead to thera-peutic benefits. Although CT has become the accepted gold standard because of its ability to show liver metastases with greater sensitivity and specificity than either ultrasound or isotope scanning, this does not imply that it is without error and should be the only noninvasive imaging modality or even the first examination of choice in the assessment of patients with suspected focal liver metastases. Recent studies by Freeny, et al, have shown that 27 percent of liver metastases confirmed at surgery went undiscovered by preop-erative CT.[58] Even with combined use of CT and ultrasound, 40 percent of preoperative plans had to be changed; in two-thirds by extended resections, in one-third by a change from cure to palliative intent.[54] Consequently, newer techniques such as MRI are being investigated. Ferrucci, et al, have shown an increase sensitivity of 14 percent for lesion detection with MRI as compared to CT.[53] Increased metastatic lesion detection via MRI has also been described independently by Reinig, et al.[59] The ultimate role that MRI will have com-pared to ultrasound or CT in the evaluation of this patient population is dependent upon ongoing clinical studies as well as considerations of time, availability, and expense.

HEPATIC INJURY

The incidence of hepatic injury secondary to blunt trauma and gunshot wound is increasing. Trauma to the liver is a common problem particularly in children because of the greater flexibility of the pediatric rib cage and the lack of surrounding fat and mesentery.[60, 61] The sonographic appearance of hematomas depends upon their age and extent. Initially there are areas of increased echogenicity due to blood clot formation. With further organiza-tion the blood clots undergo liquefaction, which is associated with progressive sonolucency and an apparent increase in the size of the hematoma. This increase in size is from increased osmotic pressure secondary to blood break-down in the products devitalized tissues.[60] With further evolution the hematoma becomes completely cystic, occasionally with the development of internal septae, and in time resolves slowly with regeneration of liver tissue. A small residual anechoic space may persist for a long period of time, but the patient usually remains asymptomatic. In addition to evaluating the liver, ultrasound is helpful in evaluating other abdominal viscera and is sensitive for the detection of hemoperitoneum. Most patients, (80 percent) with hepatic injuries require minimal or no surgical intervention.[61] Determining the exact accuracy of ultrasound in the diagnosis of hepatic injury is difficult, as there is often a lack of correlative surgical or pathologic proof.

Iatrogenic hepatic trauma, from surgery or from instrumentation, may result in the formation of a focal hematoma or a biloma. Surgical infarction of the liver is uncommon because of the dual portal and hepatic arterial blood supply; however, patients undergoing extensive upper abdominal surgery, or those with an underlying hypercoagulopathy, may develop focal or segmental regions of infarction. Sonographically, acutely infarcted liver appears either as a peripheral wedge or as a segmental region of sharply marginated hypoechogenicity (Fig. 1.14).

BENIGN HEPATIC NEOPLASMS

Benign hepatic lesions are rare with the exception of cavernous hemangiomas (CH). HA, hamartomas, FNH, and CH can be demonstrated via a variety of imaging techniques including ultrasound. Most of these are discovered incidentally in patients undergoing evaluation for unrelated causes. To date, with the exception of CH, no consistently reliable sonographic characteristics have emerged for distinguishing these benign tumors from each other or from more commonly demonstrated malignant tumors. Correlative evaluation with CT, angiography, MRI, Technetium-blood pool imaging, sulfur-colloid scintigraphy, or biopsy is frequently required for the correct diagnosis (Fig. 1.15).[62, 63] Patients without known neoplasm elsewhere, who are asymptomatic and are discovered serendipitously to have a focal echogenic lesion within the liver, can be adequately followed with a dynamic CT scan, technetium-blood pool scintigraphy, or follow-up sonography.[64] Those with a known neoplasm or who are symptomatic require further evaluation.

CAVERNOUS HEMANGIOMA

CH of the liver is reported to occur in up to 8 percent of patients with multiplicity in 10 percent of patients, representing the most common benign hepatic tumor. It is the second most common hepatic tumor in the United States, exceeded only by metastases.[62, 65, 66] The vast majority are asymptomatic with less than 13 percent producing symptoms.[67, 68] They require no treatment; however, they must be differentiated from other lesions that do require therapy. Although the sonographic appearance of hemangiomas is variable ranging from sonolucent to echogenic, several distinctive patterns have been described.[67, 69, 70] The classic description is that of a well defined,

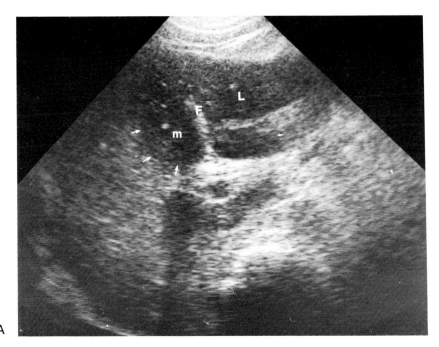

A

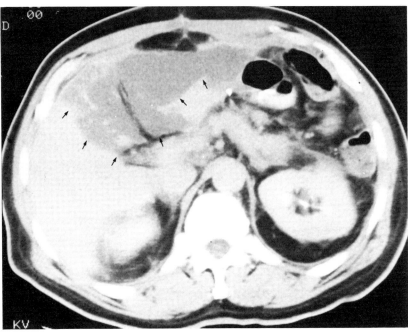

B

FIG. 1.14. Post-surgical infarction of the left lobe of the liver simulating a focal hepatic mass. (A) A transverse sonogram of the left lobe of the liver demonstrates a hypoechoic lesion involving the medial, *m*, and lateral, *L*, lobes of the liver. A vascular etiology is suggested by the geographic distribution (arrows) (*F* = falciform ligament). (B) CT scan reveals a hypodense region (small arrows) correlating to the distribution noted sonographically. This patient was status-post gastrectomy and splenectomy with inadvertent ligation of the left hepatic artery which arose from the left gastric artery and was sacrificed at surgery.

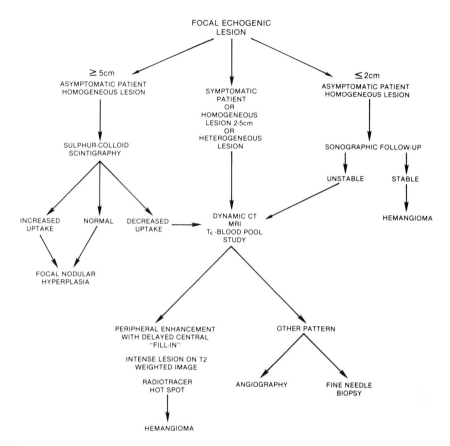

FIG. 1.15.   Investigation of focal echogenic hepatic lesions. Asymptomatic patients show no right upper quadrant symptoms and no underlying neoplasms.

echogenic, rounded, homogeneous lesion usually less than 2 cms in size (Fig. 1.16). Rarely CH may present as a hypoechoic lesion with fluid compartments or as a cystic mass making sonographic differentiation from necrotic tumors, abscesses, or hepatic cysts difficult.[69, 71, 72] Lesions may occur anywhere within the liver, although there is a tendency towards a peripheral or subcapsular location. Central hemangiomas are usually within 1 cm of the hepatic veins, are often larger than 2 cms and, because of thrombotic and fibrotic changes, may have a complex sonographic appearance (Fig. 1.17).[8, 69] CH that are larger than 2.5 cm frequently demonstrate posterior enhancement of the sound beam, a finding that is unusual in other hyperechoic masses, and probably relates to the vascularity of these lesions.[73] Although suggestive of CH, increased sound transmission is not pathognomonic, as this finding may also be observed with echogenic hypervascular metastases such as hypernephroma, carcinoid tumors, islet cell lesions, HCC,

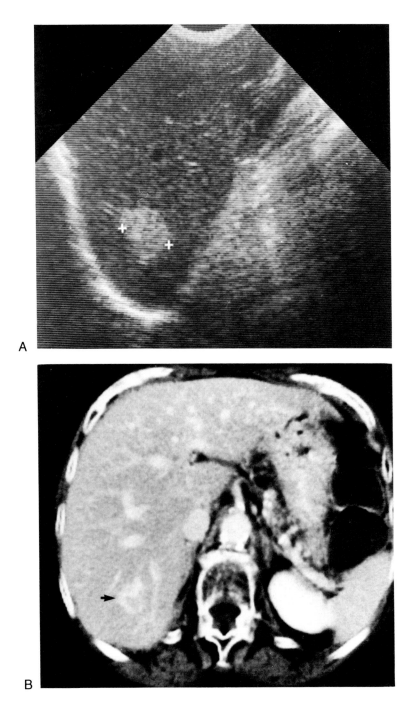

FIG. 1.16. Cavernous hemangioma. (A) Sonogram of the right lobe of the liver reveals a well defined echogenic homogeneous lesion (cursors) in the periphery of the liver. Asymptomatic patients with small peripheral-based echogenic lesions usually require no further investigation (See Fig. 1.15). (B) Dynamic CT scan of the liver demonstrates a dense focus of enhancement (black arrow) correlating to the sonographic abnormality. This CT enhancement pattern is suggestive of cavernous hemangiomas.

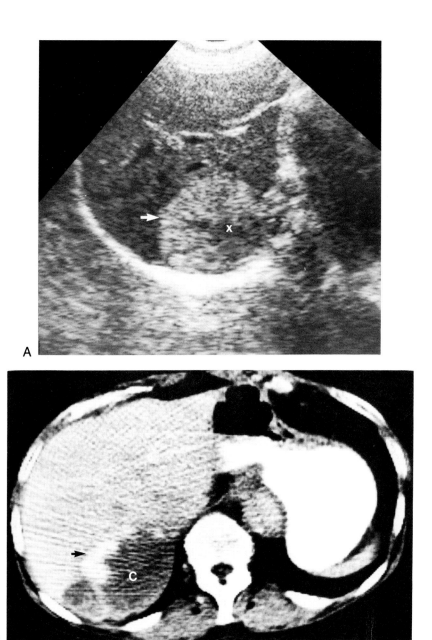

FIG. 1.17. Cavernous hemangioma with central inhomogeneity. (A) A transverse sonogram of the right lobe of the liver demonstrates a well defined echogenic lesion (white arrow) with central lucency, X. Cavernous hemangiomas tend to be homogeneous when small; however with increasing size, central inhomogeneity, as a result of hemorrhage, thrombosis, or fibrosis, can occur. These lesions are indistinguishable sonographically from HA, hepatomas and echogenic metastases, and require other imaging techniques for further delineation (See Fig. 1.5). (B) Dynamic CT scan demonstrates peripheral enhancement (black arrow) within a hypodense lesion, C, in the posterior segment of the right lobe of the liver. This peripheral CT enhancement pattern, although typical for cavernous hemangioma, is present in only 50 percent of cases.

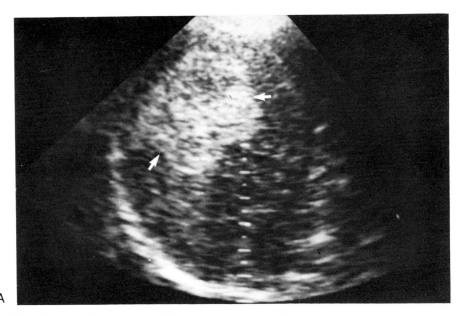

A

FIG. 1.18. (A) Ultrasound of the right lobe of the liver reveals an echogenic lesion (white arrows) with areas of inhomogeneity. (*Figure continues.*)

and metastatic choriocarcinoma. With a high frequency transducer, and using a magnified image, blood flow may sometimes be observed in the small vascular channels within the tumor. A CH may enlarge slowly and undergo degeneration with fibrosis and calcification. Lesions may occasionally cause pain and liver enlargement. Only in the cases of the classic well-defined hyperechoic lesion in an asymptomatic patient, with no underlying malignancies, can a reliable diagnosis of CH be suggested. In cases where there is doubt or an unusual ultrasound appearance, correlation with isotope red blood studies, angiography, or dynamic CT is required.[64] Biopsy of these lesions can be safely performed, provided that a fine needle is used and an optimal approach to the lesion is chosen.[71]

Isotope labeled red blood cell studies, when combined with dynamic perfusion and delayed blood pool images, have a sensitivity approaching 90 percent and a specificity of 100 percent, although sensitivity diminishes with decreasing lesion size.[62] CT, like scintigraphy, is also size sensitive, and small hemangiomas less than 1 cm in size may be difficult to evaluate because of slice offset caused by different levels of breath holding. It is these small lesions that tend to have a characteristic hyperechogenic appearance which are better suited for evaluation sonographically.[74] CT scans have other limitations as well.[74, 75] Freeney noted that only 55 percent of hemangiomas display the established CT criteria required to make a confident diagnosis.[76] MRI has been found to be more sensitive than either contrast enhanced CT or ultrasound for the detection of CH.[77] Homogeneous hyperintense signal on proton density and T2 weighted images is more than 85 percent specific for the diagnosis of CH (Fig. 1.18). Regrettably, a small percentage of vascular meta-

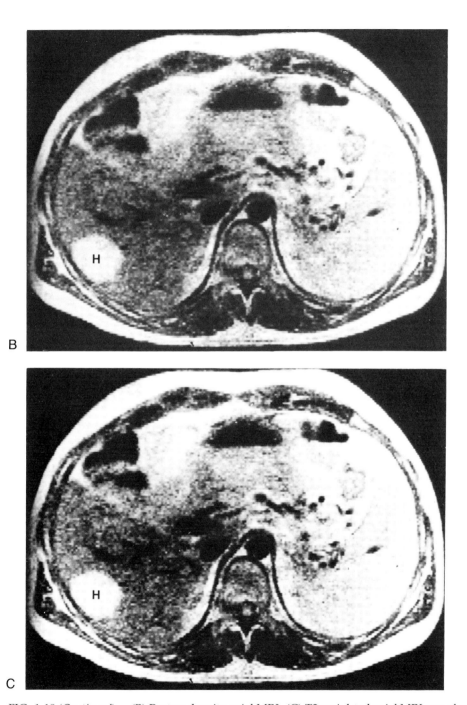

FIG. 1.18 (*Continued*).   (B) Proton density axial MRI, (C) T2 weighted axial MRI reveal a well defined intense lesion, *H*, on both imaging sequences. MRI is sensitive for the detection of cavernous hemangiomas, with this intensity pattern distinctive for cavernous hemangiomas.

static liver lesions may have a similar appearance, necessitating comparative evaluation with other modalities.[77] Angiography, which is a sensitive and specific diagnostic tool, can also be utilized for therapeutic embolization of symptomatic hemangiomas that bleed intraperitoneally.[70]

FOCAL NODULAR HYPERPLASIA

Focal nodular hyperplasia (FNH) of the liver is a rare benign tumor of unknown pathogenesis. Although primarily a disease of women in the 3rd through 5th decades of life, it occurs in both sexes and in all age groups.[78] Generally solitary, subcapsular, and nonencapsulated, averaging approximately 5 cm in diameter and multifocal in 13 percent of cases, lesions less frequently arise centrally, or are pedunculated.[79, 80] Most patients are asymptomatic, although up to 35 percent of patients may have pain, a palpable mass, or liver enlargement. Lesions of FNH tend not to bleed, but rarely patients may present with intraperitoneal hemorrhage.

Histologically, FNH of the liver consists of a central stellate or linear fibrous scar with strands of fibrosis radiating peripherally. These lesions are comprised both of normal hepatocytes and of nodular proliferating bile ducts between the radiating fibrous septa. The sonographic features of FNH are quite variable.[81] Usually the echogenicity is different from the adjacent uninvolved liver tissue and the lesions are usually homogenous, although a complex pattern may occur in rare cases complicated by hemorrhage. A discrete linear cluster of central echoes, correlating to the central fibrotic scar pathologically, although classic, is infrequently seen, and may appear similar to a linear or stellate zone of fibrosis or organized hematoma within a hepatic adenoma or CH.[67, 78, 80, 81, 82] MRI has been reported to be able to detect the central scar not detectable by ultrasound or CT (Fig. 1.19), and can differentiate FNH from metastatic lesions, CH, and primary malignant liver tumors including fibrolamellar hepatomas with central scars.[83, 84]

CT detection of FNH is dependent upon the mode of contrast administration.[81] In one series CT detected only 78 percent of the lesions and was found to be less sensitive than sonography.[79] Angiography of FNH while often diagnostic will have a typical appearance in only 75 percent of patients.

FNH, unlike other focal hepatic lesions, has Kupffer cells in addition to normal hepatocytes, and thus may concentrate radiocolloids.[79, 85] This is an important diagnostic finding in the differential evaluation of hepatic parenchymal lesions, as no other benign mass (i.e., adenomas, CH, mesenchymal, hamartomas) and no malignant liver lesions contain Kupffer cells capable of concentrating sulphur-colloids. FNH will produce a normal scintigram in 58 percent, will appear photopenic in 35 percent and will demonstrate augmented radiocolloid uptake in the remainder.[79] Scintigraphy is often the pivotal diagnostic examination unless the lesion is below scintigraphic resolution (less than 3 cm).

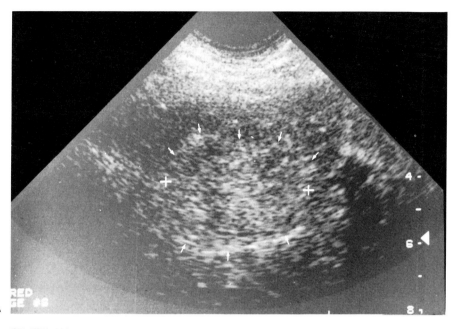

A

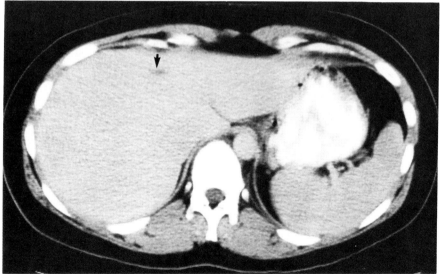

B

FIG. 1.19. (A) Transverse sonogram of the liver of a young woman referred for evaluation of vague right upper abdominal pain reveals a poorly defined region of increased echogenicity (small white arrows and cursors). (B) A CT scan initially interpreted as normal, retrospectively demonstrates a linear focus of hypodensity in the medial segment of the left lobe of the liver (black arrow). (*Figure continues.*)

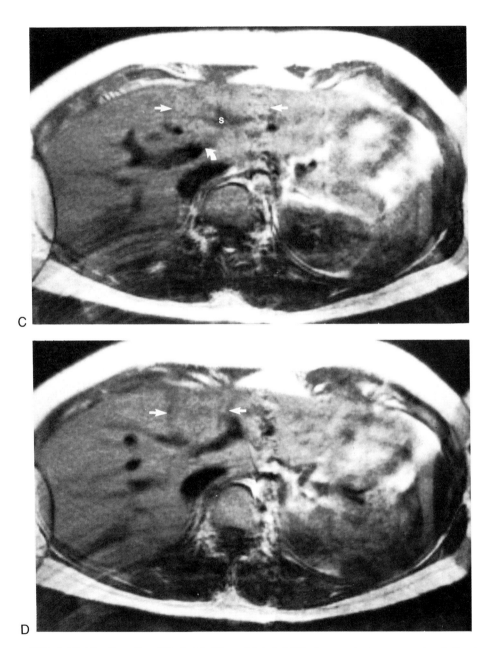

FIG. 1.19 (*Continued*). (C) Axial T1 weighted MRI demonstrates a poorly defined lesion (white arrows) with a central scar, *S,* causing effacement of the left portal vein (curved arrow). (D) T1 weighted MRI 1 cm cranial to Fig. C demonstrates a lesion (white arrow heads) straddling hepatic vascular structures. MRI has been reported to be more sensitive than either computed tomography or ultrasound for the detection of central scars of FNH. (*Figure continues.*)

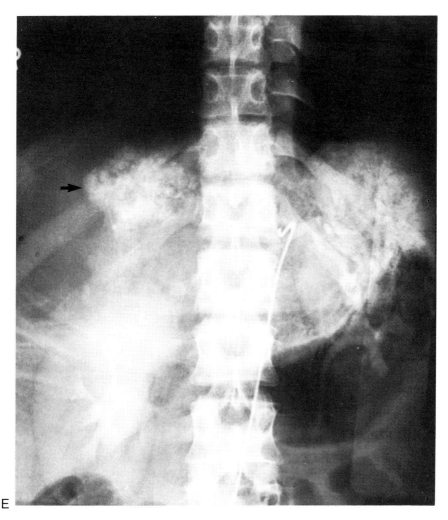

E

FIG. 1.19 (*Continued*). (E) Angiography reveals a lesion with an intense vascular stain (black arrow) typical of FNH.

HEPATIC ADENOMAS

Hepatic adenomas (HA) are solitary smooth masses that may be completely or partially encapsulated but generally lack the central scar, fibrous septa, kupffer cells, and nodularity of FNH.[86] HA are very vascular with thin-walled endothelial lined vessels dispersed throughout the lesion. Up to 50 percent of HA pathologically have areas of hemorrhage and necrosis in comparison to 6 percent of FNH. Unlike FNH which is usually clinically silent, patients with HA present with symptoms of a right upper quadrant mass, pain and hemorrhage. Hemoperitoneum may be the presenting complaint in HA in

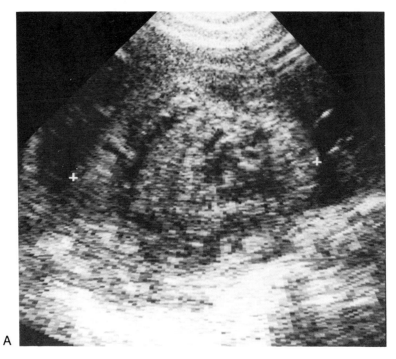

A

FIG. 1.20. Hepatic adenoma with hemorrhage and infarction. (A) Transverse sonogram of the right lobe of the liver reveals an echogenic inhomogeneous lesion (cursors) occupying most of the right lobe of the liver. There are areas of central inhomogeneity and necrosis. (*Figure continues.*)

up to a third of patients but is distinctly rare in FNH. The importance in differentiating these two lesions is due to the radical difference of patient management. FNH can be followed conservatively, while surgery is the treatment of choice for HA.[85] HA may regress following cessation of birth control pills.

There is a close association between HA and the use of oral contraceptives.[86] It has been suggested that sonography should be the first imaging method used in a young woman on oral contraceptives with pain in the right upper quadrant.[87] Biliary tract disease, which is a more frequent cause of pain in the right upper quadrant, can be simultaneously evaluated. There are no definite sonographic features that distinguish FNH from HA; however, the clinical presentation of acute onset pain in a patient at high risk of developing HA should be helpful in the differentiation from FNH and from other hepatic lesions such as metastasis, abscesses, lymphomas, CH, and hepatomas. Sonographically, HA is heterogenous, lacks a central fibrous scar, and often has foci of hemorrhage aiding in the differentiation from FNH (Fig. 1.20). CT is very sensitive in detecting fresh hemorrhage; consequentially some authors advocate the use of CT as an important adjunct to the initial screening

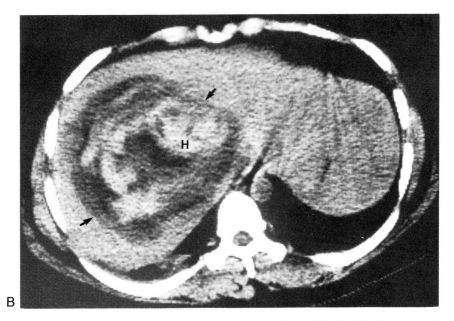

B

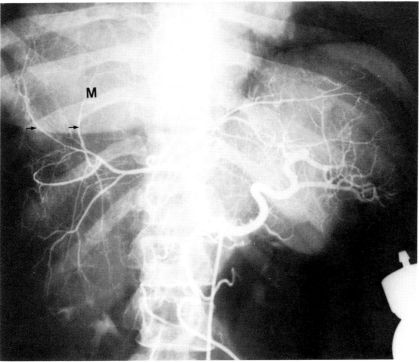

C

FIG. 1.20 (*Continued*). (B) CT scan of the liver without intravenous contrast material reveals a large inhomogeneous mass (black arrows) with central density, *H*, reflecting acute hemorrhage. (C) Celiac angiography demonstrates a large mass, *M*, causing displacement and draping of the hepatic arteries (arrows). Although usually hypervascular, this lesion appears avascular because of central hemorrhage and infarction.

ultrasound.[82] While a single imaging method will often fail to yield the correct diagnosis, the information derived from two or more tests will frequently permit discrimination between focal nodular hyperplasia and hepatic adenoma.

Glycogen storage diseases are inherited autosomal recessive metabolic disorders which result from defective mobilization of liver glycogen. Eight percent of patients with all types of these disorders are predisposed to develop HA.[88] Lesions may be solitary or multiple. Type I of the disease has reported incidences as high as 40 percent. Ultrasound is highly accurate in detecting HA in this patient population. There is often associated moderate hepatomegaly with increased hepatic echogenecity reflecting diffuse fatty or glycogen infiltration.[89] HA associated with glycogen storage diseases have a variable sonographic appearance ranging from hypo, iso, to hyperechoic and are usually well circumscribed from adjacent liver parenchyma.[88] Bowerman, et al, has described marked enhanced sound transmission through these adenomas, which is not present in adenomas unaccompanied by glycogen storage disease. Lesions demonstrating a rapidly altering sonographic appearance should be closely followed, as this may reflect hemorrhagic necrosis or malignant degeneration.[89, 90, 91]

Macroregenerating nodules are the most common hepatic masses in cirrhotic patients. Most of these lesions demonstrate a uniform parenchymal pattern of regeneration on both CT and ultrasound.[92, 93] Higher frequency transducers may be of value in delineating islands of regenerative cirrhotic tissue in parenchyma that appears uniform with lower frequency transducers. Occasionally inhomogeneous regenerative nodules, particularly if they are large, may be identified, which are indistinguishable from other focal processes (Fig. 1.21).[92] Technetium sulfur-colloid scans may show patchy uptake or may have a nodular appearance.

Mesenchymal hamartomas (MH) of the liver, which occur in young patients, are rare and appear sonographically as multiple small cysts within a solid mass, or as a multilocular cystic mass with intervening solid septa.[94, 95] These lesions probably are congenital in origin rather than being true neoplasms.[96] They are unrelated to undifferentiated embryonal sarcoma, which is a true neoplasm and is considered a separate entity, rather than malignant transformation of a MH.[97, 98] Differential diagnostic possibilities of MH in this age group include abscesses and rare cystic hepatoblastomas.[95] The intrahepatic origin of these lesions excludes other more common extrahepatic pediatric cystic abdominal masses such as mesenteric lymphangiomas, duplication cysts, cystic leiomyomas and enteric cysts.

INFECTIOUS HEPATIC LESIONS

Intrahepatic abscesses usually develop as a complication of an intraabdominal infection with direct portal venous spread to the liver.[99, 100] Common etiologic sites of infection include the biliary tract, colonic diverticulitis, and ruptured appendical abscesses. Abscesses may also result from prior abdominal sur-

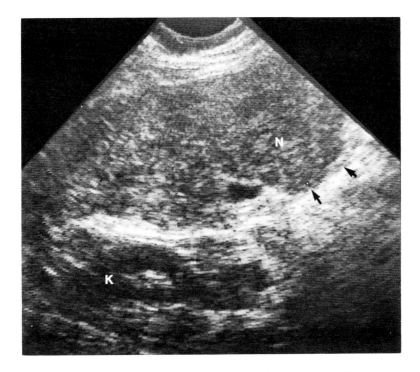

FIG. 1.21.   Macronodular cirrhosis simulating a focal neoplasm. Oblique longitudinal sonogram of the right lobe of the liver reveals diffuse distortion of the hepatic parenchymal architecture. There is expansion and convex rounding of the inferior aspect of the right lobe of the liver (arrows) simulating a focal neoplasm, N. Most nodules of macronodular cirrhosis are isoechoic with the remaining liver parenchyma. Occasionally large regenerative nodules may appear inhomogeneous simulating focal hepatic parenchymal lesions (See text) (K = kidney).

gery, trauma, neoplasm, or bacteremia in a compromised host. The mortality from untreated hepatic abscesses approaches 90 percent; consequently early diagnosis is important for prompt and appropriate therapy.[101]

The typical sonographic features are those of a spherical, slightly irregular hypoechoic lesion with distal acoustic enhancement. This pattern is present in 75 percent of cases.[102] Hyperosmolar contents are responsible for the spherical shape of abscess that if subcapsular in location will cause convex bulging of the liver surface. Fifteen to 20 percent of abscesses can be hyperechogenic compared to normal liver tissue. The hyperechogenecity is thought to result from the admixture of dissimilar liquids resulting in an inhomogeneous suspension and marked acoustic reflection.[103, 104] Another cause of hyperreflectivity is the presence of gas within the abscess.[105] Although distal acoustic enhancement, an echogenic wall, and a thin peripheral halo measuring less than 0.5 cm in thickness is suggestive of an abscess, the sonographic appearance varies greatly, depending upon the age and etiology of the infectious process (Fig. 1.22).

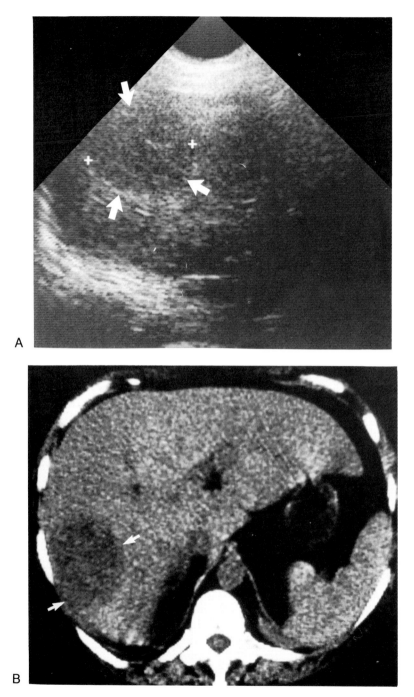

FIG. 1.22. Variable sonographic appearance of hepatic abscesses. (A) Sonogram of the right lobe of the liver demonstrates a hypoechoic lesion (cursors) and arrows with minimal enhanced posterior sound transmission. (B) CT scan of the same patient demonstrates a hypodense lesion (white arrows) in the posterior segment of the right lobe of the liver. Aspiration revealed a pyogenic abscess. (*Figure continues.*)

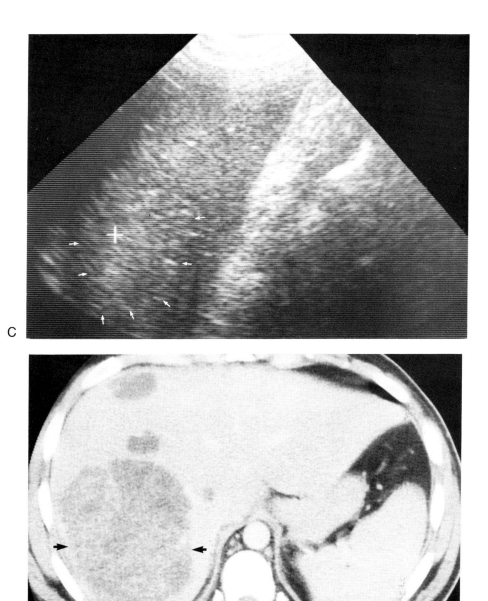

C

D

FIG. 1.22 (*Continued*). (C) (Different patient) Sonogram of the right lobe of the liver reveals a poorly defined isoechoic focus of mild alteration of the hepatic parenchymal architecture (white arrows). (D) CT of the liver of the same patient as Fig. C reveals multiple focal abscesses. The largest (black arrows) corresponding to the sonographic abnormality. Surgery confirmed multiple pyogenic abscesses. (*Figure continues.*)

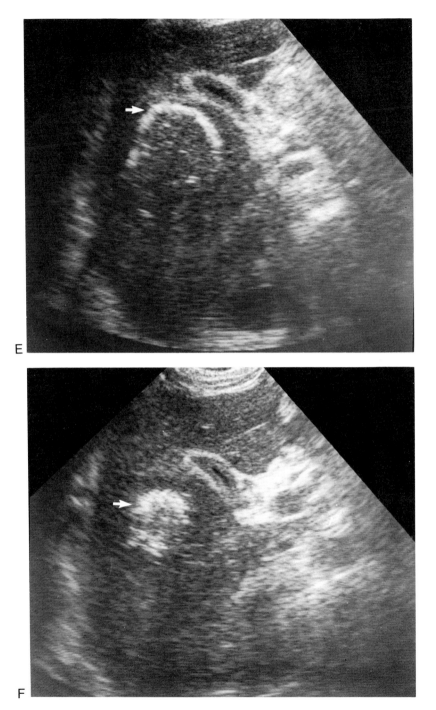

FIG. 1.22 *(Continued)*. (E) and (F) Echogenic abscess. Sonography of the right lobe of the liver reveals an echogenic focal lesion (white arrow) which at surgery was proven to be an air containing abscess. The sonographic appearance of abscesses varies and depends on their age, etiology and therapy (See text).

These variable sonographic appearances relate to their morphology and contents. There is constant change during the phases of development, organization, and repair. Most abscesses originate by pyogenic exudation within a cavity caused by inflammatory destruction of liver parenchyma. These cavities may develop septations, fluid-filled interfaces, and/or dependent debris.[99] Suppurative, fibrinopurulent, and fibroproductive products cause the varied sonographic appearance.[103] In a chronic abscess, a wall of variable thickness and definition, is generally present. Complicated hepatic cysts, necrotic tumors, echinococcal cysts, and primary and secondary hepatic malignancies may have similar appearances.[99] On a sonographic basis alone it may be impossible to distinguish between these possibilities. Where indicated, sonographically guided needle aspiration is an inexpensive, rapid procedure for establishing the correct diagnosis.[105]

Hepatic abscesses may occur outside the liver parenchyma, within any potential space or structure related to the hepatic fissures such as the falciform ligament.[106] Abscesses located high up under the dome of the diaphragm, or those associated with underlying fatty liver tissue, may be overlooked.[107] In the presence of ascending cholangitis, multiple microabscesses may be present that are below sonographic resolution. In this situation, aspiration of infected bile is suggested to establish the correct diagnosis.[107]

Sonography is helpful in detecting concurrent pleural effusions, or accompanying ascites. The presence of ascites may be an important indicator of associated peritonitis or free intraperitoneal perforation of an abscess.[102]

Echinococcus Granulosis

The liver is the organ most frequently parasitized by echinococcal disease.[108] Echinococcal disease of the liver may occur in several forms. The most prevalent, Echinococcus granulosis, represents the larval phase of the parasite present in nearly all cattle raising countries of the world. There are several sonographic appearances that may be encountered, including a solitary cyst, a cyst with one or more internal daughter cysts, a multiloculated cyst or multiple cysts.[109, 110] Hydatid cysts frequently contain sand or scolices, and internal echoes can be generated by rotating the patient during a real-time examination.[111] Cysts may vary in diameter from 1 to 20 cm. The sagging split-wall and floating undulating membrane within the cyst reflects separation of the exocyst from the pericyst and is pathognomonic for hydatid disease. A variable heterogenous echo pattern may be observed, depending upon their age and whether or not they are being treated.[112] Cysts may calcify, causing their walls to appear as thick reflecting interfaces with distal acoustic shadowing.[110] Lesions in the caudate lobe may compress the inferior vena cava, while those that arise in the upper portion of the liver may communicate with the bronchi of the lung via a transdiaphragmatic pathway resulting in an identifiable blur of the diaphragmatic contour. If there is communication with the biliary tree, biliary compression or obstruction can result.[110] If hydatid cysts become secondarily infected, their acoustic properties will change, often becoming hyperechogenic in character.[113, 109] The differential diagnosis of hydatid disease of the liver should include necrotic hepatic metastasis, chronic hematomas, abscesses, cysts of other etiologies including amebiasis, polycystic disease, and bile duct cysts.[108]

Uncomplicated percutaneous aspiration of hydatid cysts has been reported.[114] Regardless, in areas where hydatid disease is endemic, anaphylaxis as a result of post-aspiration intraperitoneal spread of scolices can be averted by prior identification of Echinococcal cysts with Casoni skin tests, or with serologic compliment fixation tests.[30]

Echinococcus Multiocularis

Echinococcus multilocularis, (EM), although rarer than the granulosis form of the disease, is endemic in many regions of the world, including central Europe, the Soviet Union, Iran, portions of Central America, and northern Canada. Sonographically there are regions within the liver that are echogenic and hyperreflective, forming a "hail-storm" pattern with foci of heterogeneous necrosis within well defined walls in 40 percent of cases.[115] Calcifications and dilated bile ducts are noted in up to 50 percent of cases. Ultrasound is useful in delineating dilated bile ducts and in demonstrating hepatic venous, vena caval, atrial, and extra-hepatic involvement. Ultrasound, because of its low cost and accuracy in countries where the disease is endemic, when utilized in conjunction with immunologic testing, is a good screening technique. Sonographically, lesions of EM may appear indistinguishable from primary and secondary hepatic neoplasms. CT can be used as an adjunctive technique to demonstrate associated microcalcifications, retroperitoneal lymph nodes, and lung base involvement.[115]

Hepatic Candidiasis

Hepatic candidiasis is uncommon and usually follows hematogenous spread of infection to the liver in an immunosuppressed patient. The classic sonographic appearance is a target lesion with a bright echogenic center. The hypoechoic outer rim is thought to be secondary to necrotic inflammatory debris and pus, while the central echogenicity is due to the presence of fungal mycelia. Less commonly, lymphoma or leukemia may have this sonographic appearance. Tissue biopsy is frequently required for definitive diagnosis.[116]

Entamoeba Histolytica

Hepatic amebic abscess formation occurs in 25 percent of patients infected with entamoeba histolytica. It is the most common nonenteric complication of amebic infection.[117, 118] Sonographically these lesions lack a significant wall,

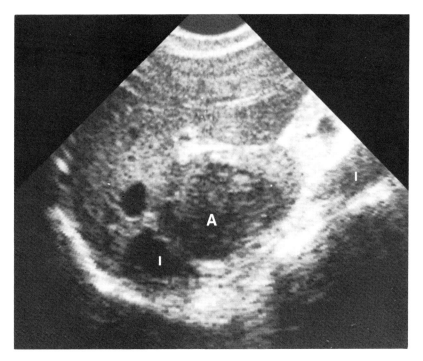

FIG. 1.23. Amebic abscess. Sonogram of the caudate lobe of the liver reveals a hypoechoic expansile mass, *A,* with medium level internal echoes (I = inferior vena cava).

are generally round or oval in configuration, and tend to be less echogenic than the normal hepatic parenchyma (Fig. 1.23). Although somewhat homogeneous in appearance, low level echoes are usually present throughout the lesions, accompanied by enhanced sound transmission. There is a tendency towards subcapsular location, and transdiaphragmatic pleural involvement, if present, can be identified sonographically.[117] When multiple abscesses are present, smaller lesions tends to be echogenic, displaying enhanced sonic transmission.[119] With successful treatment, in the short term, lesions may enlarge, remain static, or decrease in size slowly over several weeks.[120] The internal echogenicity follows a variable pattern, with the lesions eventually shrinking to develop a pattern that is usually indistinguishable from the normal surrounding hepatic parenchyma. This process may take up to 23 months, and a residual focal cystic area may persist, simulating a benign simple cyst.

HEPATOCELLULAR CARCINOMA

Hepatocellular carcinoma (HCC) is one of the most common malignancies in the world. Although relatively uncommon among Caucasians, it is one of the major malignancies in many regions throughout the world particularly in Sub-Sahara Africa and the Far East.[121] HCC accounts for 65 percent of all malignant disease in men and 31 percent of malignant tumors in women among many of the blacks of South Africa. It is the third major cause of cancer in males and the fourth among females in China. There is a close association of HCC with cirrhosis, particularly the posthepatitic macronodular variety. This is not unexpected, considering the hepatocarcinogenic properties of hepatitis B virus infection. Fifty percent of HCC are multicenteric. Forty percent are solitary and the rest are diffuse.[122, 123, 124] Portal or hepatic venous involvement is present in 25 to 40 percent of cases.[124, 125] Lymphadenopathy has been reported in up to 43 percent of cases, usually involving the porta hepatis; however, distant nodal groups may occasionally be affected.[124, 126] Rarely, hepatomas may grow directly into the bile ducts causing obstructive jaundice, producing a sonographic picture of bulky obstructing intraluminal masses in the proximal extrahepatic bile ducts.[127] Other causes of obstructive jaundice in patients with HCC include intrahepatic compression of bile ducts by tumor, and extrinsic bile duct compression by porta hepatis lymph nodes infiltrated with metastatic deposits.

The sonographic pattern of HCC is variable, usually with one of two major patterns depending upon the size and stage. Lesions are usually hypoechoic when small.[128] With advancing size they develop increased echogenicity. A small percentage of lesions are hyperechoic early in their course and these lesions tend to keep this sonographic appearance. Those that initially are hypoechoic and become secondarily hyperechoic tend to be larger in size and inhomogeneous.[128] Sheu, et al, claims that these changes relate to the microscopic structure of the underlying tumors. When small, there is a pure cell mass causing low echoes. With increasing size, lesions become necrotic, fibrotic, hemorrhagic and infiltrated with fatty metamorphosis producing high echogenicity.[128, 129] Despite the gross pathologic correlation, Shamaa, et al, were unable to detect a relationship between ultrasonic patterns of HCC and the pathologic grade.[130] During the transformation from a hypoechoic to a hyperechoic pattern, the lesion may be isoechoic with normal liver parenchyma and has the potential to be overlooked.[128]

Sonographically, lesions of HCC may be discrete, or can present with diffuse hepatomegaly and distortion of the liver architecture in the absence of an identifiable distinct mass. The appearance of the diffuse form of the disease is nonspecific and may simulate disseminated lymphoma, cirrhosis, hemochromatosis, or fatty infiltration.

Ultrasound is accurate in detecting intraluminal tumor invasion within the inferior vena cava, hepatic veins, or portal venous branches.[125] HCC can extend from the hepatic venous structures to infiltrate in 4 percent of patients into the right atrium.[131] Ultrasound is often superior to angiography in assessing vascular structures, particularly if they are obscured or are nonopacified.[125] When malignant tumors other than hepatomas affect the veins, there usually is displacement, external compression, or encasement rather than intraluminal extension, although hepatic metastases may rarely result in intraluminal tumor thrombus.[125] Documenting portal or hepatic venous involvement has important prognostic and therapeutic implications.[125]

Large screening programs have been established in endemic countries to aid in early diagnosis. The significance of early detection and early resection of HCC largely depends upon the prospect of future emergence of new lesions. In the presence of disseminated underlying liver disease, there is a risk of regenerating liver undergoing malignant transformation. The most desirable therapeutic approach would be the prevention of the progression of chronic liver disease, rather than to attempt a cure once HCC has developed.[121] The prevalence of liver disease is such that surgery will remain an important mode of therapy in patients with resectable tumors. The resectability of a hepatoma is determined by the extent of hepatic involvement, the presence of vascular invasion, and the presence of extrahepatic disease. Ultrasound, which is readily available, easy to perform and inexpensive is being utilized in areas where this neoplasm is highly endemic. Sonography is optimal in that it is sensitive, inexpensive, and can detect and localize large lesions for guiding percutaneous biopsy.[132] Some clinics in Japan and other areas of the Orient now perform screening programs on patients with established or suspected cirrhosis and chronic active hepatitis. Ultrasound examinations are performed at intervals determined by the relative risk a given patient has of developing HCC. Three to six month intervals are typical.[121] Tnaka, et al, screened over 5,000 patients at risk for developing HCC, and noted that ultrasound had more than 90 percent overall diagnostic accuracy.[133] In comparative studies, Kudo, et al, determined that ultrasound was more precise in the detection and characterization of HCC than isotope studies, CT or angiography.[134] Holm, et al, determined that with experienced staff and modern real-time equipment, ultrasound has a predictive diagnostic value of 97 and 96 percent for positive and negative findings respectively in the detection of all types of malignant hepatic disease.[4]

Forty-six percent of patients with proven HCC ranging in size from 3 to 5 cm were found to have normal serum alphafetoprotein (AFP) levels, implying that ultrasound is more sensitive, since early HCC detection as lesions must reach a minimum size limit before developing elevated AFP levels.[135] Some authors have nonetheless advocated the combined use of sonography and AFP surveillance in patients with chronic hepatitis in order to improve early diagnosis.[136, 137, 132]

Laberge, et al, has found both CT and ultrasound equally accurate in the detection of HCC.[138] CT, however, demonstrated more extensive hepatic parenchymal involvement (Fig. 1.24), and was more accurate in detecting extrahepatic spread of tumor, although vascular invasion was more frequently seen with ultrasound. Consequentially, if a lesion is detected sonographically within multiple hepatic segments or within the hepatic or portal venous systems, the workup can be terminated. In these cases ultrasound guided needle biopsy is an accurate and high yield procedure for confirming the presence and extent of tumor.[139] If the ultrasound findings are equivocal or if the lesion appears resectable on ultrasound, then CT should be performed for further delineation of lesions that would otherwise be missed sonographically, and for evaluation of extrahepatic disease (Fig. 1.25).[138, 140, 124]

There is considerable interest in evaluating the diagnostic accuracy of MRI

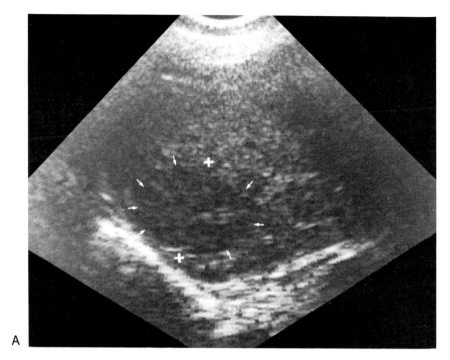

A

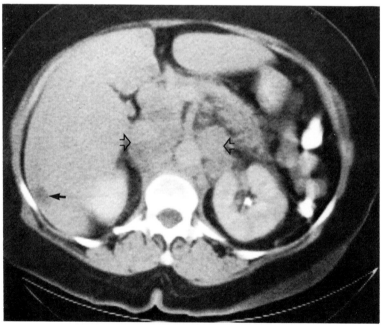

B

FIG. 1.24. Hepatoma. (A) Sonogram of the right lobe of the liver reveals a poorly defined hypoechoic mass (arrows) in the posterior segment of the right lobe of the liver. (B) Although a CT scan of the same region reveals a smaller area of hepatic parenchymal involvement (solid black arrow), it is helpful in delineating extra hepatic disease (Open black arrows = retroperitoneal adenopathy).

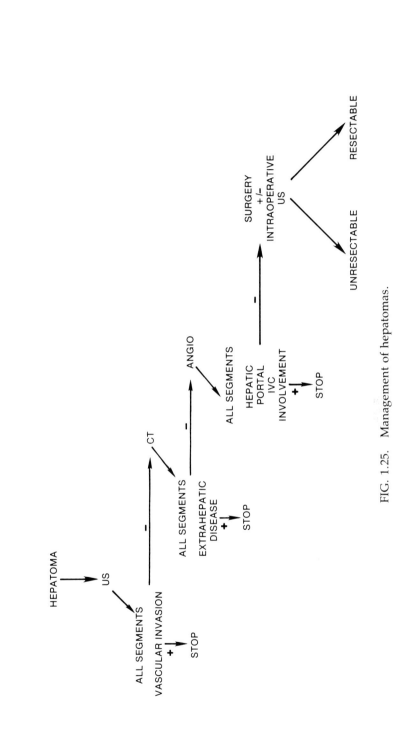

FIG. 1.25.　Management of hepatomas.

for HCC lesion detection because of its increased tissue contrast resolution. Although the ultimate role of MRI is presently undefined, newer pulse sequences are promising. Ebara, et al, noted that MRI and CT had comparable sensitivities, although ultrasound in this series was more sensitive than either technique.[141] The diagnostic sensitivity of MRI appears to be size related, with lesions less than 2 cm in size detected with sensitivities diminishing to 33 percent.[125]

PRIMARY INTRAHEPATIC CHOLANGIOCARCINOMA

Sonographically, intrahepatic cholangiocarcinomas present with a dilated intrahepatic biliary tree and normal extra hepatic bile ducts. Occasionally, an apparent intraductal mass at the confluence of the right and left hepatic ducts (Klatskin tumor), or a mass at the porta hepatis may be seen.[142, 143] If associated with large portal lymph nodes the sonographic appearance may be indistinguishable from other causes of portal lymphadenopathy such as lymphoma or metastatic disease; bulky portal lymphadenopathy may simulate a central parenchymal mass.[144]

Comparative studies have been performed between ultrasound, CT and MRI. Although cholangiocarcinoma, in one series, was better delineated with MRI than it was with either CT or ultrasound, ultrasound was superior to MRI in the delineation of intrahepatic biliary duct dilatation.[143] Cholangiography remains the test of choice for delineating bile duct anatomy and tumor extent.

PEDIATRIC HEPATIC LESIONS

Malignant lesions of the liver in childhood are ten times more common than primary benign lesions.[145, 146, 147, 148] Hematogenous extension from primary neoplasms such as neuroblastoma, Wilms tumor, rhabdomyosarcoma, focal lymphoma, or leukemia are the most common metastatic lesions. Hepatoblastoma, HCC, and primary hepatic rhabdomyosarcoma are the most common primary malignant tumors. Benign lesions, which are less common, include multiple hemangiomas, adenomas of glycogen storage disease, choledochal cysts, FNH, abscesses, and cystic hepatoblastomas.[147] Ultrasound is recommended as the initial imaging procedure because of its low cost, lack of ionizing radiation, and accuracy in separating cystic from solid lesions. Most pediatric focal hepatic lesions cannot be differentiated on the basis of their sonographic appearance alone. Correlative information with clinical data as well as with information derived from ancillary imaging modalities, such as scintigraphy and CT, are almost always required.[145, 146, 147]

Vascular lesions such as hemangiomas, hemangioendotheliomatosis, and mesenchymal hamartomas are usually associated with dilatation of the proximal abdominal aorta and hepatic veins. This aids in their differentiation from hepatoblastomas and hepatomas which, despite their vascularity, are usually not associated with dilatation of these vessels.[149]

The differential diagnosis of a cystic mass in a child should include a mesenchymal hamartoma, embryonal cell sarcoma (Fig. 1.26), a cystic hepatoblas-

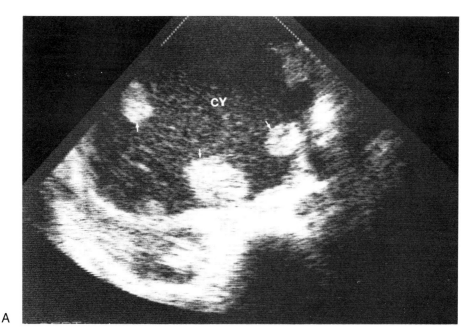

A

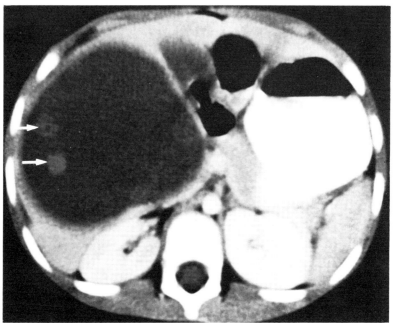

B

FIG. 1.26. Embryonal sarcoma. (A) Transverse sonogram of the right lobe of the liver of a 4-year-old patient who presented with right upper quadrant pain. There is a predominately cystic lesion, *CY*, with internal echoes and multiple large echogenic nodular masses (arrows). (B) CT scan of the same region demonstrates the cystic mass in the right lobe of the liver with internal solid components (arrows). (Courtesy of Bruce Markle, M.D., National Children's Hospital Center, Washington, D.C.)

toma, abscess, hydatid cyst, or necrotic metastases. If solid, a hepatoblastoma, infantile hemangioendothelioma, HCC, or metastatic lesion should be considered.[97]

Ultrasound cannot consistently distinguish between benign and malignant hepatic tumors, although invasion or amputation of portal venous radicals is indicative of malignant disease rather than benign disease where simple compression of venous structures is generally found.[147] CT and scintigraphy are often required as complementary procedures adding functional and morphologic information. CT is also helpful in the assessment of the remainder of the abdomen including the retroperitoneum and intraperitoneal viscera. Tcm^{99-}HIDA may reveal radiotracer uptake in benign lesions such as FNH, and choledochal cysts. Tcm^{99}RBCs will often show increased flow in CH and in infantile hemangioendotheliomatosis.[150, 151]

NEW DEVELOPMENTS

Quantitative microstructural sonography, although still currently experimental, utilizes frequency as well as amplitude of ultrasound echoes in a spectral analysis technique.[152] There is some promise that this technique may be able to distinguish tumors from other forms of underlying disseminated parenchymal disease such as might be found in alcoholic liver disease.

Improvements in transducer design have resulted in the development of small, easily manipulated, high frequency probes that can be adapted for intraoperative use. Intraoperative ultrasound has been reported to be of value in localizing focal hepatic lesions for excision, drainage or biopsy.[153] This method clearly shows the portal and hepatic veins around a tumor, making it easier for the surgeon to optimize vascular ligation points during a portal-branch oriented segmental hepatectomy.[154] Intraoperative sonography can also detect intravascular tumor more accurately than preoperative imaging techniques, and is more accurate in assessing the internal characteristics of space occupying lesions.

SUMMARY

Despite rapid technologic advances, and the introduction of new, competitive imaging techniques, ultrasound, although a mature modality, remains a versatile and indispensible technology. Ease, access, low cost, and accuracy will assure its central role in the investigation of localized hepatic lesions for the foreseeable future.

ACKNOWLEDGEMENT

We wish to extend our gratitude to Kathleen Jensen for her invaluable assistance in the preparation of this manuscript.

REFERENCES

1. Federle MP, Filly RA, Moss AA: Cystic hepatic neoplasms: complementary roles of CT and sonography. AJR 136:345, 1981

2. Sexton CC, Zeman RK: Correlation of computed tomography, sonography, and gross anatomy of the liver. AJR 141:711, 1983

3. Marks WM, Filly RA, Callen PW: Ultrasonic anatomy of the liver: a review with new applications. J Clin Ultrasound 7:137, 1979

4. Holm J, Jacobsen B: Accuracy of dynamic ultrasonography in the diagnosis of malignant liver lesions. J of Ultrasound Med 5:1, 1986

5. Bernardino ME: Radiology: Diagnosis/imaging/intervention. Taveras JM, Ferrucci JT (eds): Vol 4, Lippincott, New York, 1986

6. Thompson JN, Gibson R, Czerniak A, Blumgart LH: Focal liver lesions: a plan for management. Brit Med J 290:1643, 1985

7. Scheible W: A diagnostic algorithm for liver masses. Semin Roentgenol 18:84, 1983

8. Zeman RK, Paushter DM, Schiebler ML, et al: Hepatic imaging: current status. Rad Clin of North Am 23:473, 1985

9. Tylen U: Radiological diagnosis of liver tumours. Annales Chirurgiae et Gynaecologiae 75:35, 1986

10. Pagani JJ: Intrahepatic vascular territories shown by computed tomography (CT). Radiology 147:173, 1983

11. Goldsmith NA, Woodburne RT: The surgical anatomy pertaining to liver resection. Surg Gynecol Obstet 105:310, 1957

12. Graif M, Manor A, Itzchak Y: Sonographic differentiation of extra- and intrahepatic masses. AJR 141:553, 1983

13. Gore RM, Callen PW, Filly RA: Displaced retroperitoneal fat: sonographic guide to right upper quadrant mass localization. Radiology 142:701, 1982

14. Auh YH, Rubenstein WA, Zirinsky K, et al: Accessory fissures of the liver: CT and sonographic appearance. AJR 143:565, 1984

15. Mitchell SE, Gross BH, Spitz HB: The hypoechoic caudate lobe: an ultrasonic pseudolesion. Radiology 144:569, 1982

16. Prando A, Goldstein HM, Bernardino ME, Green B: Ultrasonic pseudolesions of the liver. Radiology 130:403, 1979

17. Auh YH, Pardes JG, Chung KB, et al: Posterior hepatodiaphragmatic interposition of the colon: ultrasonographic and computed tomographic appearance. J Ultrasound Med 4:113, 1985

18. Skwarok DJ, Goiney RC, Cooperberg PL: Hepatic pseudotumors in patients with ascites. J Ultrasound Med 5:5, 1986

19. Gosink BB: Intrahepatic gas: differential diagnosis. AJR 137:763, 1981

20. Pardes JG, Haaga JR, Borkowski G: Focal hepatic fatty metamorphosis secondary to trauma. J Comput Assist Tomogr 6:769, 1982

21. Quinn SF, Gosink BB: Characteristic sonographic signs of hepatic fatty infiltration. AJR 145:753, 1985

22. Scott WW, Jr., Sanders RC, Siegelman SS: Irregular fatty infiltration of the liver: diagnostic dilemmas. AJR 135:67, 1980

23. Kawashima A, Suehiro S, Murayama S, Russell WJ: Focal fatty infiltration of the liver mimicking a tumor: sonographic and CT features. J Comput Assist Tomogr 10:329, 1986

24. Bashist B, Hecht HL, Harley WD: Computed tomographic demonstration of rapid changes in fatty infiltration of the liver. Radiology 142:691, 1982

25. Yates CK, Streight RA: Focal fatty infiltration of the liver simulating metastatic disease. Radiology 159:83, 1986

26. Patel S, Sandler CM, Rauschkolb EN, McConnell BJ: [133]Xe uptake in focal hepatic fat accumulation: CT correlation. AJR 138:541, 1982

27. Halvorsen RA, Korobkin M, Ram PC, Thompson WM: CT appearance of focal fatty infiltration of the liver. AJR 139:277, 1982

28. Brick SH, Hill MC, Lande IM: The mistaken or indeterminate CT diagnosis of hepatic metastases: the value of sonography. AJR 148:723, 1987

29. Barnes PA, Thomas JL, Bernardino ME: Pitfalls in the diagnosis of hepatic cysts by computed tomography. Radiology 141:129, 1981

30. Roemer CE, Ferrucci JT, Jr, Mueller PR, et al: Hepatic cysts: diagnosis and therapy by sonographic needle aspiration. AJR 136:1065, 1981

31. Spiegel RM, King DL, Green WM: Ultrasonography of primary cysts of the liver. AJR 131:235, 1978

32. Hill M, Sanders RC: Gray scale B scan characteristics of intraabdominal cystic masses. J of Clin Ultrasound 6:215, 1978

33. Weaver RM, Jr, Goldstein HM, Green B, Perkins C: Gray scale ultrasonographic evaluation of hepatic cystic disease. AJR 130:849, 1978

34. Forrest ME, Cho KJ, Shields JJ, et al: Biliary cystadenomas: sonographic-angiographic-pathologic correlations. AJR 135:723, 1980

35. Frick MP, Feinberg SB: Biliary cystadenoma. AJR 139:393, 1982

36. Marchal GJ, Desmet VJ, Proesmans WC, et al: Caroli disease: high-frequency US and pathologic findings. Radiology 158:507, 1986

37. Lieberman E, Salinas-Madrigal L, Gwinn JL, et al: Infantile polycystic disease of the kidneys and liver: clinical, pathological and radiological correlations and comparisons with hepatic fibrosis. Medicine 50:277, 1971

38. Mittelstaedt CA, Volberg FM, Fischer GJ, McCartney WH: Caroli's disease: sonographic findings. AJR 134:585, 1980

39. Sorensen KW, Glazer GM, Francis IR: Diagnosis of cystic ectasia of intrahepatic bile ducts by computed tomography. J Comput Assist Tomogr 6:486, 1982

40. Austin RM, Sussman S, McArdle CR, et al: Computed tomographic and ultrasound appearances of a solitary intrahepatic choledochal cyst. Clin Rad 37:149, 1986

41. Cancer facts and figures. American Cancer Society, New York, 1985

42. Adson MA: Canon lecture-hepatic metastases in perspective. AJR 140:695, 1983

43. Malt RA: Current concepts-surgery for hepatic neoplasms. N Engl J Med 31:1591, 1985

44. Scheible W, Gosink BB, Leopold GR: Gray scale echographic patterns of hepatic metastatic disease. AJR 129:983, 1977

45. Marchal GJ, Pylyser K, Tshibwabwa-Tumba EA, et al: Anechoic halo in solid liver tumors: sonographic, microangiographic, and histologic correlation. Radiology 156:479, 1985

46. Marchal G, Tshibwabwa-Tumba E, Oyen R, et al: Correlation of sonographic patterns in liver metastases with histology and microangiography. Invest Rad 20:79, 1985

47. Bernardino ME, Green B: Ultrasonographic evaluation of chemotherapeutic response in hepatic metastases. Radiology 133:437, 1979

48. Ginaldi S, Bernardino ME, Jing BS, Green B: Ultrasonographic patterns of hepatic lymphoma. Radiology 136:427, 1980

49. Burgener FA, Hamlin DJ: Histiocytic lymphoma of the abdomen: radiographic spectrum. AJR 137:337, 1981

50. Nyberg DA, Jeffrey RB, Jr, Federle MP, et al: AIDS-related lymphomas: evaluation by abdominal CT. Radiology 159:59, 1986

51. Lepke R, Pagani JJ: Sonography of hepatic chloromas. AJR 138:1176, 1982

52. Callen PW, Filly RA, Marcus FS: Ultrasonography and computed tomography in the evaluation of hepatic microabscesses in the immunosuppressed patient. Radiology 136:433, 1980

53. Ferrucci JT: MR imaging of the liver. AJR 147:1103, 1986

54. Gunven P, Makuucki M, Takayasu K, et al: Preoperative imaging of liver metastases. Comparison of angiography, CT scan, and ultrasonography. Ann Surg 202:573, 1985

55. Alderson PO, Adams DF, McNeil BJ, et al: Computed tomography, ultrasound, and scintigraphy of the liver in patients with colon or breast carcinoma: a prospective comparison. Radiology 149:225, 1983

56. Prando A, Wallace S, Bernardino ME, Lindell MM, Jr.: Computed tomographic arteriography of the liver. Radiology 130:697, 1979

57. Matsui O, Kadoya M, Suzuki M, et al: Work in progress: dynamic sequential computed tomography during arterial portography in the detection of hepatic neoplasms. Radiology 146:721, 1983

58. Freeny PC, Marks WM, Ryan JA, Bolen JW: Colorectal carcinoma evaluation with CT: preoperative staging and detection of postoperative recurrence. Radiology 158:347, 1986

59. Reinig JW, Dwyer AJ, Miller DL, et al: Liver metastasis detection: comparative sensitivities of MR imaging and CT scanning. Radiology 162:43, 1987

60. Lam AH, Shulman L: Ultrasonography in the management of liver trauma in children. J Ultrasound Med 3:199, 1984

61. Moon KL, Jr, Federle MP: Computed tomography in hepatic trauma. AJR 141:309, 1983

62. Engel MA, Marks DS, Sandler MA, Shetty P: Differentiation of focal intrahepatic lesions with ^{99m}Tc-red blood cell imaging. Radiology 146:777, 1983

63. Bree RL, Schwab RE, Neiman HL: Solitary echogenic spot in the liver: is it diagnostic of a hemangioma? AJR 140:41, 1983

64. Pen JH, Pelckmans PA, van Maercke YM, et al: Clinical significance of focal echogenic liver lesions. Gastrointest Radiol 11:61, 1986

65. Johnson CM, Sheedy PF, Stanson AW, et al: Computed tomography and angiography of cavernous hemangiomas of the liver. Radiology 138:115, 1981

66. Ishak KG, Rabin L: Benign tumors of the liver. Med Clin North Am 59:995, 1975

67. Wiener SN, Parulekar SG: Scintigraphy and ultrasonography of hepatic hemangioma. Radiology 132:149, 1979

68. Park WC, Phillips R: The role of radiation therapy in the management of hemangiomas of the liver. JAMA 212:1496, 1970

69. Mirk P, Rubaltelli L, Bazzocchi M, et al: Ultrasonographic patterns in hepatic hemangiomas. J Clin Ultrasound 10:373, 1982

70. Freeny PC, Vimont TR, Barnett DC: Cavernous hemangioma of the liver: ultrasonography, arteriography, and computed tomography. Radiology 132:143, 1979

71. Solbiati L, Livraghy T, L De Pra, et al: Fine-needle biopsy of hepatic hemangioma with sonographic guidance. AJR 144:471, 1985

72. Barnett PH, Zerhouni EA, White RI, Siegelman SS: Computed tomography in the diagnosis of cavernous hemangioma of the liver. AJR 143:439, 1980

73. Taboury J, Porcel A, Tubiana JM, Monnier JP: Cavernous hemangiomas of the liver studied by ultrasound. Radiology 149:781, 1983

74. Itai Y, Ohtomo K, Araki T, et al: Computed tomography and sonography of cavernous hemangioma of the liver. AJR 141:315, 1983

75. Barnett PH, Zerhouni EA, White RI, Jr, Siegelman SS: Computed tomography in the diagnosis of cavernous hemangioma of the liver. AJR 134:439, 1980

76. Freeny PC, Marks WM: Hepatic hemangioma: dynamic bolus CT. AJR 147:711, 1986
77. Glazer GM, Aisen AM, Francis IR, et al: Hepatic cavernous hemangioma: magnetic resonance imaging. Radiology 155:417, 1985
78. Scatarige JC, Fishman EK, Sanders RC: The sonographic "scar sign" in focal nodular hyperplasia of the liver. J Ultrasound Med 1:275, 1982
79. Rogers JV, Mack LA, Freeny PC, et al: Hepatic focal nodular hyperplasia: angiography, CT, sonography, and scintigraphy. AJR 137:983, 1981
80. Fishman EK, Farmlett E, Kadir S, Siegelman SS: Computed tomography of benign hepatic tumors. J Comput Assist Tomogr 6:472, 1982
81. Welch TJ, Sheedy PF, Johnson CM: Radiographic characteristics of benign liver tumors: focal nodular hyperplasia and hepatic adenoma. RadioGraphics 5:673, 1985
82. Welch TJ, Sheedy PF, Johnson CM, et al: Focal nodular hyperplasia and hepatic adenoma: comparison of angiography, CT, US, and scintigraphy. Radiology 156:593, 1985
83. Butch RJ, Stark DD, Malt RA: MR imaging of hepatic focal nodular hyperplasia. J Comput Assist Tomog 10:874, 1986
84. Mattison GR, Glazer GM, Quint LE, et al: MR imaging of hepatic focal nodular hyperplasia: characterization and distinction from primary malignant hepatic tumors. AJR 148:711, 1987
85. Sandler MA, Petrocelli RD, Marks DS, Lopez R: Ultrasonic features and radionuclide correlation in liver cell adenoma and focal nodular hyperplasia. Radiology 135:393, 1980
86. Klatstein G: Hepatic tumors: possible relationships to use of oral contraceptives. Gastroenterology 73:386, 1977
87. Quinn SF, Hanks J, Shaffer H: Sonographic diagnosis of a liver cell adenoma. Southern Med J 79:372, 1986
88. Brunelle F, Tammam S, Odievre M, Chaumont P: Liver adenomas in glycogen storage disease in children. Ultrasound and angiographic study. Pediatr Radiol 14:94, 1984
89. Bowerman RA, Samuels BI, Silver TM: Ultrasonographic features of hepatic adenomas in type I glycogen storage disease. J Ultrasound Med 2:51, 1983
90. Mason HH, Anderson DH: Glycogen disease of the liver (von Gierke's disease) with hepatomata. Pediatrics 16:785, 1955
91. Grossman H, Ram PC, Coleman RA, et al: Hepatic ultrasonography in type I glycogen storage disease (von Gierke's disease): detection of hepatic adenoma and carcinoma. Radiology 141:753, 1981
92. Laing FC, Jeffrey RB, Federle MP, Cello JP: Noninvasive imaging of unusual regenerating nodules in the cirrhotic liver. Gastrointest Radiol 7:245, 1982
93. Freeman MP, Vick CW, Taylor KJW, et al: Regenerating nodules in cirrhosis: sonographic appearance with anatomic correlation. AJR 146:533, 1986
94. Rosenbaum DM, Mindell HJ: Ultrasonographic findings in mesenchymal hamartoma of the liver. Radiology 138:425, 1981
95. Ros PR, Goodman ZD, Ishak KG, et al: Mesenchymal hamartoma of the liver: radiologic-pathologic correlation. Radiology 158:619, 1986
96. Edmondson HA: Differential diagnosis of tumors and tumor-like lesions of liver in infancy and childhood. AMA J Dis Child 91:168, 1956
97. Ros PR, Olmsted WW, Dachman AH, et al: Undifferentiated (embryonal) sarcoma of the liver: radiologic-pathologic correlation. Radiology 160:141, 1986
98. Stocker JT, Ishak KG: Undifferentiated (embryonal) sarcoma of the liver. Report of 31 cases. Cancer 42:336, 1978
99. Kuligowska E, Connors SK, Shapiro JH: Liver abscess: sonography in diagnosis and treatment. AJR 138:253, 1982

100. Silver S, Weinstein A, Cooperman A: Changes in the pathogenesis and detection of intrahepatic abscess. Am J Surg 137:608, 1979

101. Freeny PC: Acute pyogenic hepatitis: sonographic and angiographic findings. AJR 135:388, 1980

102. Terrier F, Becker CD, Triller JK: Morphologic aspects of hepatic abscesses at computed tomography and ultrasound. Acta Radiologica Diagnosis 24:129, 1983

103. Subramanyam BR, Balthazar EJ, Raghavendra BN, et al: Ultrasound analysis of solid-appearing abscesses. Radiology 146:487, 1983

104. Powers TA, Jones TB, Karl JH: Echogenic hepatic abscess without radiographic evidence of gas. AJR 137:159, 1981

105. Schwerk WV, Durr HK: Ultrasound gray-scale pattern and guided aspiration puncture of abdominal abscesses. J Clin Ultrasound 9:389, 1981

106. Sones PJ, Jr, Thomas BM, Masand PP: Falciform ligament abscess: appearance on computed tomography and sonography. AJR 137:161, 1981

107. Rubinson HA, Isikoff MB, Hill MC: Diagnostic imaging of hepatic abscesses: a retrospective analysis. AJR 135:735, 1980

108. Choliz JD, Olaverri FJL, Casas TF, Zubieta SO: Computed tomography in hepatic echinococcosis. AJR 139:699, 1982

109. Hadidi A: Ultrasound findings in liver hydatid cysts. JCU 7:365, 1979

110. Gharbi HA, Hassine W, Brauner MW, Dupuch K: Ultrasound examination of the hydatic liver. Radiology 139:459, 1981

111. Lewall DB, McCorkell SJ: Hepatic echinococcal cysts: sonographic appearance and classification. Radiology 155:773, 1985

112. Bezzi M, Teggi A, De Rosa F, et al: Abdominal hydatid disease: US findings during medical treatment. Radiology 162:91, 1987

113. Lewall DB, McCorkell SJ: Hepatic echinococcal cysts: sonographic appearance and classification. Radiology 155:773, 1985

114. Mueller PR, Dawson SL, Ferrucci JT, Jr., Nardi GL: Hepatic echinococcal cyst: successful percutaneous drainage. Radiology 155:627, 1985

115. Didier D, Weiler S, Rohmer P, et al: Hepatic alveolar echinococcosis: correlative US and CT study. Radiology 154:179, 1985.

116. Ho B, Cooperberg PL, Li DKB, et al: Ultrasonography and computed tomography of hepatic candidiasis in immunosuppressed patients. J Ultrasound Med 1:157, 1982

117. Ralls PW, Colletti PM, Quinn MF, Halls J: Sonographic findings in hepatic amebic abscess. Radiology 145:123, 1982

118. DeBakey ME, Ochsner A: Collective review. Hepatic amebiasis. A 20 year experience and analysis of 263 cases. Int Abstr Surg 92:209, 1951

119. Sukov RJ, Cohen LJ, Sample WF: Sonography of hepatic amebic abscesses. AJR 134:911, 1980

120. Ralls PW, Quinn MF, Boswell WD, Jr, et al: Patterns of resolution in successfully treated hepatic amebic abscess: sonographic evaluation. Radiology 149:541, 1983

121. Okuda K: Early recognition of hepatocellular carcinoma. Hepatology 6:729, 1986

122. Kamin PD, Bernardino ME, Green B: Ultrasound manifestations of hepatocellular carcinoma. Radiology 131:459, 1979

123. Broderick TW, Gosink B, Menuck L, et al: Echographic and radionuclide detection of hepatoma. Radiology 135:149, 1980

124. Teefey SA, Stephens DH, James EM, et al: Computed tomography and ultrasonography of hepatoma. Clinical Radiology 37:339, 1986

125. Subramanyam BR, Balthazar EJ, Hilton S, et al: Hepatocellular carcinoma with venous invasion. Radiology 150:793, 1984

126. Longmaid HE, Seltzer SE, Costello P, Gordon P: Hepatocellular carcinoma presenting as primary extrahepatic mass on CT. AJR 146:1005, 1985

127. vanSonnenberg E, Ferrucci JT, Jr: Bile duct obstruction in hepatocellular carcinoma (hepatoma)—clinical and cholangiographic characteristics. Radiology 130:7, 1979

128. Sheu JC, Chen DS, Sung JL, et al: Hepatocellular carcinoma: US evolution in the early stage. Radiology 155:463, 1985

129. Tanaka S, Kitamura T, Imaoka S, et al: Hepatocellular carcinoma: sonographic and histologic correlation. AJR 140:701, 1983

130. Shamaa SS, El-Desoky I, El-Diasty T, et al: Primary hepatocellular carcinoma: clinical, ultrasonic, and pathological patterns and correlations. Cancer Detect Prevent 9:227, 1986

131. Morimoto K, Matsui K, Hashimoto T: Intraatrial extension of hepatocellular carcinoma detected with ultrasound. JCU 14:466, 1986

132. Maringhini A, Cottone M, Sciarrino E, et al: Ultrasonographic and radionuclide detection of hepatocellular carcinoma in cirrhotics with low alpha-fetoprotein levels. Cancer 54:2924, 1984

133. Tanaka S, Kitamura T, Ohshima A, et al: Diagnostic accuracy of ultrasonography for hepatocellular carcinoma. Cancer 58:344, 1986

134. Kuda M, Hirasa M, Takakuwa H, et al: Small hepatocellular carcinomas in chronic liver disease: Detection with SPECT. Radiology 159:697, 1986

135. Sheu JC, Sung JL, Chen DS, et al: Early detection of hepatocellular carcinoma by real-time ultrasonography. Cancer 56:660, 1985

136. Liaw YF, Tai DI, Chu CM, et al: Early detection of hepatocellular carcinoma in patients with chronic type B hepatitis. Gastroent 90:263, 1986

137. Takashima T, Matsui O, Suzuki M, Ida M: Diagnosis and screening of small hepatocellular carcinomas. Radiology 145:635, 1982

138. LaBerge JM, Laing FC, Federle MP, et al: Hepatocellular carcinoma: assessment of resectability by computed tomography and ultrasound. Radiology 152:485, 1984

139. Tanaka S, Kitamura T, Kasugai H, et al: Early diagnosis of hepatocellular carcinoma: usefulness of ultrasonically guided fine-needle aspiration biopsy. JCU 14:11, 1986

140. Chen DS, Sheu JC, Sung JL, et al: Small hepatocellular carcinoma—a clinicopathological study in thirteen patients. Gastroent 83:1109, 1982

141. Ebara M, Ohto M, Watanabe Y, et al: Diagnosis of small hepatocellular carcinoma: correlation of MR imaging and tumor histologic studies. Radiology 159:371, 1986

142. Carr DH, Hadjis NS, Banks LM, et al: Computed tomography of hilar cholangiocarcinoma: a new sign. AJR 145:53, 1985

143. Dooms GC, Kerlan RK, Jr., Hricak H, et al: Cholangiocarcinoma: imaging by MR. Radiology 159:89, 1986

144. Machan L, Muller NL, Cooperberg PL: Sonographic diagnosis of Klatskin tumors. AJR 147:509, 1986

145. Miller JH, Greenspan BS: Integrated imaging of hepatic tumors in childhood. Part 1: Malignant lesions (primary and metastatic) Radiology 154:83, 1985

146. Miller JH, Greenspan BS: Integrated imaging of hepatic tumors in childhood. Part 2: Benign lesions (congenital, reparative, and inflammatory) Radiology 154:91, 1985

147. Brunelle F, Chaumont P: Hepatic tumors in children: ultrasonic differentiation of malignant from benign lesions. Radiology 150:695, 1984

148. Miller JH: The ultrasonographic appearance of cystic hepatoblastoma. Radiology 138:141, 1981

149. Abramson SJ, Lack EE, Teele RL: Benign vascular tumors of the liver in infants: sonographic appearance. AJR 138:629, 1982

150. Pardes JG, Bryan PJ, Gauderer MWL: Spontaneous regression of infantile hemangioendotheliomatosis of the liver: demonstration by ultrasound. J Ultrasound Med 1:349, 1982

151. Dachman AH, Lichtenstein JE, Friedman AC, Hartman DS: Infantile hemangioendothelioma of the liver: a radiologic-pathologic-clinical correlation. AJR 140:1091, 1983

152. King DL, Lizzi FL, Feleppa EJ, et al: Focal and diffuse liver disease studied by quantitative microstructural sonography. Radiology 155:457, 1985

153. Glen PM, Noseworthy J, Babcock DS: Use of intraoperative ultrasonography to localize a hepatic abscess. Arch Surg 119:347, 1984

154. Igawa S, Sakai K, Kinoshita H, Hirohashi K: Intraoperative sonography: clinical usefulness in liver surgery. Radiology 156:473, 1985

2 Diffuse Benign Liver Disease

LAURENCE NEEDLEMAN

Ultrasound is commonly performed to evaluate suspected hepatobiliary disease. It is a well established means to diagnose biliary dilatation and masses involving the liver, pancreas, or bile ducts, but less established to evaluate hepatocellular diseases. It is important to understand the strengths and weaknesses of sonography to both diagnose the presence of these diseases and to evaluate complications which may occur in those with parenchymal liver disease.

TECHNIQUE

Static scans are most accurate to obtain measurements of the liver and to evaluate the overall organ. In practice, most examinations are done adequately with real-time ultrasound. Its advantages are its shorter examination time and its ability to evaluate the liver in multiple planes.

The liver should be evaluated in at least two planes, usually longitudinal and transverse. Power and time gain compensation are considered optimal when parenchymal echoes are as bright as possible and fluid-filled structures are as anechoic as resolution permits.

Longitudinal views of the liver and the right kidney together are helpful to compare the echogenicity of the two organs. Increased echogenicity of the liver may appear as closely packed and fine or inhomogeneous and coarsened. In addition to the overall echogenicity of the liver, the texture should be evaluated for homogeneity of the parenchymal echoes, definition of the portal venule walls, and attenuation of the sound beam by the liver.

The normal liver (Fig. 2.1) shows a homogeneous parenchyma with echogenicity slightly greater than the normal renal cortex. The walls of the larger portal venules and of several smaller branches, especially those in the focal zone, should be relatively bright. In normal sized subjects, the parenchyma should have similar echogenicity from anterior to posterior. In larger patients some attenuation of the sound beam may be noted.

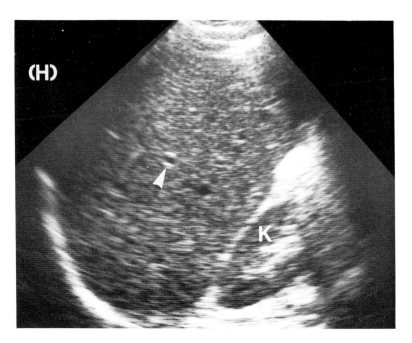

FIG. 2.1. Normal liver. Longitudinal sonogram of the right lobe of the liver and the right kidney, *K*. The parenchymal echogenicity is homogeneous. The portal venule walls (arrowhead) exhibit normal brightness, particularly in the focal zone. The attenuation is normal with a normal appearance of the liver posteriorly. (*H*) = toward patient's head.

A complete study should include evaluation of the bile ducts and the spleen. The size of the portal and splenic vein should be noted and ascites and varices should be searched for when appropriate.

LIVER SIZE

Based on its use in nuclear medicine, several investigators have used the longitudinal length of the liver to determine if hepatomegaly is present. Gosink and Leymaster found a length of 15.5 cm in the midclavicular line 87 percent accurate to determine hepatomegaly. A normal length was 13 cm or less. Twenty-five percent of their patients had indeterminate values (13.0 to 15.5 cm).[1]

Niederau, et al. evaluated 915 normals and found longitudinal diameters adequate in most cases. Anteroposterior dimensions were also useful in very slender or very heavy subjects. In thin persons the longitudinal dimension is exaggerated while it is smaller in fat subjects. A follow-up clinical study of abnormal subjects showed the longitudinal midclavicular diameter was a reasonable single measure.[3] The 95th percentile value for this measure was 12.6 cm (the mean ± S.D. was 10.5 ± 1.5 cm).[2] Receiver operating characteristic (ROC) curves were established to determine hepatomegaly in acute viral hepatitis and increased alcohol consumption.[3]

By determining and adding the area on sequential static scans, liver volume can be determined with reasonable accuracy,[4] however, this technique is more complicated and time consuming than linear measurements and is clinically impractical in most situations.

FATTY INFILTRATION OF THE LIVER

Fatty infiltration of the liver (FIL) can occur from a variety of causes including alcohol intake, diabetes mellitus, obesity, steroid use, drugs, trauma, toxic substances, Reye's syndrome, inborn errors of metabolism, and others.[5] In many cases it is reversible, and the degree or presence of FIL can change over time. This can be rapid, usually occurring over months, but may even change over days.[6, 7]

FIL produces increased echogenicity of the liver which may be fine (Fig. 2.2) or coarsened (Fig. 2.3).[5, 8–11] Fine echogenicity is said to be more typical.[5] Attenuation of the sound beam is a feature of FIL. The presence of fat, but

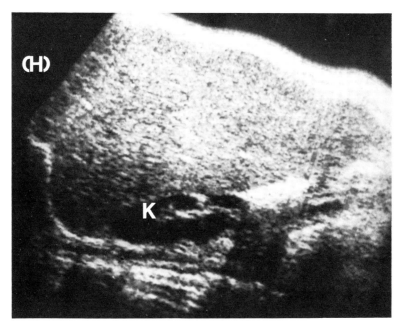

FIG. 2.2. Fatty infiltration in an infant due to glycogen storage disease. Longitudinal sonogram of the right lobe of the liver and right kidney, K. The liver is enlarged and the parenchymal echogenicity is increased compared to the kidney. The parenchyma exhibits fine homogeneously increased echoes and no portal venule walls are defined. There is distal attenuation of the sound beam. (H) = toward patient's head.

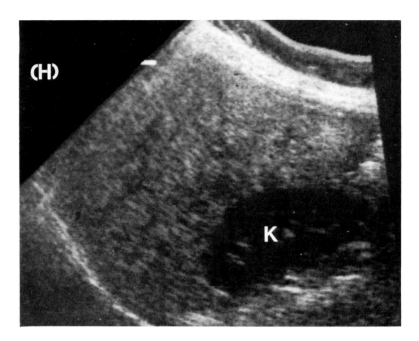

FIG. 2.3. Fatty infiltration. Longitudinal sonogram of the right lobe of the liver and right kidney, K. The parenchymal echogenicity is increased, making the normal kidney appear hypoechoic. The parenchyma exhibits coarsened increased echoes and no portal venule walls are defined. There is no significant attenuation of the sound beam. (H) = toward patient's head.

not fibrosis, has been shown to correlate with attenuation in both clinical[12] and tissue characterization studies.[13, 14]

Liver enlargement is helpful to determine if fatty change is present since cirrhosis shows a normal or small liver. In one study, 75 to 80 percent of patients with moderate to severe FIL had hepatomegaly.[5]

Sonography is a good test to detect FIL with sensitivities exceeding 90 percent in many studies[5, 15] and accuracies reported to 85 to 97 percent.[5] Moderate to severe fatty infiltration virtually always produces an abnormal liver texture.[5, 11, 15]

Focal Fatty Infiltration

Diagnostic difficulties may occur with FIL because the process need not be uniform nor diffuse through the liver.[16, 17] Usually FIL has a diffuse, lobar or segmental distribution.[18] This pattern of distribution leads to angulated or geometric boundaries between normal and affected liver and can suggest the diagnosis.[19] Fatty replaced liver, unlike focal masses, will have little or no mass effect. Vessels can be seen to course through involved portions of the liver without displacement.[20] Interdigitating margins of normal and echogenic fatty liver may also be characteristic[19] (Fig. 2.4). Rare presentations of

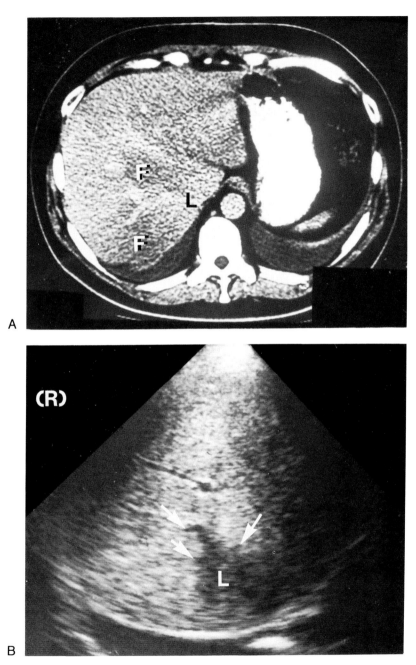

FIG. 2.4. Focal fatty infiltration. (A) Computed tomography (CT) shows high attenuation normal liver, *L*, mixed with lower attenuation fatty replaced liver, *F*. (B) Transverse sonogram of the area labelled on the CT shows the normal liver, *L*, surrounded by the echogenic fatty liver. There are interdigitating finger-like projections (arrows) forming the border between the two. (*R*) = toward patient's right.

focal fatty liver may be of single or multiple echogenic nodules which may simulate metastases[21, 22] (Fig. 2.5).

Another diagnostic problem created by focal FIL occurs when there is nearly generalized fatty change with only small normal regions of liver. The spared areas may simulate hypoechoic masses. A common location for the spared area is the quadrate lobe anterior to the portal vein bifurcation or related to the gallbladder bed[23, 24, 25] (Fig. 2.6). Its shape is typically ovoid but may be spherical to sheet-like. Subcapsular spared areas of normal liver have also been described.[23] The location of the areas led Marchal and coworkers to hypothesize that the cause of the sparing is alteration of blood flow in these areas. Systemic veins, not available to the rest of the liver, supply collaterals to these regions and protect them from fatty infiltration.[23]

HEPATITIS

Acute Hepatitis

Kurtz, et al[26] described a liver texture associated with acute hepatitis. These livers exhibited portal venule walls which were brighter than normal (Fig. 2.7). In some, parenchymal echogenicity was also decreased. This pattern has been called the centrilobular (CL) pattern.

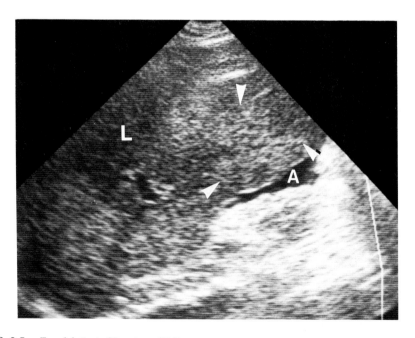

FIG. 2.5. Focal fatty infiltration. Oblique sonogram shows normal liver, L, and multiple discrete echogenic nodules, one of which is delineated by arrowheads. The echogenic areas represented focal regions of fatty replacement. A = Ascites at the edge of liver.

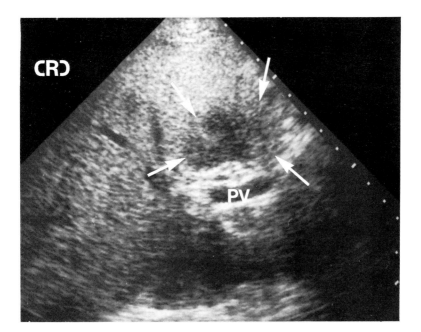

FIG. 2.6. Focal sparing in diffuse fatty infiltration. Transverse sonogram. A focal periportal hypoechoic "mass" (outlined by arrows) represents normal liver surrounded by echogenic fatty replaced liver. Its location is typical, being anterior to the portal vein, *PV*, and related to the gallbladder bed (not shown). (*R*) = toward patient's right.

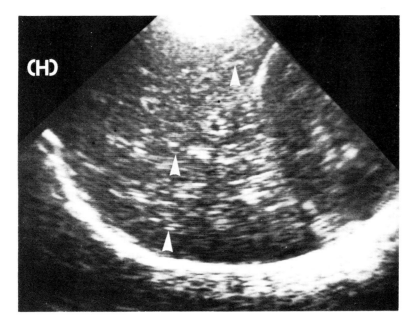

FIG. 2.7. Centrilobular pattern in acute hepatitis. Longitudinal sonogram show abnormally bright portal venule walls in the near field, focal zone, and far field (arrowheads) of the liver. (*H*) = toward patient's head.

In 13 cases with pathology consistent with the CL pattern, ultrasound detected 69 percent, missing only mild cases. Those with the CL pattern differed significantly from both normals and those with echogenic livers.[11]

Giorgio, et al[27] studied a large number of patients with acute viral hepatitis and did not find a significant difference between those with a CL pattern with hepatitis (32 percent) and those without (31 percent).[27] A correlation was found between the presence of a CL pattern and thinness.[27] While our group has identified normal patients with a CL pattern it has not been on the order of 31 percent but rather less than 2 percent. Subjective differences in the criteria of this pattern may explain the discrepant results between the studies. In the study by Giorgio, et al, an echogenic texture, rather than the CL pattern, was seen in some of their patients. These patients with acute hepatitis had significant vacuolar cellular degeneration without fatty infiltration at biopsy.[27]

The centrilobular pattern has been described in rare cases of leukemic infiltration of the liver[26] and in one case of toxic shock syndrome.[28] This pattern has also rarely been seen in diffuse lymphomatous involvement of the liver.

In processes which produce the CL pattern, edema or infiltration occurs in the cells or lobules. Presumably, this accentuates the acoustical mismatch between the liver and portal tracts and makes protal venule walls stand out.[26]

Acute alcoholic hepatitis displays a bright liver pattern.[29] The pattern is likely the result of coexistent fatty infiltration.

Chronic Hepatitis

Chronic hepatitis is another cause of increased liver echogenicity. The definition of portal venule walls is lost. Attenuation is not a feature of chronic hepatitis.[26] The loss of definition of portal walls is explained by the location of the pathologic changes in chronic hepatitis. These diseases have fibrotic and inflammatory processes surrounding the lobules and abutting the portal vein radicles. The acoustical mismatch between the portal vein walls and diseased liver is therefore lost and the venule walls lose their definition.[30]

CIRRHOSIS

Cirrhosis is a chronic liver disease characterized by parenchymal destruction, fibrosis, and nodular regeneration. Complications of cirrhosis are related to hepatocellular failure and portal hypertension.

There is no single sonographic texture indicative of cirrhosis. The parenchyma is usually heterogeneous with increased echogenicity (Fig. 2.8). The pattern is typically coarse, although fine homogeneously increased echogenicity can also be seen. Sandford et al showed a correlation of cirrhosis with

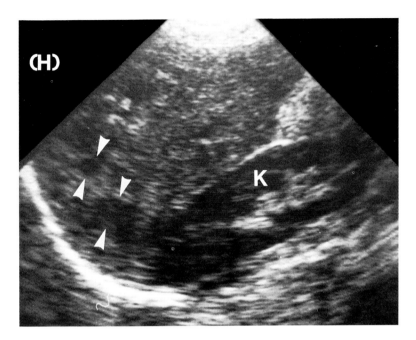

FIG. 2.8.   Cirrhosis. Longitudinal scan of the right lobe of the liver and right kidney, K. The parenchyma is very inhomogeneous and coarsened. Nodules of varying sizes are identified, two of which we marked by arrowheads. At the time of pathological analysis, the liver showed multiple regenerative nodules corresponding to the nodules. The parenchymal echogenicity between the nodules is increased compared to the kidney and the portal venule walls are not well defined. (*H*) = toward patient's head.

both increased echogenicity and loss of detail.[12] The definition of portal venule walls is variable and may be decreased[9, 11, 12] or normal.[15]

   Heterogenicity may be quite striking, even suggesting the presence of focal masses[31] or may be quite subtle (Fig. 2.9). The appreciation of heterogenicity is improved if scans of normal livers using the same machine are available for comparison. Some of the heterogenicity of the cirrhotic liver may be due to small regenerative nodules scattered through the liver (Fig. 2.8).

   Confusion in the literature has resulted from the thought that fibrosis in cirrhosis caused attenuation of the sound beam. It appears that fat, and not fibrosis, causes attenuation.[12–14] Some of the confusion has resulted because fatty change and fibrosis are often present together, particularly in those with alcoholic liver disease.

   Liver morphology may help establish the diagnosis of cirrhosis. A small liver is typical of advanced disease, although a cirrhotic liver may be normal sized. Nodules on the surface can also be characteristic. Harbin, et al have described CT and sonographic changes in the size of the lobes in cirrhosis. There is shrinkage of the right lobe and relative enlargement of the caudate lobe.[34] A ratio of $\geq$ 0.65 between the caudate and right lobe to diagnose

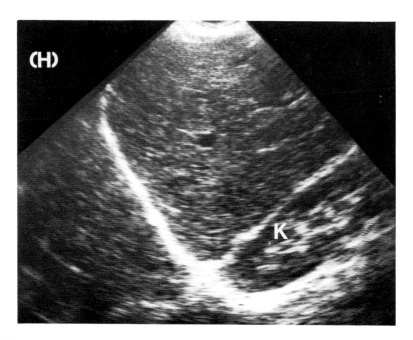

FIG. 2.9. Primary biliary cirrhosis. Longitudinal scan of the liver and right kidney, K. Abnormal liver texture is identified by the mild heterogenicity of the parenchyma. The echogenicity is normal compared to the kidney and the portal venule walls are of normal brightness. Compare this case to Figure 2.1 which was performed on the same machine and the same transducer. (H) = toward patient's head.

cirrhosis had 84 percent sensitivity, 100 percent specificity and 94 percent accuracy. Normal livers had a ratio of <0.6. Giorgio, et al, using the same criteria, confirmed the high specificity (100 percent) but found lower sensitivity (43 percent). They showed the sensitivity varied on the etiology of the cirrhosis. The ratio was most sensitive in cirrhosis due to hepatitis B virus (66 percent) and less for other types of cirrhosis (34 percent).[35] This is compatible with the striking shrinkage of the liver that can be seen with hepatitis B associated cirrhosis. The ratio is least sensitive in alcoholic cirrhosis.[35]

The liver usually displays some sonographic abnormality in cirrhosis. Sensitivity of liver texture alone has varied between studies from 65 to 100 percent.[11, 32, 33] In one study macronodular cirrhosis was abnormal in only 20 percent. Other authors have noted difficulty detecting primary biliary cirrhosis.[15] Primary biliary cirrhosis is more likely to exhibit a heterogeneous texture, sometimes subtle, with preserved portal vasculature (Fig. 2.9) rather than increased echogenicity or poorly defined portal venule walls.

Portal Hypertension

In the United States cirrhosis is the leading cause of portal hypertension. The complications of portal hypertension produce much of the morbidity and mortality seen in this disease.

The sonographic manifestations of portal hypertension are related to changes in size and flow through the portal system, congestive splenomegaly, and the development of collateral pathways.

The portal vein and its branches increase in size in portal hypertension. A portal vein of ≥1.3 cm is highly specific (100 percent) for portal hypertension but is seen in only 57 percent of cases[36] (Fig. 2.10). Dilatation of the splenic or superior mesenteric vein of >1 cm during inspiration is more sensitive but less specific for portal hypertension.[36] In evaluating this technique, Zoli, et al found the best result by summing the diameter of the superior mesenteric and splenic veins in expiration. If the sum exceeded 1.8 cm and was corrected for body surface, the results were excellent with sensitivity equal to 91 percent and a negative predictive value of 92 percent.[37] The size of the portal vessels do not bear a direct relationship to either the degree of portal hypertension or the presence of collaterals.[38] In fact the portal vein may decrease in size as collaterals open and divert blood flow away from it.[38]

In portal hypertension the splanchnic veins respond abnormally during respiration. Normally, their caliber increases 50 to 100 percent during inspiration. In portal hypertension this response is absent or slight. Bolondi, et al found that blunting or loss of respiratory variation was sensitive (80 percent) and specific (100 percent) for portal hypertension.[39]

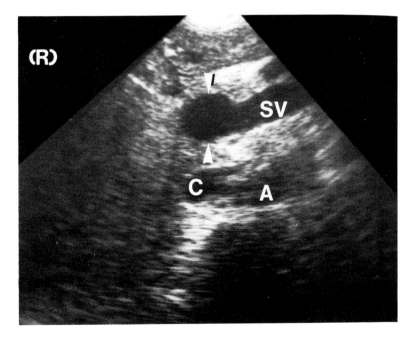

FIG. 2.10. Portal hypertension. Transverse sonograms of the splenic vein, SV, and splenoportal confluence (arrowheads). The portal vein is measured in front of the inferior vena cava, C. The portal vein is dilated measuring 2.4 cm as is the splenic vein which measures 1.6 cm. A = aorta. (R) = toward patient's right.

These findings may offer a noninvasive means to follow some patients with portal hypertension. In one study of patients who were treated for portal hypertension, the return of normal respiratory variation and a decrease of the caliber of the splanchnic veins correlated significantly with a reduction of the portal pressure.[40]

The most common portosystemic collaterals are the coronary vein, esophageal varices, splenorenal and gastrosplenic collaterals, patent paraumbilical veins, hemorrhoid veins, and retroperitoneal shunts. Collaterals detected by ultrasound may be seen in up to 88 percent of those with portal hypertension.[41]

Esophageal varices are important sources of complications due to their propensity to bleed. They are best imaged anterior to the aorta by angling toward the diaphragm. Collaterals in this location and elsewhere appear as serpiginous tubular structures (Fig. 2.11).

The coronary vein originates from the superior aspect of the portal or splenic vein near the splenoportal confluence. In portal hypertension the vein dilates above its normal 4 mm size.[41] This vessel supplies collateral flow to gastric and esophageal varices.

The ligamentum teres is usually echogenic or may have a small anechoic center. As collaterals in the ligamentum teres open, the center becomes sonolucent centrally producing a bull's-eye appearance in the transverse plane[42, 43] (Fig. 2.12). A central vascular channel exceeding 3 mm is a specific sign of

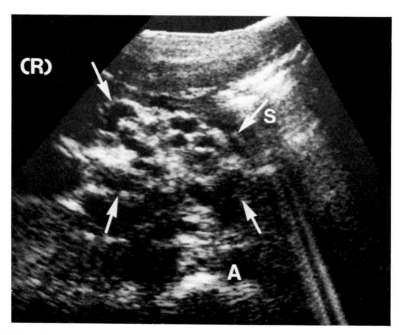

FIG. 2.11. Gastro-esophageal varices. Transverse sonogram shows a mass of serpiginous echofree structures (outlined by arrows) representing varices filling the region between the left lobe of the liver and the great vessels. A = aorta. S = shadow from stomach gas. (R) = toward patient's right.

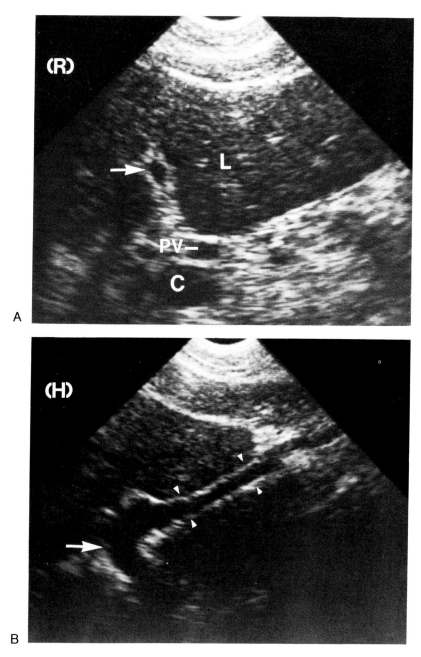

FIG. 2.12. Patent paraumbilical vein. (A) Transverse sonogram of left lobe of the liver, *L*, shows the echo-free collateral in the ligamentum teres (arrow) producing a "bull's eye" appearance. *PV* = portal vein. *C* = inferior vena cava. (*R*) = toward patient's right. (B) Longitudinal sonogram shows paraumbilical collateral (arrowheads) arising from the left portal vein (arrow).

portal hypertension.[44] Doppler ultrasound can be helpful to demonstrate that the flow in the patent ligamentum teres is hepatofugal.[45] Lafortune and his coworkers have shown that the collateral does not represent a recanalized umbilical vein but rather patent paraumbilical veins.[46]

Many descriptions of the wide variety of collaterals that may be present in portal hypertension have appeared in the sonographic literature.[41, 47–50] Their recognition is usually straightforward, as their location and tubular or serpiginous shape suggest their vascular origin. Rarely, varices may simulate a cystic or lymphomatous mass.[51] Duplex Doppler can demonstrate the vascular nature of these lesions, showing typical portal waveforms within them.[52]

Worldwide, schistosomiasis is a major cause of portal hypertension. It is a massive health problem affecting 200 million people.[53] As the parasite implants along portal vein branches, a granulomatous reaction ensues. This produces marked thickening and fibrosis along the portal tracts ("pipe-stem" fibrosis). Sonographically increased echogenicity and thickening of the portal vein walls are noted.[53] The presence of wall thickening, which is usually marked, distinguishes this from the centrilobular pattern. Splenomegaly is constant, and the portal vein is dilated in 73 percent. The parenchymal echogenicity is normal probably due to the preservation of the lobules seen pathologically.[53]

Cirrhosis and Hepatocellular Carcinoma

Cirrhosis is a risk factor for hepatocellular carcinoma. In a group of 1,200 cirrhotics Cottone, et al found 5 percent to have hepatocellular carcinoma at first presentation and 12 percent to develop the tumor during a four year follow-up.[54] The risk is highest for those with cirrhosis due to hepatitis B virus or hemochromatosis but alcoholic and cryptogenic cirrhosis also carry an increased risk.[55]

Ultrasound appears to be an effective screening test to detect the tumor. In two studies the sensitivity and specificity of ultrasound were 86 and 99 percent[31] and 90 and 93 percent[52] respectively. Okazaki, et al found ultrasound to be significantly better than alpha fetoprotein screening.[31]

Of the 27 hepatocellular carcinomas detected by Cottone, et al 59 percent were echogenic, 26 percent anechoic, and 15 percent exhibited mixed echogenicity. One-third of the patients had solitary tumors while in two-thirds, tumors were multiple.[52] False positive diagnoses were frequently due to regenerative nodules or areas of massive necrosis.[31, 52]

CONCLUSIONS

Although liver biopsy is the primary means to diagnose hepatocellular diseases, ultrasound does have a role to play in their evaluation. Ultrasound is relatively sensitive for most processes. Detection is more likely in moderate or severe disease and some pathologically mild cases have normal sonograms. Sonographic grading does not correlate to strict histologic severity.

There are two abnormal sonographic liver textures which are significantly different from one another and from normal: the centrilobular pattern and the "echogenic" liver. The centrilobular pattern is usually seen in acute hepatitis. An echogenic liver may be seen in fatty infiltration as well as chronic hepatitis, cirrhosis, and vacuolar degeneration.

Often a distinction between fatty livers and those with other processes (e.g., cirrhosis) cannot be made. This is particularly true when the liver exhibits increased echogenicity (whether fine or coarsened), and decreased definition of portal venule walls, but no significant attenuation. If attenuation is clearly present it is likely that there is fatty change. This does not exclude the possibility that underlying cirrhosis or fibrosis is also present. If heterogenicity of the parenchyma is present, particularly if it is striking or the portal venule walls are preserved, cirrhosis is the most likely diagnosis. Liver size and morphology may also suggest a diagnosis of either fatty change or cirrhosis.

In cirrhotics, ultrasound can be useful in several ways. Ascites can be easily detected. Specific findings exist to determine if there is portal hypertension. Ultrasound can evaluate for the presence of collaterals and splenomegaly and is an accurate screening test to detect hepatocellular carcinoma complicating the disease.

ACKNOWLEDGEMENT

The author thanks Alfred B. Kurtz, M.D. for his helpful discussions and Emily N. Pompetti for her preparation of this manuscript.

REFERENCES

1. Gosink BB, Laymaster CE: Ultrasonic determination of Hepatomegaly. JCU 9:37, 1981
2. Niederau C, Sonnenberg A, Muller JE, et al: Sonographic measurements of the normal liver, spleen, pancreas, and portal vein. Radiology 149:537, 1983
3. Niederau C, Sonnenberg A: Liver size evaluated by ultrasound: ROC curves for hepatitis and alcoholism. Radiology 153:503, 1984
4. VanThiel DH, Hagler NG, Schade RR, et al: In vivo hepatic volume determination using sonography and computed tomography. Gastroenterology 88:1812, 1985
5. Scatarige JC, Scott WW, Donovan PJ, et al: Fatty infiltration of the liver: Ultrasonographic and computed tomographic correlation. J Ultrasound Med 3:9, 1984
6. Clain JE, Stephens DH, Charboneau JW: Ultrasonography and computed tomography in focal fatty liver. Report of two cases with special emphasis on changing appearances over time. Gastroenterology 87:948, 1984
7. Bashist B, Hecht HL, Harley WD: Computed tomographic demonstration of rapid changes in fatty infiltration of the liver. Radiology 142:691, 1982
8. Behan M, Kazam E: The echographic characteristics of fatty tissues and tumors. Radiology 129:143, 1978
9. Gosink BB, Lemon SK, Scheible W, Leopold GR: Accuracy of ultrasonography in diagnosis of hepatocellular disease. AJR 133:19, 1979

10. Foster KJ, Dewbury KC, Griffith AH, Wright R: The accuracy of ultrasound in the detection of fatty infiltration of the liver. Br J Radiol 53:440, 1980

11. Needleman L, Kurtz AB, Rifkin MD, et al: Sonography of diffuse benign liver disease: Accuracy of pattern recognition and grading. AJR 146:1011, 1986

12. Sandford NL, Walsh P, Matis C, et al: Is ultrasonography useful in the assessment of diffuse parenchymal liver disease? Gastroenterology 89:186, 1985

13. Taylor KJ, Riely CA, Hammers, L, et al: Quantitative US attenuation in normal liver and in patients with diffuse liver disease: Importance of fat. Radiology 160:65, 1986

14. Garra BS, Insana MF, Shawker TH, Russell MA: Quantitative estimation of liver attenuation and echogenicity: Normal state versus diffuse liver disease. Radiology 162:61, 1987

15. Saverymuttu SH, Joseph AEA, Maxwell JD: Ultrasound scanning in the detection of hepatic fibrosis and steatosis. Br Med J 292:13, 1986

16. Mulhern CB, Arger PH, Coleman BG, Stein GN: Nonuniform attenuation in computed tomography study of the cirrhotic liver. Radiology 132:399, 1979

17. Scott WW Jr, Sanders RC, Siegelman SS: Irregular fatty infiltration of the liver: Diagnostic dilemmas. AJR 135:67, 1980

18. Tang-Barton P, Vas W, Weissman J, et al: Focal fatty liver lesions in alcoholic liver disease: A broadened spectrum of CT appearances. Gastrointest Radiol 10:133, 1985

19. Quinn SF, Gosink BB: Characteristic sonographic signs of hepatic fatty infiltration. AJR 145:753, 1985

20. Halvorsen RA, Korobkin M, Ram PC, Thompson WM: CT appearance of focal fatty infiltration of the liver. AJR 139:277, 1982

21. Swobodnik W, Wechsler JG, Manne W, Ditschuneit H: Multiple regular circumscript fatty infiltrations of the liver. JCU 13:577, 1985

22. Kawashima A, Suehiro S, Murayama S, Russell WJ: Case Report Focal fatty infiltration of the liver mimicking a tumor: Sonographic and CT features. J Comput Assist Tomogr 182:329, 1986

23. Marchal G, Tshibwabwa-Tumba E, Verbeken E, et al: "Skip areas" in hepatic steatosis: A sonographic-angiographic study. Gastrointest Radiol 11:151, 1986

24. Sauerbrei EE, Lopez M: Pseudotumor of the quadrate lobe in hepatic sonography: A sign of generalized fatty infiltration. AJR 147:923, 1986

25. White EM, Simeone JF, Mueller PR, et al: Focal periportal sparing in hepatic fatty infiltration: A cause of hepatic pseudomass on US. Radiology 162:57, 1987

26. Kurtz AB, Rubin CS, Cooper HS, et al: Ultrasound findings in hepatitis. Radiology 136:717, 1980

27. Giorgio A, Amoroso P, Fico P, et al: Ultrasound evaluation of uncomplicated and complicated acute viral hepatitis. JCU 14:675, 1986

28. Lieberman JM, Bryan PJ, Cohen AM: Toxic shock syndrome: Sonographic appearance of the liver. AJR 137:606, 1981

29. Shepherd DFC, Dewbury KC: Sequential imaging of the progress of acute alcoholic hepatitis with ultrasound and isotopes. Br J Radiol 53:163, 1980

30. Kurtz AB, Dubbins PA, Rubin CS: Echogenicity: analysis, significance, and masking. AJR 137:471, 1981

31. Okazaki N, Yoshida T, Yoshino M, Matue H: Screening of patients with chronic liver disease for hepatocellular carcinoma by ultrasonography. Clin Onc 10:241, 1984

32. Dewbury KC, Clark B: The accuracy of ultrasound in the detection of cirrhosis of the liver. Br J Radiol 32:945, 1979

33. Debongnie JC, Pauls C, Fievez, Wibin E: Prospective evaluation of the diagnostic accuracy of liver ultrasonography. Gut 22:130, 1981

34. Harbin WP, Robert NJ, Ferrucci JT, Jr: Diagnosis of cirrhosis based on regional changes in hepatic morphology. A radiological and pathological analysis. Radiology 135:273, 1980

35. Giorgio A, Amoroso P, Lettieri G, et al: Cirrhosis: Value of caudate to right lobe ratio in diagnosis with US. Radiology 161:443, 1986

36. Bolondi L, Mazziotti A, Arienti V, et al: Ultrasonographic study of portal venous system in portal hypertension and after portosystem shunt operations. Surgery 95:(3)261, 1984

37. Zoli M, Dondi C, Marchesini G, et al: Splanchnic vein measurements in patients with liver cirrhosis: A case-control study. J Ultrasound Med 4:641, 1985

38. Lafortune M, Marleau D, Breton G, et al: Portal venous system measurements in portal hypertension. Radiology 151:270, 1984

39. Bolondi L, Gandolfi L, Arienti V, et al: Ultrasonography in the diagnosis of portal hypertension: Diminished response of portal vessels to respiration. Radiology 142:167, 1982

40. Zoli M, Marchesini G, Marzocchi A, et al: Portal pressure changes induced by medical treatment: US detection. Radiology 155:763, 1985

41. Subramanyam BR, Balthazar EJ, Madamba MR, et al: Sonography of portosystemic venous collaterals in portal hypertension. Radiology 146:161, 1983

42. Schabel SI, Ritten GM, Javid LH, et al: The "bull's-eye" falciform ligament: A sonographic finding of portal hypertension. Radiology 136:157, 1980

43. Glazer GM, Laing FC, Brown TW, Gooding GAW: Sonographic demonstration of portal hypertension: The patent umbilical vein. Radiology 136:161, 1980

44. Saddekni S, Hutchinson DE, Cooperberg PL: The sonographically patent umbilical vein in portal hypertension. Radiology 145:441, 1982

45. Salmi A, Paterlini A: Sonographic patent umbilical vein: Lack of specificity for portal hypertension. Am J Gastroenterol 81(7):556, 1986

46. Lafortune M, Constantin A, Breton G, et al: The recanalized umbilical vein in portal hypertension: A myth. AJR 144:549, 1985

47. Dokmeci AK, Kimura K, Matsutani S, et al: Collateral veins in portal hypertension: demonstration by sonography. AJR 137:1173, 1981

48. Juttner H-U, Jenney JM, Ralls PW, et al: Ultrasound demonstration of portosystemic collaterals in cirrhosis and portal hypertension. Radiology 142:549, 1982

49. Kane RA, Katz SG: The spectrum of sonographic findings in portal hypertension: A subject review and new observations. Radiology 142:453, 1982

50. DiCandio G, Campatelli A, Mosca F, et al: Ultrasound detection of unusual spontaneous portosystemic shunts associated with uncomplicated portal hypertension. J Ultrasound Med 4:297, 1985

51. Needleman L, Rifkin MD: Vascular ultrasonography: abdominal applications. Radiol Clin North Am 24:(3)461, 1986

52. Smith DF, Lawson TL: Abdominal applications of Doppler ultrasound, p 105. In Jaffe CC (ed): Vascular and Doppler Ultrasound. Clinics in Diagnostic Ultrasound. Vol. 13. Churchill Livingstone, New York, 1984

53. Cerri GG, Alves VAF, Magalhaes A: Hepatosplenic schistosomiasis mansoni: Ultrasound manifestations. Radiology 153:777, 1984

54. Cottone M, Marceno MP, Maringhini A, et al: Ultrasound in the diagnosis of hepatocellular carcinoma associated with cirrhosis. Radiology 147:517–9, 1983

55. Scharschmidt BF: Hepatic Tumors. p. 848. In Wyngaarden JB, Smith LH, Jr (eds): Cecil Textbook of Medicine, 17th Ed. WB Saunders, Philadelphia, 1985

3 The Biliary System

ROBERT A. KANE

Since the publication of the first volume of *"Clinics in Diagnostic Ultrasound,"* *Diagnostic Ultrasound in Gastrointestinal Disease*, in 1979, ultrasonography has become widely used and firmly entrenched as the principle imaging modality for assessment of the biliary tract, so much so that other once competitive imaging procedures, such as intravenous cholangiography and oral cholecystography, are seldom performed. While excellent results were obtained by experienced investigators using static gray-scale ultrasound units, the development and perfection of real-time instrumentation, as well as a more thorough understanding of anatomy and pathophysiology of the biliary tract and improved training of residents and fellows in ultrasonography, has resulted in much more widespread success in diagnostic imaging of the biliary tract by ultrasonography. In the following pages, a review of normal and pathological anatomy in the biliary tract is presented along with an update of the latest advances in ultrasonographic biliary imaging.

GALLBLADDER SONOGRAPHY

Normal Anatomy

The gallbladder is an ovoid or pear-shaped, fluid-filled organ, normally situated in the anterior aspect of the right upper quadrant of the abdomen along the visceral surface of the liver, where there is often an indentation or fossa to accommodate the gallbladder. The gallbladder fossa is typically sited along the visceral surface of the right lobe of the liver near its junction with the medial segment of the left lobe. In fact, an imaginary plane of section running from the gallbladder fossa anteriorly to the sulcus for the inferior vena cava posteriorly forms one of the major surgical landmarks to define the relatively avascular plane between the right lobe and medial left lobe.[1] The neck of the gallbladder is situated quite close to the junction of the first and second portions of the duodenum, which may in fact be indented by the gallbladder. The cystic duct arises from the neck of the gallbladder and enters into the common bile duct, but because of the small size and convoluted course of this structure, the cystic duct is seldom completely imaged unless dilated.

The neck of the gallbladder is usually deeper and more cephalad in position relative to the fundus which is often quite anterior in position, at times extending to the anterior peritoneal reflection. The hepatic flexure of the colon is often in close proximity to the fundus of the gallbladder and the apex of the duodenum lies posterior to the neck of the gallbladder. The exact position and orientation of the gallbladder is quite variable and depends on such factors as body habitus, the size and contour of the liver, the presence of scoliosis, and the position of the diaphragm. Despite this variability, true aberrant positions of the gallbladder are uncommon, but occasionally a completely intrahepatic gallbladder may be present. Agenesis of the gallbladder also occurs rarely.

The gallbladder is a thin-walled, fluid-filled, cystic-appearing structure by ultrasonography. The wall is generally no more than 2 mm in thickness and has a uniform, moderately echogenic texture. The bile contained within the lumen of a normally-functioning gallbladder is completely anechoic. Gallbladder size and volume varies considerably; however, in most patients the width of the gallbladder will not exceed 5 cm and the length will be no more than 8 to 10 cm. There are numerous exceptions; most notably in diabetics, patients with pancreatitis or chronic debilitating illnesses, during recuperation from major abdominal surgery, and in patients on narcotics and anticholinergic medications.[2] An increase in gallbladder volume has also been noted during pregnancy, possibly related to incomplete emptying which was noted in the first trimester, while overall gallbladder enlargement was only seen in the second and third trimesters.[3] Most of these large but otherwise normal gallbladders will maintain an oval, pear-shaped configuration as opposed to a gallbladder with obstruction of the cystic duct, which will often assume a more rounded and tense appearance since the distention is caused by increased intraluminal pressure.[4] Not all obstructed gallbladders will show this tense contour, and at times a functional test may be required to establish the presence or absence of cystic duct obstruction. This might be further evaluated by administration of an oral fatty meal or intravenous cholecystokinin, or alternatively by a radionuclide biliary scan.

The gallbladder frequently folds back upon itself at the neck where it narrows rapidly prior to the origin of the cystic duct. Occasionally the neck of the gallbladder may be quite large, forming what has been termed a "Hartmann's pouch" (Fig. 3.1). This is important for two reasons. If cut transversely, the fold between the body and neck of the gallbladder may simulate the appearance of a true septation within the gallbladder, which indeed is a very rare occurrence. By rotating the scan head from the short axis to the long axis of the gallbladder, the true nature of the Hartmann's pouch can be demonstrated. A large neck of the gallbladder must be carefully assessed since it is a frequent site for stone formation and is not easily imaged due to numerous refractive shadows in this region. Occasionally a fold or pseudoseptation may occur in the gallbladder fundus, forming the Phrygian cap,[5]

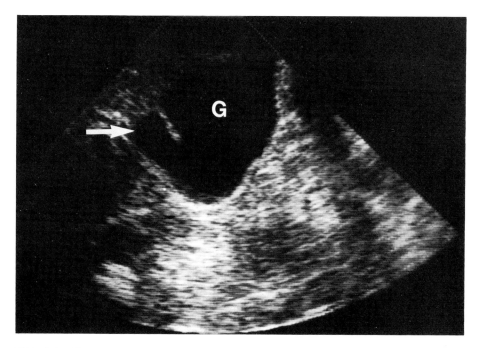

FIG. 3.1. Prominent gallbladder neck forming a Hartmann's pouch (arrow). G = gallbladder.

and this is another site where small gallstones are apt to be missed without careful attention to scanning technique.

The gallbladder wall is generally 1 to 2 mm in thickness and of uniform, moderately echogenic texture. At times the wall may be imperceptible where it sits adjacent to the liver parenchyma. When the gallbladder is contracted, its uniform texture changes and three components of the wall can be recognized: (1) a relatively hyperechoic inner margin corresponding to the redundant mucosa, (2) a hypoechoic middle layer probably corresponding to the submucosal and muscular layers, and (3) a hyperechoic outer margin which may represent serosal or pericholecystic fatty layer.[6] This three-layer appearance should not be confused with gallbladder wall edema or other forms of pathological thickening of the gallbladder wall, since it is only seen in the contracted state and will disappear as the gallbladder distends with fasting.

In many patients, a persistent hyperechoic linear structure is seen extending from the region of the neck of the gallbladder to the right portal vein. This represents the chief or main lobar fissure of the liver[7] and can be seen due to the presence of fat and/or collagen within this fissure. This marks the avascular plane between the right and medial left lobes of the liver. Frequently there is short linear echogenic structure along the posterior wall of the gallbladder at the junction of the neck and body. This is the so-called junctional fold (Fig. 3.2) and is a normal finding caused by the folding back

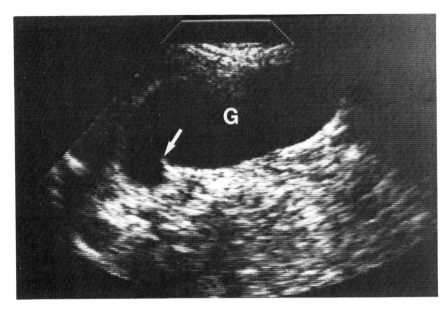

FIG. 3.2. The junctional fold (arrow) projecting into the gallbladder, G, lumen.

of the gallbladder neck upon the body.[8] It could occasionally be confused with a small stone, as a refractive shadow may emanate from this region, but careful scanning will elucidate its true nature. The junctional fold may vary or disappear with change in patient position from supine to decubitus or upright. Acoustic shadows may also be seen emanating from the spiral valves of Heister[9] and make evaluation of the neck of the gallbladder somewhat more difficult. Refractive shadows may also be seen in short axis scans where the ultrasound beam strikes tangentially along the circumference of the gallbladder.[10]

Technique

The gallbladder should be scanned following an 8 to 12 hour fast in order to ensure good distention. Scans should be performed in the long and short axis, both while the patient is supine as well as in the left lateral decubitus position. This change in patient position may result in better imaging of portions of the gallbladder which have been obscured by gas and may also cause small stones which are poorly visualized in the neck of the gallbladder to change position into the body or fundus and hence be more readily recognized. In addition, erect scans may also be of value in certain patients when the gallbladder is poorly visualized in the recumbent positions due to excessive bowel gas, obesity, or a high position of the liver and gallbladder beneath the rib cage. The gallbladder may be imaged directly or by using the liver as an acoustic window. In very obese patients, coronal scanning through the liver is often the best way to visualize the gallbladder. If the patient has undergone a proper 8 to 12 hour fast, there should be virtually 100 percent success in visualizing the gallbladder using modern real-time instrumentation. Complete nonvisualization of the gallbladder should at first raise the question of possible prior surgery, either cholecystectomy or cholecystoenteric anastomosis. If there is no history or evidence of previous surgery and the gallbladder remains nonvisualized despite using all of the anatomic landmarks, this should be an indication of pathology of some sort, such as a chronic scarred gallbladder containing stones and no bile, or replacement of the gallbladder by tumor. One other possibility is agenesis of the gallbladder which is a rare condition that will occasionally be encountered. This cannot be definitively diagnosed sonographically, but could be suggested and perhaps further evaluated by radionuclide biliary scanning. Nonvisualization of the gallbladder was associated with gallbladder pathology in 96 percent of cases in one surgical series which was done largely with static scanning.[11] The vast majority of these cases are small scleroatrophic gallbladders with stones and devoid of bile.

In average and small-sized patients, most gallbladders can be successfully imaged using a 5 MHz transducer while larger patients may require the use of a 3.5 MHz crystal. Since the confident diagnosis of cholelithiasis depends in most cases on demonstration of an acoustic shadow, meticulous scanning technique is essential and there are several factors which are important in optimal demonstration of acoustic shadowing (Table 3.1). Since a high resolution crystal has a narrower beam profile, a 5 MHz transducer will allow demonstration of acoustic shadows in stones as small as 2 to 3 mm, which well may not be demonstrable using a 3.5 MHz crystal. Also, since the ultrasound beam is narrowest within the focal zone, it is imperative to choose a transducer with the correct focal zone which will encompass the gallbladder or to reposition the patient such that the gallbladder falls within the focal zone, otherwise subtle acoustic shadowing may be missed because the beam width is broader than the diameter of the small stone. Since maximal reflection of the ultrasound beam occurs at an incident angle of 90 degrees, scanning in the perpendicular plane to a small stone will enhance the ability

TABLE 3.1. Requirements for optimal demonstration of acoustic shadowing from stones

High frequency (preferably 5 MHz)
Stone in focal zone
Perpendicular scanning plane
Low gain setting
Suspended respiration
Multiple patient positions

to demonstrate subtle acoustic shadowing. Similarly, the overall gain setting should be kept as low as possible in order to avoid obscuring a subtle acoustic shadow by the increased noise generated at higher gain settings. While suspended respiration is optimal for depicting and freezing an acoustic shadow for hard copy imaging, at times the most subtle acoustic shadowing is better appreciated in real time when a thin, pencil-like shadow can be seen to move in conjunction with the tiny stone as the gallbladder changes position with respiration. Finally, as mentioned earlier, the patient must be examined in several different positions in order to completely evaluate areas such as the fundus and neck of the gallbladder, which may be obscured by gas-filled bowel structures, reverberation artifacts, or refractive shadows.

PATHOLOGY

Cholelithiasis

The classic appearance of a gallstone is that of a rounded, echogenic structure situated dependently within the lumen of the gallbladder, casting a clean, acoustical shadow posteriorly due to absorption and reflection of sound at the surface of the gallstone (Fig. 3.3). This appearance is diagnostic of cholelithiasis virtually 100 percent of the time and is also the most common appearance for gallstones. Large stones typically have a curvilinear contour but smaller stones, less than 1 cm in diameter, may appear either rounded or more linear in configuration (Fig. 3.4). Because of the absorption of sound

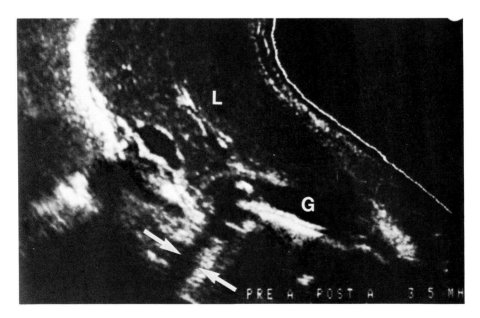

FIG. 3.3. Curvilinear gallstone with posterior acoustic shadowing (arrows). G = gallbladder, L = liver.

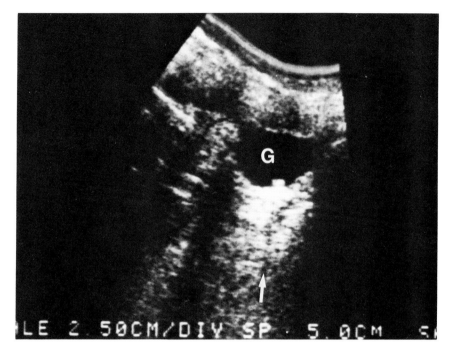

FIG. 3.4.   Small, linear-appearing gallstone, *G*, with pencil-thin acoustic shadow (arrow).

within the stone, the acoustic shadow is usually sharp and "clean," that is, free of echoes. This is contrasted with the shadows emanating from bowel gas, which are caused purely by reflection of the sound beam. As a result these shadows frequently are less well defined and "dirty" because of numerous reverberation artifacts.[12, 13] The distinction between clean and dirty shadows is important to avoid overcalling gallstones as a results of shadows from the adjacent gas-filled duodenum or hepatic flexure of the colon.

Extremely small acoustic shadows may not be completely free of echoes due to averaging which may occur when the stone is equal or slightly smaller in size than the width of the focal zone. Similarly, noise within the system may cause some apparent echoes within the acoustic shadow, but this should be recognizable.

Most stones move freely within the gallbladder lumen unless so large as to extend from the anterior to the posterior wall or unless impacted in the neck of the gallbladder.

In vitro studies have demonstrated that all gallstones cast acoustic shadow regardless of composition, presence or absence of calcification, and size or shape.[14, 15] As a practical matter, stones smaller than 2 to 3 mm in size will seldom demonstrate a clear-cut acoustic shadow in vivo, because the beam width may in fact be wider than the diameter of the stone (Fig. 3.5), consequently allowing some sound to pass unabsorbed around the stone and

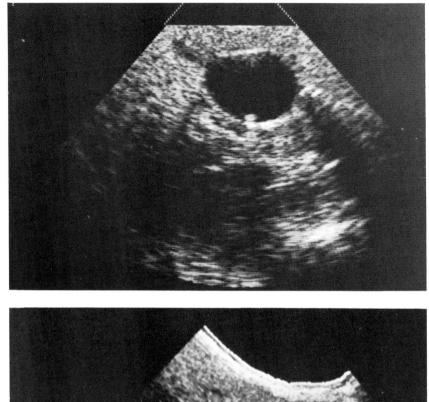

A

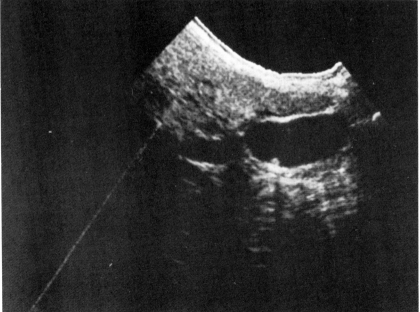

B

FIG. 3.5. (A) 3.5 MHz real-time scan, demonstrating a tiny gallstone but no acoustic shadow. (B) 5 MHz static scan of the same stone successfully demonstrates an acoustic shadow due to the narrower beam width.

obliterate the shadow.[16] Intraoperative ultrasonography using higher frequency transducers (7.5 to 10 MHz) has been shown to be effective in demonstrating tiny gallstones and producing clear-cut acoustic shadows which could not be demonstrated preoperatively using lower frequency transducers.[17]

While an acoustic shadow cannot reliably be produced from tiny gallstones, if the stones are multiple in number and can be collected along one wall or one segment of the gallbladder, a summation affect may occur such that the conglomerate grouping of tiny stones casts an acoustic shadow (Fig. 3.6).[18] This conglomeration can sometimes be accomplished by sitting the patient upright. Tiny stones may disperse themselves within the bile in the gallbladder lumen and may require some time to settle out. When this occurs the bile-filled gallbladder may have a "snowstorm" appearance due to perturbation of the stones. If this is recognized, having the patient lie still for several minutes may allow time for the stones to settle dependently and enable an acoustic shadow to be produced.

Some gallstones are of extremely low density, less than that of the concentrated liquid bile, and in that setting the stones will float within the lumen of the gallbladder. This presents a classical ultrasound appearance of linear echogenic densities suspended within the lumen of the gallbladder, with the line being parallel to the gravitational field (Fig. 3.7). This appearance is also essentially 100 percent diagnostic for gallstones whether an acoustic shadow is present or not. The level at which the stones float depends upon their density relative to the density of the bile within the gallbladder and may vary from the lower or middle third of the gallbladder up to near the

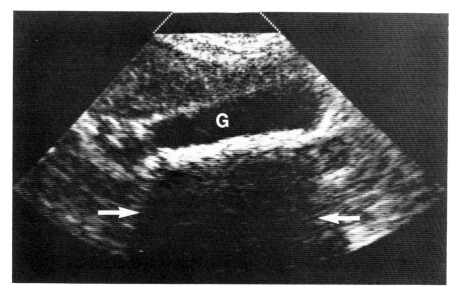

FIG. 3.6.   Conglomeration of hundreds of tiny gallstones producing a broad acoustic shadow (arrows). G = gallbladder.

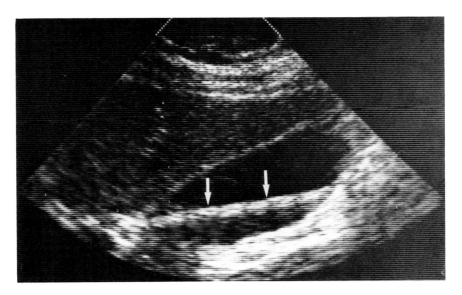

FIG. 3.7. Linear echogenic densities in the gallbladder lumen (arrows) caused by tiny floating gallstones. Note the denser, more echogenic bile dependent to the floating gallstones.

neck in the upright position, or near the anterior wall when supine. While some low density gallstones will be of sufficiently low density to float by themselves,[19] others can be made to float following oral cholecystography, because the contrast material within the gallbladder is somewhat denser than normal bile.[20] In these patients the stones may float in the presence of contrast material but may be situated dependently in the absence of contrast.

Occasionally stones without clear-cut acoustic shadowing can actually be seen to move within the gallbladder lumen with changes in patient position. Thus a stone may be seen to "roll" over itself in real time as the patient rolls from left decubitus to supine or from an erect position to supine.[2] This is also a highly accurate diagnosis for cholelithiasis, approaching 100 percent, although theoretically, tumefactive sludge might also have a capacity to move within the gallbladder lumen as the gravitational field changes.[21] This distinction is of some importance since tumefactive sludge may progress to the formation of stones but may also resolve completely, leaving a normal gallbladder lumen. Consequently if tumefactive sludge is a possibility, it is probably advisable to re-examine the patient in a few weeks time to confirm or disprove the diagnosis of cholelithiasis. Of course, an impacted stone in the gallbladder neck or fundus will not move (Fig. 3.8).

Occasionally in the presence of cholelithiasis and chronic cholecystitis, the gallbladder becomes so scarred and contracted that it presents as a thick-walled structure with echogenic stones casting acoustic shadow but little or no visible bile (Fig. 3.9). This is the so-called scleroatrophic gallbladder and it can be a source of confusion since the paucity of bile may lead the sonogra-

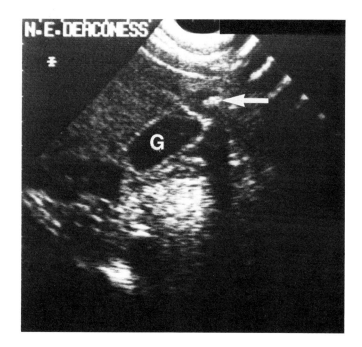

FIG. 3.8.   Impacted gallstone within a Phrygian cap (arrow). *G* = body of gallbladder.

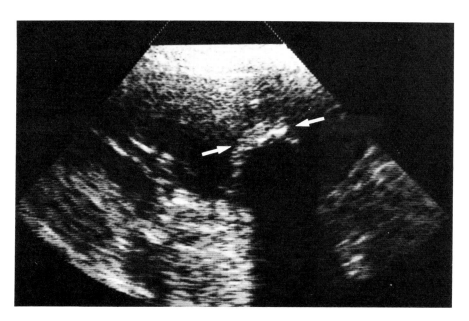

FIG. 3.9.   Scleroatrophic gallbladder with echogenic stones (arrows) and acoustic shadowing but no visible bile.

pher to the erroneous conclusion that the gallbladder is not visualized. The acoustic shadows may be interpreted as emanating from adjacent bowel. There are several observations which will help avoid this pitfall. If the chief fissure of the liver can be identified, it may be seen to extend directly to this persistent area of acoustic shadowing, thereby identifying it as the scarred gallbladder. In addition, since the gallbladder arises in a fossa indenting the underside of the liver, if the acoustic shadow also arises from this fossa then it is unlikely to be emanating from bowel loops which will not indent the liver. Of course the acoustic shadow should also be a clean type shadow when arising from a scleroatrophic gallbladder filled with stones. Finally, careful scanning will usually allow one to demonstrate a separation between the echogenic wall of the gallbladder and the echogenic surface of the gall-stones by a thin hypoechoic rim representing minimal residual bile in the lumen or a hypoechoic portion of the gallbladder wall. Complete acoustic shadowing is seen distal to the inner most curvilinear hypoechoic structure. This observation has been termed the wall-echo-shadow (WES) triad[22] or double-arc-shadow sign,[23] and can be demonstrated in most patients with a scleroatrophic gallbladder leading to a confident diagnosis of cholelithiasis (Fig. 3.10). At times, a WES sign may be demonstrated in patients with gallstones in whom the gallbladder volume is normal and the wall is not especially thickened. This probably results from large stones which almost completely fill the lumen of the gallbladder or might conceivably occur with

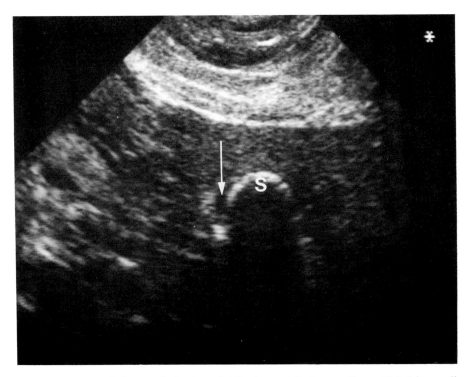

FIG. 3.10. A small hypoechoic rim of bile (arrow) between the gallbladder wall and the large gallstone, *S*, establishes the confident diagnosis of cholelithiasis.

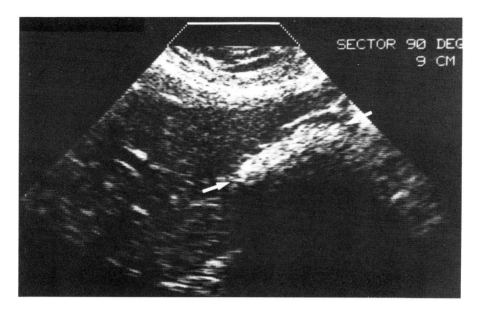

FIG. 3.11.   WES sign caused by milk of calcium bile filling the gallbladder lumen (arrows).

multiple, very low-density, floating stones which abut the anterior surface of the gallbladder. Nevertheless the sign is very useful in confidently predicting the presence of cholelithiasis.

A similar appearance of persistent acoustic shadow emanating from a gallbladder fossa with nonvisualization of a bile-filled gallbladder lumen may also be seen with milk of calcium bile (Fig. 3.11)[24, 25] or with calcification of the gallbladder wall (porcelain gallbladder).[26] Milk of calcium bile may be recognized by its gravity dependance if upright scans are obtained (Fig. 3.12). Otherwise, plain films of the abdomen will readily demonstrate these two entities.

Nonshadowing echogenic structures within the gallbladder lumen present a more difficult problem. If echogenic material in the gallbladder can not be made to demonstrate acoustic shadowing despite all the maneuvers mentioned previously, the possibility of cholelithiasis cannot be excluded, but biliary sludge or thick, concentrated bile may have a similar appearance. Since sludge is not necessarily an indicator of gallbladder disease and may be seen in normal individuals after a prolonged fast, it is essential to attempt to make this distinction. Both sludge and stones will assume a dependant position in the gallbladder and will move with changes in the patient's position. However while stones usually move rapidly and may even be seen in motion, biliary sludge is quite viscous and hence accommodates more slowly to the changes in gravity. Therefore with a rapid change in patient position, the sludge may be caught midway between its original location and the new dependant portion of the gallbladder.

Biliary sludge is a homogeneous substance with low to moderate echogenic-

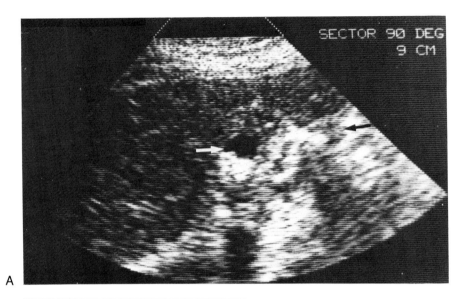

A

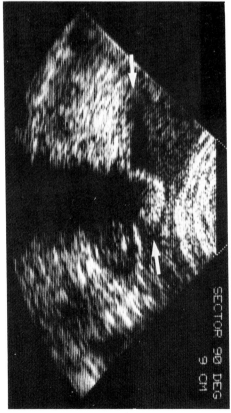

B

FIG. 3.12. (A) Supine scan with milk of calcium bile dependently along the posterior gallbladder wall. (B) Erect scan shows a shift of the milk of calcium bile to the gallbladder fundus. Arrows denote gallbladder.

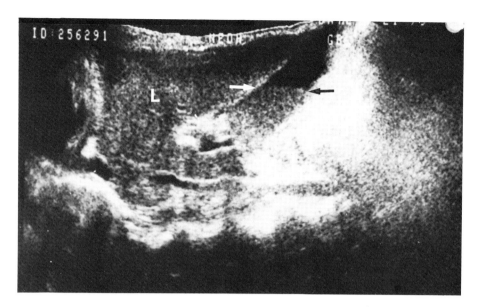

FIG. 3.13.   Bile-sludge level within the gallbladder (arrows). Note the homogeneity and moderate echogenicity of the sludge, similar to the echogenicity of the liver parenchyma. L = liver.

ity (Fig. 3.13). Its composition consists principally of calcium bilirubinate pigment granules, although smaller amounts of cholesterol crystals have also been found within sludge.[27] While it usually lacks structure, occasionally it may round up and form sludge balls or tumefactive sludge.[21] Sludge and stones may coexist, and typically when this occurs the homogeneity of the sludge is interrupted by larger, more echogenic material corresponding to the stones.[2] When this pattern is recognized, careful scanning will usually allow acoustic shadows to be demonstrated, thereby establishing the diagnosis of stones (Fig. 3.14). In a prospective series, when the typical homogeneous appearance of sludge was seen, there was only a ten percent incidence of cholelithiasis at surgery, whereas, if there were focal nonshadowing structures in the gallbladder lumen measuring less than 5 mm in size, this group had an 81 percent incidence of cholelithiasis.[28] Since this is still not sufficient for a definitive diagnosis, when focal nonshadowing opacities are demonstrated, further maneuvers are warranted, such as reexamination after fatty meal or cholecystokinin. If the diagnosis still cannot be confidently made, the study is reported as equivocal and generally the patient is rescheduled for a repeat ultrasound examination in several weeks time, at which time the diagnosis usually becomes clear.

Acute Cholecystitis

The normal gallbladder wall is smooth, thin, and hyperechoic, measuring no more than 2 mm in thickness. Increased thickness of the gallbladder wall can be seen in both acute and chronic cholecystitis, but also in a variety

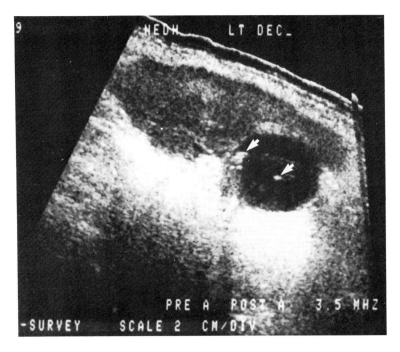

FIG. 3.14.   Inhomogeneous sludge containing focal hyperreflective areas corresponding to stones (arrows).

of other clinical conditions without intrinsic gallbladder disease. Wall thickening must be assessed with the gallbladder distended, as redundant mucosa
may simulate the thickened wall when the gallbladder is collapsed (Fig. 3.15).[6]
The most common reason for wall thickening in the absence of gallbladder
pathology is the presence of low serum albumin due to shift of fluid from
the intravascular to the extravascular space resulting in edema of the gallbladder wall (Fig. 3.16).[29] Similarly, edema may be produced by severe congestive
heart failure and renal failure with fluid overload. Wall thickening is also
described with ascites.[30] Some of the wall thickening which occurs in this
condition is due to the concomitant hypoalbuminemia occurring in most
cirrhotics, and some of it may indeed be artifactual due to beam angulation.[31]
Edema has also been described from obstruction of the lymphatic drainage
of the gallbladder,[32] and in hepatitis,[33] and anaphylactic reactions.[2]

   Nevertheless, edema of the gallbladder wall, that is the presence of a
continuous hypoechoic rim or halo or a more focal sonolucent zone, is one
of the two major criteria for the ultrasonographic diagnosis of acute cholecystitis,[34, 35] providing that hypoalbuminemia and the other conditions mentioned
above can be excluded (Table 3.2). The lucent zones probably represent accu-
mulations of edema, inflammatory exudate and/or hemorrhage. The sonolucent halo may be at times quite subtle and is best demonstrated by using a
5 MHz transducer (Fig. 3.17). The halo is best judged between the liver

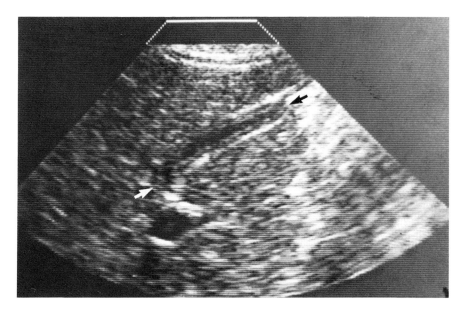

FIG. 3.15.   Normal contracted gallbladder (arrows) demonstrating hyperechoic mucosal and serosal layers surrounding the echo poor submucosal and muscular layer.

parenchyma and wall of the gallbladder, since the free wall may lie adjacent to bowel and the hypoechoic bowel wall might be mistaken for a positive halo sign. Gallbladder edema may also be markedly eccentric and may at times involve only a portion of the gallbladder wall (Fig. 3.18).

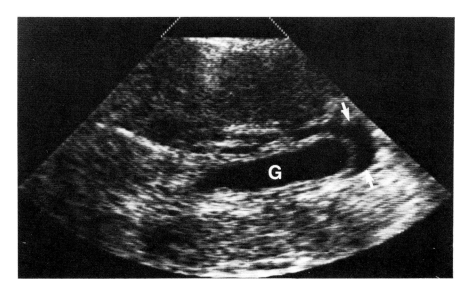

FIG. 3.16.   Normal gallbladder, G, with a hypoechoic halo of edema (arrows) around the fundus secondary to hypoalbuminemia.

TABLE 3.2. Sonographic signs of acute cholecystitis

Primary
  Gallbladder wall edema (halo)
  Gallbladder tenderness (Murphy's sign)
  Gas in gallbladder wall
Secondary
  Rounded, tense distention
  Pericholecystic fluid
  Gallstones

A second major diagnostic finding in acute cholecystitis is the sonographic Murphy's sign.[36] This is considered positive when the point of maximum tenderness is seen when pressing on the gallbladder with the transducer or by pressing the transducer into the subcostal region at the level of the gallbladder and having the patient attempt a deep inspiration, which will be arrested when the pressure from the transducer is transmitted to the gallbladder. This is a very useful sign and helps to discriminate tenderness arising from the gallbladder from other causes of right upper quadrant or generalized abdominal tenderness. This is a highly specific sign of acute cholecystitis (92 percent in Ralls' series)[37] but should be made by the physician himself or herself in real time.

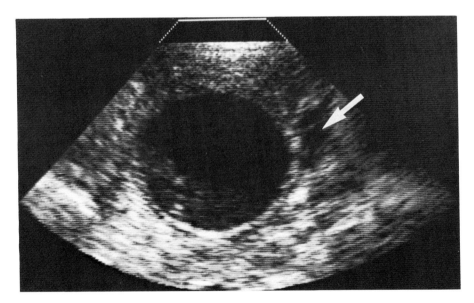

FIG. 3.17.   Acute cholecystitis with a subtle hypoechoic rim or halo due to edema in the wall. Note also the tense distended gallbladder contour, rounded on transverse view, and the small pericholecystic fluid collection (arrow).

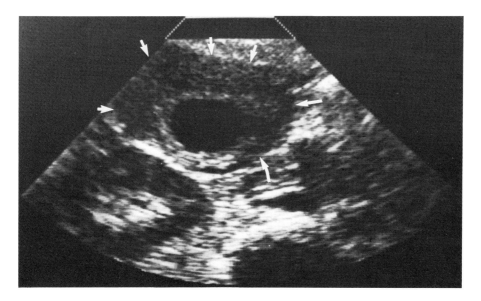

FIG. 3.18.   Acalculous cholecystitis with eccentric wall thickening and edema (arrows).

Clinically, most patients with acute cholecystitis have right upper quadrant pain and tenderness, fever, leukocytosis with a left shift, elevated alkaline phosphatase, and sometimes elevated bilirubin. However, many patients do not exhibit all of the classic clinical findings and occasionally you may encounter patients with no significant fever or leukocytosis, even patients without pain or tenderness. This is particularly true in the elderly debilitated population, in diabetics, and in patients recuperating from major surgery. Similarly, a small percentage of patients will not exhibit a positive Murphy's sign or may not show edema of the gallbladder wall. Thus, there is still a role for a radionuclide biliary scanning in patients with clinical suspicion of acute cholecystitis and a negative ultrasound study.

There are several secondary signs of acute cholecystitis (Table 3.2), which may increase the confidence level of the diagnosis. Distention of the gallbladder is a useful secondary sign, particularly when the gallbladder wall assumes a rounded or tense configuration suggesting the presence of fluid under pressure (Fig. 3.17). This tense configuration is more useful than mere measurements of gallbladder size, since the gallbladder may be enlarged due to prolonged fasting, diabetes, effects of certain medications, and a variety of other conditions unrelated to acute cholecystitis.

Small pericholecystic fluid collection are often seen in association with cholecystitis (Fig. 3.17). These may be small bile collections as a result of microperforations, but they are frequently caused merely by localized peritonitis. Care should be taken not to mistake fluid in the duodenum for a pericholecystic fluid collection.

We do not consider the presence of gallstones, per se, to be a primary

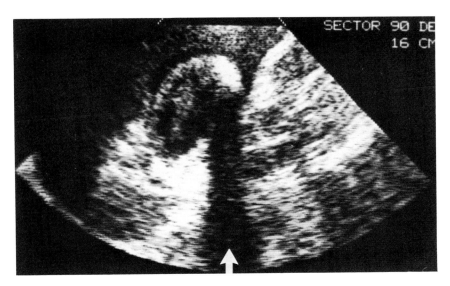

FIG. 3.19. Emphysematous cholecystitis with highly echogenic focus of gas in the gallbladder wall with "dirty" acoustic shadowing (arrow).

criterion for the diagnosis of acute cholecystitis (unless the stone is impacted in the gallbladder neck), since the prevalence of cholelithiasis is great in the general population. In addition, since acalculous cholecystitis occurs in approximately 10 percent of cases,[38, 39] the absence of stones does not mitigate against the diagnosis of cholecystitis.

One other primary sign of acute cholecystitis is the presence of gas within the wall or lumen of the gallbladder.[40, 41] Emphysematous cholecystitis is a result of gas production by bacterial organisms, such as clostridia, *E. coli*, and anaerobic streptococcus. Bacterial invasion of the gallbladder wall is a result of ischemia, which may be secondary to distention of the gallbladder wall from a cystic duct obstruction, resulting in venous obstruction and vascular engorgement. However, it may occur in the absence of gallstones, particularly in diabetics, and some speculate that ischemia due to arterial insufficiency may be a primary cause of emphysematous cholecystitis in this group of patients. Because the process is essentially ischemic, a high percentage of patients will evolve into gangrenous cholecystitis and even perforation with pericholecystic abscess.[42]

The ultrasonographic appearance of gas in the gallbladder wall is that of an intensely hyperechoic focus with posterior acoustic shadowing (Fig. 3.19). The shadow is not "clean" however due to numerous reverberation artifacts caused by reflection of the sound beam at the gas interface. In real time, the gas collections are sometimes seen to shimmer or scintillate as the gallbladder moves with respiratory activity. Calcification in the wall of the gallbladder may similarly appear hyperechoic, but the acoustic shadow is "clean" due to predominant absorption of sound at the calcified wall. At times, only tiny foci of gas can be seen in the wall, within small microabscesses. This has a typical appearance of bright echogenic foci with comet-tail reverbera-tions, but this appearance can also be seen in adenomyomatosis of the gall-bladder, in which deposits of cholesterol crystals in the dilated sinuses may result in a similar appearance.[43]

Complications of Acute Cholecystitis

Most cases of acute cholecystitis are now detected relatively early, due to the success of both ultrasonography and radionuclide biliary scanning in diagnosing this disorder. Because of the intense hyperemia in the gallbladder wall as a result of the acute inflammation, frank hemorrhage into the gallblad-der lumen may occur with formation of an intraluminal thrombus. This will appear as a moderately echogenic organized focus within the lumen of the gallbladder (Fig. 3.20) with structural integrity rather than gravity dependence as might be seen with sludge. The clot shows no acoustic shadowing.[44, 45] A similar appearance might be seen tumefactive sludge or with polypoid intraluminal tumors of the gallbladder, but clinical context usually will serve to distinguish a clot from these other entities. Hemorrhage into the gallblad-der may also be seen following blunt or penetrating trauma to the liver, including following needle biopsy, as well as rupture of an hepatic aneurysm. The resulting hemobilia may present clinically with gastrointestinal (GI) bleeding.

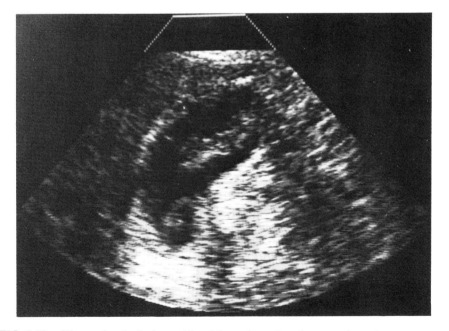

FIG. 3.20.   Hemorrhagic cholecystitis with moderately echogenic thrombus projecting centrally into the lumen of the gallbladder.

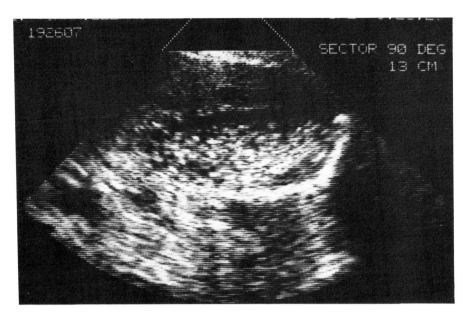

FIG. 3.21. Gengrenous gallbladder filled with highly viscous pus and fibrinous exudate. Note the absence of acoustic shadowing or dependent layering.

Acute cholecystitis may progress to empyema or gangrene if left untreated. There are specific ultrasonographic findings which may indicate gangrenous cholecystitis, including the presence of inhomogeneous, moderately echogenic material that fills the gallbladder lumen (Fig. 3.21) but does not show

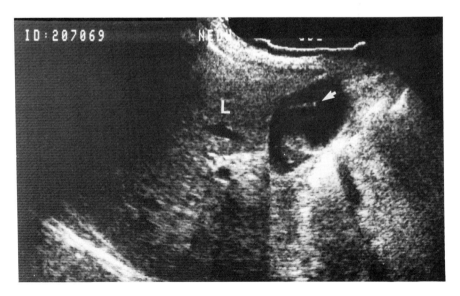

FIG. 3.22. Gangrenous cholecystitis with desquamation of the mucosa (arrow) into the gallbladder lumen. L = liver.

dependent layering or acoustic shadowing.[46] This appearance is caused by the presence of extremely thick purulent material and fibrinous exudate within the gallbladder lumen. Other sonographic signs suggestive of gangrene include the presence of intraluminal membranes (Fig. 3.22) as a result of desquammation of the gallbladder mucosa,[47, 48] and marked irregular thickening of the gallbladder wall due to ulceration, hemorrhage, and necrosis. Unfortunately, gangrene may occur with none of these ultrasonographic findings, and, in fact, the gallbladder wall may appear thin and unremarkable even as it is in the process of disintegration (Fig. 3.23). The diagnosis of gangrene cannot, of course, be made in these cases, but, if any of the other observations are made, this is an indication for immediate surgical or percutaneous drainage of the gallbladder in order to avoid the inevitable life-threatening sequelae of frank perforation, pericholecystic abscess, bile peritonitis, and septicemia.

With dissolution of the gallbladder wall, frank bile leakage may result in the formation of a biloma (a walled-off collection of bile) or in generalized bile peritonitis. Since the bile is infected, a pericholecystic abscess will form. This abscess has an appearance in some ways similar to that of gangrene or empyema of the gallbladder, in that there is a confined collection of thick echogenic material which may not layer out (Fig. 3.24). The difference is that there is no longer any perceptible gallbladder wall surrounding the pericholecystic abscess.[46] The ultrasound appearance can be quite variable ranging from predominantly hypoechoic, to predominantly echogenic with an

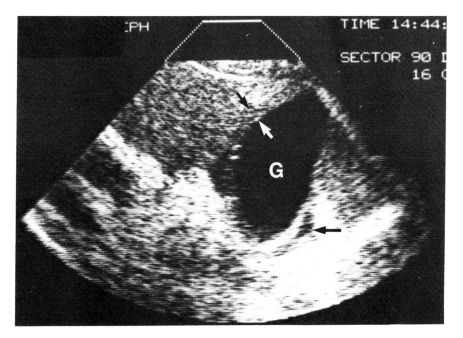

FIG. 3.23. Gangrenous gallbladder, *G*, with minimal sonographic changes of eccentric wall edema (arrows) and minimal pericholecystic fluid (arrowhead).

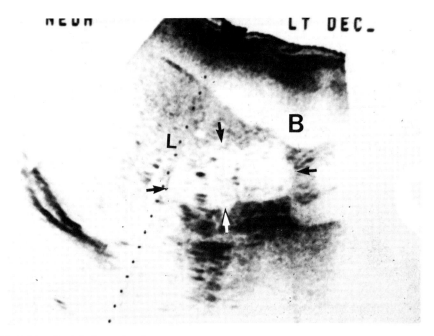

FIG. 3.24. Pericholecystic abscess (arrows). Note the echogenic purulent material suspended within the abscess and the absence of any defined gallbladder wall. The fluid anterior to the liver is a biloma, *B,* resulting from free rupture of the gallbladder wall. *L* = liver.

almost solid appearance, although generally increased through transmission would be recognized.[49, 50] The appearance depends entirely on the composition of the abscess. If the perforation occurs into the liver substance or is covered by omentum, a chronic abscess may result and the clinical presentation may be much more occult, with smoldering low-grade fevers, pain, and abnormal liver function tests. The ultrasound appearance, however, is not substantially different from the more typical acute pericholecystic abscesses. Percutaneous ultrasound or CT-guided catheter drainage can often be successful in treating these conditions.

Hyperplastic Cholecystoses

There are two principle hyperplastic diseases of the gallbladder, cholesterolosis and adenomyomatosis. The typical "strawberry gallbladder" of cholesterolosis is not usually recognized sonographically because of the small size of the granular deposits of cholesterol crystals. In the polypoid form, however, the aggregates of cholesterol are larger in size, forming small mucosal polyps which can be identified sonographically as small echogenic foci attached to the wall of the gallbladder.[51, 52] These can be either single or multiple and generally do not cast acoustic shadows (Fig. 3.25) and are not

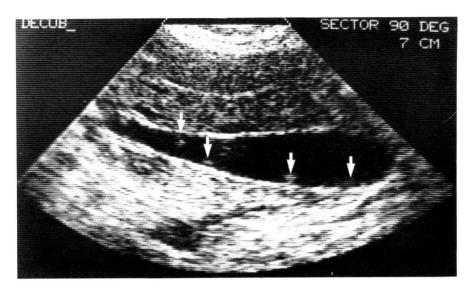

FIG. 3.25. Cholesterol polyps (arrows) of the gallbladder appear as brightly echogenic nondependent foci which do not usually cast acoustic shadows.

dependent but rather affixed to the wall and hence, will not move with changes in patient position. This allows distinction between polyps and tiny stones. Adenomatous and inflammatory polyps have a similar appearance and all three types of polyps can be single or multiple and are indistinguishable sonographically,[53] but cholesterol polyps are more common.

Adenomyomatosis may occur focally in the tip of the gallbladder fundus, but this form is seldom recognized sonographically due to its peripheral location along the curving surface of the fundus. Generalized adenomyomatosis causes a diffuse thickening of the gallbladder wall as a result of muscular hypertrophy and proliferation of mucosa into the muscular wall.[54-56] The wall thickening involves the body and fundus but to some extent spares the neck of the gallbladder, resulting in a somewhat characteristic hourglass configuration (Fig. 3.26). Within the thickened wall, there are numerous dilated Rokitansky-Aschoff sinuses. When fluid-filled, these can be visualized as discrete, tiny, anechoic foci in the gallbladder wall. Frequently, the dilated sinuses are filled with cholesterol crystals resulting in the presence of numerous hyperechoic foci in the wall of the gallbladder (Fig. 3.27) which frequently show comet-tail reverberation artifacts posteriorly.[46] These crystal deposits may simulate gas within microabscesses, but the patients with adenomyomatosis have a mild clinical course, unlike patients with acute cholecystitis. Finally, the gallbladders with this condition are frequently spastic and if challenged with a fatty meal, will often show complete obliteration of the lumen in the affected segments of the gallbladder, while the unaffected neck of the gallbladder will remain relatively unchanged. The ultrasound appearance of adenomyomatosis is sufficiently characteristic for a confident diagnosis to be made in the vast majority of the cases.

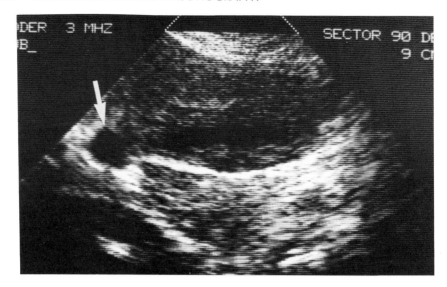

FIG. 3.26.   Adenomyomatosis with wall thickening in the body and fundus of the gallbladder but no thickening in the neck (arrow).

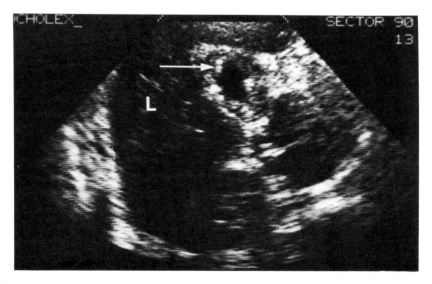

FIG. 3.27.   Adenomyomatosis with multiple echogenic foci in the wall due to deposition of cholesterol crystals in the dilated sinuses. Note the comet-tail reverberations (arrow). L = liver.

NEOPLASTIC DISEASE

Benign Tumors

Benign neoplasms of the gallbladder are uncommon and generally epithelial in origin consisting of both papillomas and adenomas.[53] The papilloma is a pedunculated mass with a multiple branching configuration pathologically.

These branches are not usually visible sonographically, and the mass merely appears as an intraluminal, echogenic structure which does not layer out or cast any acoustic shadow. This appearance may be simulated by tumefactive sludge and organized thrombus within the gallbladder lumen. Adenomas are usually more broad-based and sessile, and sonographically have an appearance similar to hyperplastic and cholesterol polyps: small, echogenic densities arising from the gallbladder wall which remain fixed in place with changes in patient position and which do not cast acoustic shadows (Fig. 3.28). Adenomatous polyps may be single or multiple. The inability to distinguish adenomatous polyps from hyperplastic or cholesterol polyps is not clinically significant, since none of these lesions is thought to predispose to the development of carcinoma.

Malignant Tumors

Carcinoma of the gallbladder is a fairly uncommon but highly malignant tumor, the fifth most common malignancy of the GI tract, affecting females by a 4 to 1 ratio over males. It occurs principally in the elderly and has a high correlation with coexistent gallstones (80 to 90 percent) and chronic

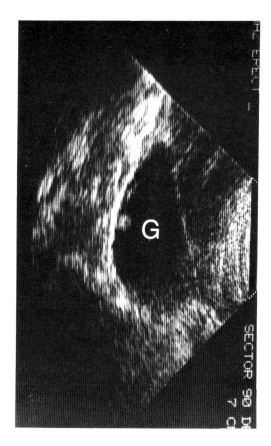

FIG. 3.28. Adenomatous polyp along the posterior of wall of the gallbladder, *G,* simulating a non-shadowing, small gallstone which did not move with a change in the patient's position.

cholecystitis, suggesting that chronic irritation of the gallbladder mucosa may result in a dysplasia initially and ultimately in a neoplastic transformation. These tumors are usually clinically silent until well advanced, often associated with a large invasive mass of the liver or metastatic lymphadenopathy. Therefore, the prognosis is quite poor with approximately 20 percent one-year survival and less than 5 percent five-year survival. The ultrasonographic appearance of gallbladder carcinoma has been categorized into three types.[57] Most commonly, there is a large solid mass filling the gallbladder bed and obliterating the lumen of the gallbladder (Fig. 3.29). This is a nonspecific appearance and can be simulated by any hepatic mass, the only clues being lack of visualization of a normal gallbladder lumen and perhaps identification of stones engulfed by the tumor. Occasionally the tumor may not only invade the liver but lead to a localized intrahepatic perforation, resulting in a bizarre complex appearance of a solid and cystic intrahepatic mass which might simulate an abscess.

The other two types of gallbladder carcinoma include a polypoid fungating intraluminal mass (Fig. 3.30) and focal or diffuse thickening of the gallbladder wall (Fig. 3.31), or a combination of these two findings.[58, 59] These appearances are considerably less common than the first type. The intraluminal mass simulates the appearance of gallbladder clot, benign papillomas, and even metastatic disease to the gallbladder. The infiltrative wall-thickening pattern may simulate chronic cholecystitis, adenomyomatosis, gangrenous or xanthogranulomatous cholecystitis.[60] The clinical presentation usually

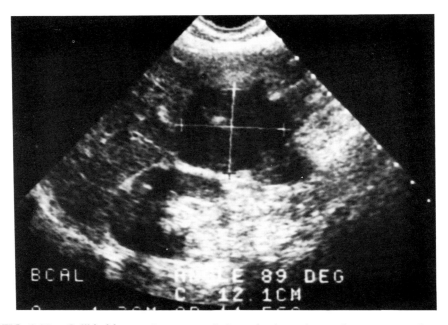

FIG. 3.29. Gallbladder carcinoma consisting of a large hypoechoic mass replacing the gallbladder (denoted by markers).

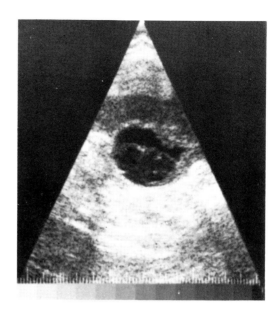

FIG. 3.30. Gallbladder carcinoma presenting as a hypoechoic intraluminal mass.

serves to distinguish these various lesions, but sonographically the appearance may be quite similar (Fig. 3.32).

Calcification of the gallbladder wall (porcelain gallbladder) is an infrequent development occurring in less than 1 percent of all cholecystectomy specimens. This occurs much more commonly in women by a 5 to 1 ratio, is seen typically in the 5th through 8th decades of life, and is associated with cholelithiasis in over 95 percent of cases. It is postulated that the calcification results from either chronic cystic duct obstruction with precipitation of calcium carbonate salts, dystrophic calcification as a result of chronic infection and ischemia, or as a result of chronic irritation of the gallbladder wall by stones. It is extremely important to recognize the appearance of a porcelain gallbladder since there is a high association with gallbladder carcinoma, which may occur as frequently as 10 to 20 percent. Since the prognosis for gallbladder carcinoma is so poor, prophylactic cholecystectomy is recommended when a diagnosis of porcelain gallbladder is made.

Three sonographic patterns of calcification have been described.[26] The most common pattern consists of a curvilinear, hyperechoic structure with complete acoustic shadowing, simulating the appearance of a scleroatrophic gallbladder filled with stones (Fig. 3.33). The distinction between these two entities can only be made by obtaining a plain film of the abdomen to assess for curvilinear calcification. Milk of calcium bile within the gallbladder may have a similar appearance as well, but this can be distinguished by erect scans in which the milk of calcium will settle out dependently, forming a bile-liquid calcium layer.

The second sonographic pattern consists of biconvex echogenic lines representing both the anterior and posterior walls with posterior shadowing (Fig.

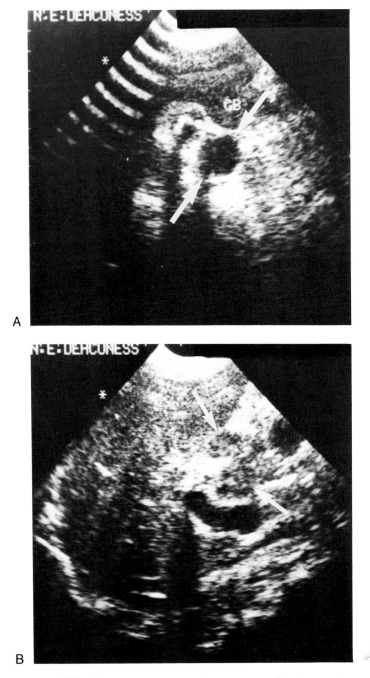

FIG. 3.31.   (A) Gallbladder carcinoma occurring as an exophytic mass (arrows) arising from a small scarred and stone-containing gallbladder. (B) Metastatic lymphadenopathy in the porta hepatis (arrows).

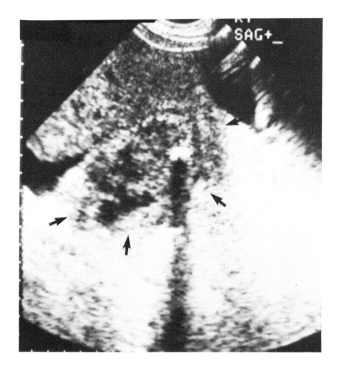

FIG. 3.32. Carcinoma of the gallbladder with cholelithiasis, focal wall thickening, and intraluminal echogenic material simulating the sonographic appearance of gangrenous cholecystitis (arrows).

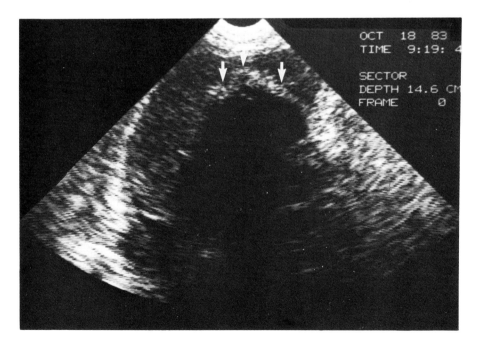

FIG. 3.33. Porcelain gallbladder (arrows) with complete acoustic shadowing posterior to the calcified wall. Note the similarity in appearance to a contracted, stone-filled gallbladder as shown in Fig. 3.9.

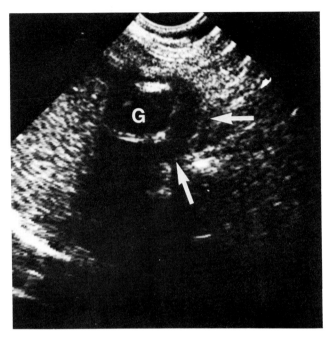

FIG. 3.34. Type 2 gallbladder wall calcification with visualization of both anterior and posterior calcified walls despite acoustic shadowing. Note the eccentric wall thickening (arrows) due to an associated gallbladder carcinoma. G = gallbladder lumen.

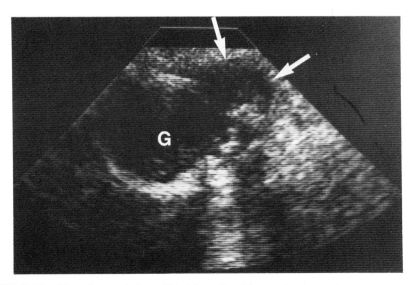

FIG. 3.35. Type 2 porcelain gallbladder, G, with exophytic carcinoma (arrows).

3.34). These gallbladders are larger in size and filled with bile, allowing sufficient sound penetration through the calcified anterior wall to enable visualization of the calcified posterior wall as well. The third pattern of calcification consists of an irregular clump of echogenic material, again with acoustic shadowing. This may also simulate a scarred and contracted gallbladder filled with stones.

Signs of development of carcinoma within a porcelain gallbladder include local or diffuse thickening of the gallbladder wall external to the calcified portion (Fig. 3.34), an eccentric mass arising from the gallbladder wall (Fig. 3.35), as well as any signs of biliary obstruction, portal or peripancreatic lymphadenopathy, or liver metastases. Since Types 1 and 3 simulate the appearance of cholelithiasis in a scarred and empty gallbladder, it is imperative to obtain plain films on all patients with this appearance in order to detect those who have calcification of the gallbladder wall. The Type 2 calcifications are essentially pathognomonic by their sonographic appearance, with the exception of possible confusion with air within the gallbladder wall, which can be distinguished by the reverberation artifacts created by the gas.

Metastatic disease is frequently seen in the gallbladder, but can have similar features to primary gallbladder carcinoma, such as asymmetric wall thickening, a polypoid intraluminal mass (Fig. 3.36), or obliteration of the gallbladder

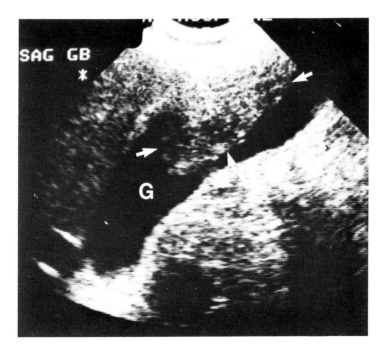

FIG. 3.36.   Metastatic melanoma to the gallbladder lumen, presenting as a polypoid mass (arrows). (Courtesy of Dr. Joseph Simeone, Massachusetts General Hospital.) G = gallbladder.

by mass.[61, 62] Melanoma is the most common source of metastases. Clinical presentation may mimic cholecystitis or the patient may be asymptomatic.

BILE DUCTS

Normal Anatomy

The common bile duct is formed by the confluence of the main left and right intrahepatic ducts at the porta hepatis just anterior and lateral to the confluence of the main right and left portal veins. It then exits the liver and runs along the hepatoduodenal ligament coursing caudally, medially, and posteriorly, crossing under the apex of the duodenal bulb and entering the head of the pancreas where it runs for several centimeters prior to entering the ampulla of Vater. The common hepatic duct, which is that segment between the confluence and the entry of the cystic duct, is well seen in nearly all individuals as the anterior tubular structure in the porta hepatis, with the undivided right portal vein situated posteriorly and the right hepatic artery between these two structures. The common hepatic duct is the most anterior and lateral of these three structures at the porta. The entry point of the cystic duct is seldom visualized sonographically. Below this point, however, the common bile duct can be seen descending in an anterior to posterior direction and crossing the hepatic artery and portal vein. The hepatic artery remains much more anterior in position relative to the common bile duct, with the portal vein being somewhat intermediate between the two.[63]

Various patient maneuvers, such as scanning in the supine and left lateral decubitus positions, ingestion of water, and scanning with the patient erect, will usually allow satisfactory visualization of both the common hepatic and the common bile duct. Obesity and excessive gassiness may hinder the ability to visualize the distal common bile duct. The common hepatic duct is most often well visualized by sagittal, oblique, subcostal scans with the patient either supine or in the left lateral decubitus position,[64] but the distal common bile duct is often better seen by transverse imaging of the head of the pancreas.[65] Under optimal conditions, the confluence of the common bile duct and pancreatic duct can be imaged in the immediate periampullary portion of the pancreas.

The intrahepatic bile ducts are usually not visualized, although portions of normal-sized main right and left hepatic ducts can occasionally be visualized just anterior to the corresponding main right and left portal veins.[63] These are generally quite small in size and are seen only over a short distance. Beyond the initial bifurcation, the bile ducts are never visualized when normal in caliber, being below the limits of resolution of conventional ultrasound systems. Normally, in the periphery of the liver, the only portion of the portal triad that can be visualized as a fluid-filled structure is the portal venous branch.

Technique

It is useful to conceive of the biliary tree as having separate segments in order to analyze the level of obstruction when present and to narrow the differential diagnosis. For this type of analysis the common duct is divided into distal (intrapancreatic) and proximal (suprapancreatic) portions, and the intrahepatic ducts separated into proximal (hilar or periportal) and peripheral segments.

The distal intrapancreatic segment of the common duct is best evaluated by transverse scans through the head of the pancreas and uncinate process (Fig. 3.37), with the patient supine or in an RPO position to minimize the amount of gas in the distal antrum and duodenum.[65] Erect transverse scans of the pancreas are also useful and if persistent gas is a problem, ingestion of water and rescanning may help displace bowel gas and provide an acoustic window to the pancreas. The proximal common duct is best evaluated by subcostal oblique or parasagittal scans (Fig. 3.38) with the patient supine or more usually in the LPO position.[64] The proximal duct is usually well visualized for a distance of several centimeters even in gassy or obese patients, although at times it may be necessary to image in the coronal plane by scanning in the intercostal spaces in the mid axillary line.

The central intrahepatic ducts are usually also best visualized in the transverse plane by imaging the main trunks of the right and left portal vein

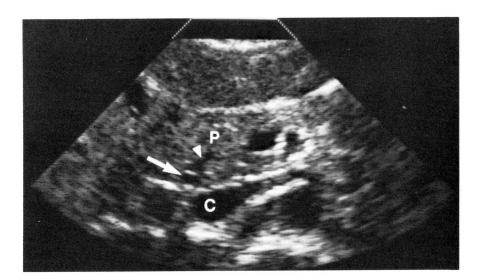

FIG. 3.37.   Common bile duct (arrow) in cross-section situated posteriorly within the low head of the pancreas. Note the adjacent obliquely oriented pancreatic duct (arrowhead), thus indicating the section is quite near the ampulla of Vater. P = pancreas, C = inferior vena cava.

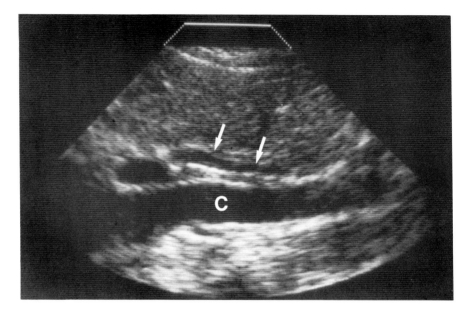

FIG. 3.38. Common duct in long axis coursing obliquely from the porta hepatis anterolaterally to the head of the pancreas posteromedially (arrows). C = inferior vena cava.

(Fig. 3.39). The left main hepatic duct is seen just anterior to the bifurcation of the left portal vein into its medial and lateral branches. The right hepatic duct is seen situated anterior to the undivided right portal vein (Fig. 3.40) which pursues a horizontal course into the right lobe of the liver.[63] The peripheral ducts, as mentioned, cannot be directly visualized when normal in size but are assessed by scanning through the hepatic parenchyma, usually in sagittal orientation, observing the number and position of the various portal and hepatic venous structures in each slice.

PATHOLOGY

Biliary Obstruction

Obstruction of the biliary tract is detected with considerable accuracy by ultrasonography, making it the imaging method of choice to assess for biliary obstruction. The common duct has a normal diameter of 5 mm or less at the porta[66] and may be 1 to 2 mm larger in the hepatoduodenal ligament,[67] subsequently tapering again as it courses through the pancreas. It has been established that there is some increase in the diameter of the normal common duct with advancing age,[68] such that at age 70 the average diameter of the normal common duct is closer to 7 mm, while at age 50 the average diameter is 5 mm and at age 30, approximately 4 mm. In addition, a certain percentage of patients will show an increase in the diameter of the common duct following cholecystectomy, where one may see diameters up to 10 mm in an unobstructed system.[69, 70] This again more often occurs in the elderly population than in younger patients. Finally, if there has been a previous episode of biliary obstruction, the duct may remain dilated despite resolution of the obstruction. One of the useful ways of assessing equivocal dilatation of the common duct is by administration of an oral fatty meal[71] or intravenous injection of cholecystokinin.[72] This results in contraction of the gallbladder, relaxation of the sphincter of Oddi, and increased bile flow from the liver parenchyma. In normal patients, the caliber of the bile duct will either remain the same or decrease up to 3 mm. An increase in the diameter of the common duct following challenge with fat or cholecystokinin is an indication of an obstructive abnormality, which may be due to a fixed lesion such as a fibrous stricture, an impacted stone, small tumor, or a functional disorder due to spasm of the sphincter of Oddi.

Central intrahepatic bile duct dilatation is assessed by imaging the main right and left hepatic ducts immediately anterior to the main right and left portal veins. While normally much smaller, with biliary obstruction the central ducts dilate and become equal or greater in diameter than the adjacent portal vein, giving rise to the "shotgun" sign[73] or the "parallel channel"

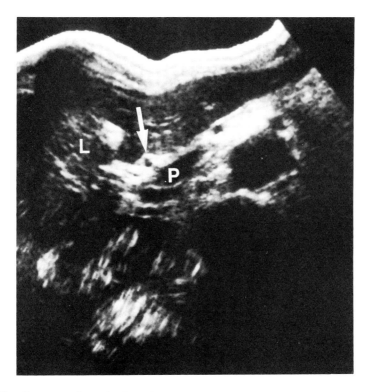

FIG. 3.39. Common hepatic duct in cross-section (arrow) located anteriorly and laterally to the main portal vein, *P*, at the level of the porta hepatis. *L* = liver.

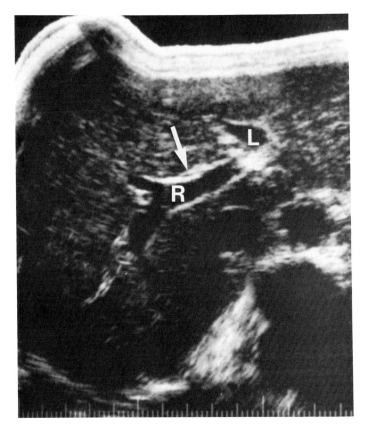

FIG. 3.40. Main right, R, and left, L, portal veins. A short segment of the main right hepatic duct is seen anterior to the right portal vein (arrow).

sign.[74] In addition to having an increased diameter when obstructed, the ducts are also seen over a greater length (over 2 cm) and tortuosity of the duct walls may also be observed. Peripheral intrahepatic bile duct dilatation has several manifestations,[75] including an abnormal stellate branching pattern with three, four and five branches seen converging together. Undulating, irregular walls can be seen with dilated bile ducts, and there is also an increased number of tubular structures in the periphery of the liver, the so-called too many tubes sign. Finally when grossly dilated, acoustic enhancement may be seen through the dilated ducts.

It should always be kept in mind that one may have acute obstruction of the common duct, usually by an impacted stone, with no detectable ductal dilatation but with symptoms of biliary colic and often associated cholangitis. This occurs infrequently but will contribute some false negative ultrasound studies.[76] Fortunately most of these patients will not go undetected because of their symptom complex and since the vast majority will have elevations of alkaline phosphatase and often bilirubin as well. Thus, further direct cholangiographic studies will generally reveal the obstruction. Acute biliary obstruction due to distal impacted stones may present with nondilated ducts in up to 30 percent of patients.[77, 78] The only other clinical entity that typically may present with obstructive ducts and nondilatation is sclerosing cholangitis. Whereas the lack of dilatation due to stone disease is due to either the acuteness of the obstruction with lack of time for the ducts to dilate or an intermittent ball-valve type of obstruction,with sclerosing cholangitis the ducts are often incapable of dilatation due to the intense desmoplastic reaction surrounding them.

In another group of patients the bile duct dilatation may precede the clinical evidence of biliary obstruction and indeed may even be seen before the bilirubin is elevated.[79, 80] There may be dilatation of the common duct only or occasionally dilatation of the central intrahepatic ducts. This group of patients may have only partial obstruction or intermittent obstruction, but even in the presence of near total obstruction it may take several days before the clinical and laboratory findings confirm the ultrasound diagnosis, although the alkaline phosphatase level again is nearly always elevated. Clear cut biliary dilatation by sonography should be investigated further regardless of the patient's symptoms or bilirubin level.

Finally one may occasionally encounter patients in whom the common duct changes rapidly in size, even changing in real time.[81] This may occur following interventional procedures such as surgical or endoscopic sphincterotomy and occasionally due to ball-valve type obstructions. We have encountered a patient in whom there was an afferent loop obstruction following a Billroth 2 procedure in whom the duct changed rapidly during the real-time examination (Fig. 3.41) in spite of there being no biliary obstruction per se but rather an obstruction of the duodenum. Because of the potentially rapid changes in the biliary tree, it is prudent ot obtain information regarding the duct caliber immediately prior to planned surgical, endoscopic, or percutaneous intervention.

Assessment of the gallbladder can be helpful in delineating the level of biliary obstruction, but often the state of the gallbladder may be misleading. Obviously a grossly distended Courvoisier-type gallbladder is indicative of a chronic obstruction of the distal common duct, but many patients will not show gallbladder dilation in this setting because of intrinsic disease in the gallbladder wall from cholelithiasis and chronic cholecystitis, thereby preventing dilatation in the face of a high grade obstruction. Similarly an empty gallbladder in the presence of dilated central and peripheral intrahepatic ducts is a helpful sign to indicate obstruction at or near the bifurcation or at least proximal to the cystic duct insertion. Since the site of cystic duct entry into the common duct is variable and can seldom be demonstrated, the precise level of obstruction in this type case is better determined by evaluation of the proximal and distal common duct directly.

Choledocholithiasis

With proper scanning technique, which includes assessment of the distal common duct by scanning through the head of the pancreas in transverse

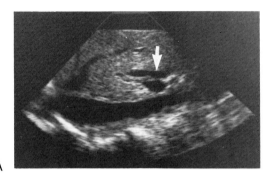

A

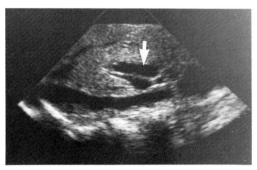

B

FIG. 3.41. Rapid change in caliber of the common duct (arrow) on scans obtained within seconds of one another.

orientation, ultrasound can achieve an overall sensitivity of approximately 75 percent in the detection of choledocholithiasis.[65] Most common duct stones are located in the distal common duct, frequently at or near the ampulla. This can only be seen well in the scans designed to show the low head of the pancreas and uncinate process, either with the patient supine, RPO or erect. According to Laing's series, 70 percent of distal common duct stones can be successfully imaged sonographically, while almost 90 percent of proximal stones are successfully imaged. Most common duct stones have a familiar appearance of an echogenic structure with posterior acoustic shadowing (Fig. 3.42), but approximately 10 percent of common duct stones may not exhibit any acoustic shadowing. This phenomenon may be due to the small size (Fig. 3.43) or to the varying composition of common duct stones, some of which are merely conglomerations of soft sludge and others which may be very porous in consistency (Fig. 3.44). These type stones may not exhibit the typical acoustic shadow and often appear less brightly echogenic than the more typical hard stones. Nonshadowing stones cannot be distinguished from other intraluminal lesions, such as clot, tumor, or parasitic infestation.

It is important to recognize that in approximately 20 to 25 percent of cases with acute biliary obstruction, there may be no intrahepatic bile duct dilatation and in a smaller percentage, the extrahepatic biliary tree may also be nondilated. These occurrences are usually seen in the presence of very small stones which intermittently obstruct at the ampulla.[77, 78] Most of these patients will have elevation of alkaline phosphatase and often bilirubin levels, and most

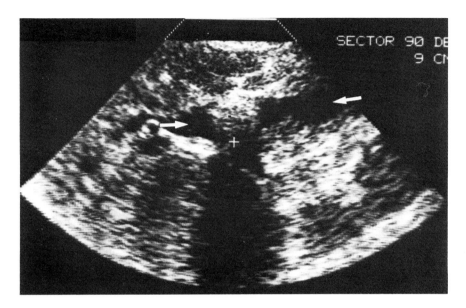

FIG. 3.42.   Large stone in the mid common duct with posterior acoustic shadowing. White arrows denote enlarged common bile duct.

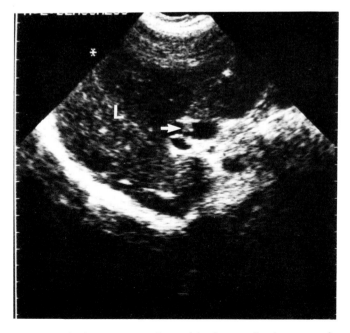

FIG. 3.43.   Small nonshadowing stone (arrow) in the proximal common hepatic duct. L = liver.

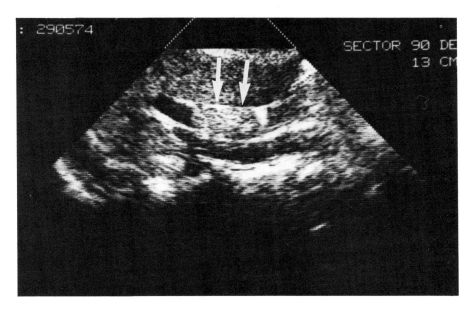

FIG. 3.44.   Large nonshadowing common duct stone (arrows). This was very soft and sludge-like in consistency at surgery.

of them will also experience typical colicky right upper quadrant pain and often fever and chills as well. Thus in patients with this clinical presentation, the lack of direct visualization of common duct stones or ductal dilatation does not allow one to exclude the diagnosis of choledocholithiasis, and further testing is indicated either with radionuclide biliary scanning or CT, or by direct cholangiographic procedures such as endoscopic retrograde cholangio-pancreatography (ERCP) or transhepatic cholangiography.

It is also important whenever possible to demonstrate the intraluminal stone in two projections 90° to one another in order to be certain that the lesion identified as a stone is truly within the duct rather than adjacent to it (Fig. 3.45). It is not uncommon for an apparent stone or a mass to be seen at the distal end of the duct in sagittal orientation but by rotating the real time transducer into an axial plane, the lesion can be seen to lie immediately adjacent to the duct but not within the lumen (Fig. 3.46). One other potential pitfall involves the common duct which is filled with stones, such that all that is imaged sonographically is acoustic shadowing. This can be easily mistaken for gas in the duodenum, which is the most common reason for failure to visualize the duct. Scanning in the RPO position will help to recognize this phenomenon, since gas in the duodenum should move either back into the stomach or into the more distal duodenum with the right side dependent. If the shadowing remains in this position, one should think of the possibility of a stone-filled duct. Another point to remember is that acoustic shadowing from small stones is optimally produced when the beam

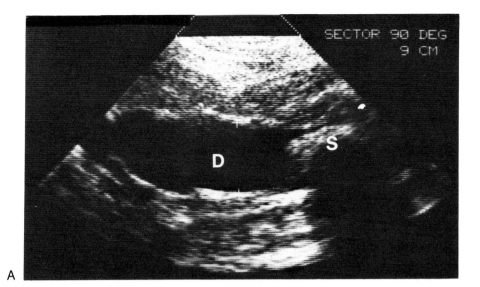

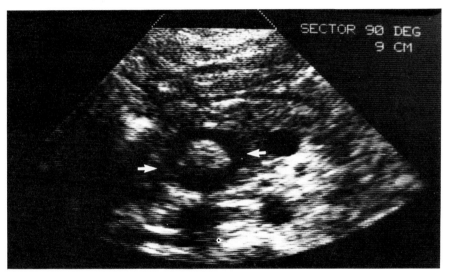

FIG. 3.45. (A) Grossly dilated common duct, *D*, with an echogenic focus (*S* = stone) with acoustic shadowing at the distal end of the duct on sagittal view. (B) Axial scan confirms the intraluminal location of this distal common duct stone. (Arrows denote duct.)

is perpendicular to the stone rather than coming at a tangential angle where refraction may obscure the acoustic shadow.

When there is an acutely impacted stone at the ampulla, even optimal display of the entire extrahepatic ductal system may fail to be diagnostic since the stone may be impossible to recognize due to the surrounding duodenum and its gas. One can only, at this point, diagnose a distal periampullary

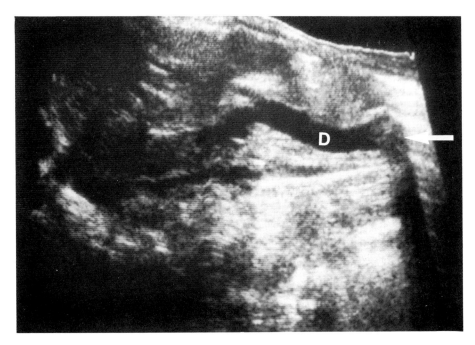

FIG. 3.46. Common duct pseudo-calculus. The sagittal view of the dilated common duct, *D,* appears to end in an echogenic focus with acoustic shadowing (arrow) simulating a stone. This focus arose from gas in the duodenum and there were no stones in the duct.

obstruction and include choledocholithiasis in a differential with stricture, pancreatitis, and small, strategically-located tumors of the pancreas and ampulla. Approximately 30 percent of distal stones are still missed even with optimal scanning technique, and it is these distally-impacted stones that are usually missed.[65] One may occasionally see dilatation of the pancreatic duct due to a distally-impacted gallstone and resultant pancreatitis and spasm, although double duct dilatation is more often seen with tumors and may also be seen with chronic pancreatitis and strictures.

Stones may also be present in the intrahepatic ducts[82] and complete biliary evaluation includes thorough scanning of the entire liver. Intrahepatic stones are generally easily recognized due to their brightly echogenic appearance and acoustic shadowing. It is important to remember that stones may occur proximal to an obstruction from another cause, such as chronic stricture, pancreatitis, or even slow-growing neoplastic lesions. Stones may also be occasionally seen in association with sclerosing cholangitis, particularly if the extrahepatic common duct is involved.

Pancreatitis

Dilatation of the common duct may occur with acute pancreatitis, but intrahepatic ductal dilatation is seldom seen. Ductal dilatation often occurs in association with pancreatic pseudocyst, but it should not be assumed that the pseudocyst is necessarily the cause of the obstruction, as it has been well recognized that drainage of the pseudocyst will not necessarily result in relief of the bile duct dilatation. The biliary obstruction often results from stricturing secondary to the acute inflammation rather than to a pressure effect from the expanding pseudocyst. The ductal dilatation seen with acute pancreatitis may resolve completely after resolution of the acute episode, and the ducts may return to normal (Fig. 3.47). Occasionally, however, the

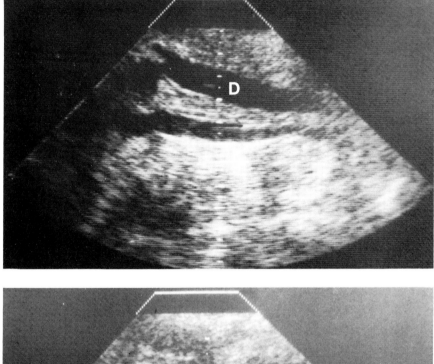

FIG. 3.47. (A) Acute pancreatitis causing marked dilatation of the common duct, *D*, due to distal stricture. (B) Two months later the common duct (arrows) is now normal in caliber following resolution of the pancreatitis, thereby excluding a fibrous stricture.

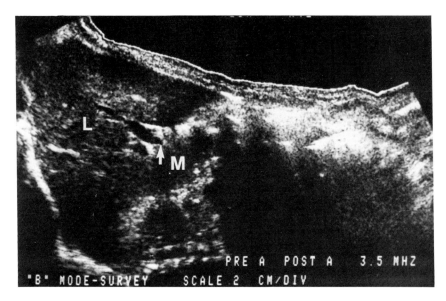

FIG. 3.48. Focal chronic pancreatitis with common duct dilatation and a tapered stricture of the duct (arrow). A solid mass, *M*, was seen at the site of the stricture and could not be distinguished from carcinoma of the pancreas. *L* = liver.

ducts may remain dilated even after resolution of the obstruction, presumably due to loss of elasticity. Consequently, in a patient who has had previously documented biliary obstruction, the mere presence of ductal dilatation alone is not necessarily diagnostic of continued obstruction. This group of patients might be challenged with fat or cholecystokinin to look for dynamic changes in the ducts, but frequently a more functional evaluation using a radionuclide biliary scan or other cholangiographic imaging procedure is necessary to assess for the presence or absence of obstruction.

Focal chronic pancreatitis may also result in ductal dilatation (Fig. 3.48) and may be indistinguishable sonographically from cancer of the pancreas, since both appear as focal masses usually hypoechoic to surrounding pancreatic tissue. Other signs, such as pancreatic calcifications, might suggest chronic pancreatitis, but this is not infallible, as carcinoma may arise in a setting of chronic pancreatitis. Often a needle biopsy is the only means to make this distinction, since the CT appearance is also quite similar. If biopsy is entertained it should be done following decompression of the biliary tree, in order to avoid potentially puncturing an obstructed biliary system which could lead to bile leakage and peritonitis.

BENIGN NEOPLASMS

Benign tumors of the bile ducts include papillomas, adenomas, cystadenomas, and granular cell myoblastomas. All of these are extremely uncommon lesions, and are indeed much less common than primary carcinoma of the bile ducts.[83] Papillomas and solid adenomas appear generally as intraluminal solid filling defects, usually of low to moderate echogenicity and without acoustic shadowing. These lesions mimic the appearance of biliary sludge, soft stones, and clot. Biliary cystadenomas are lesions usually seen in young females and tend to present as very large bulky masses. The typical appearance is that of a multiloculated cystic mass (Fig. 3.49), usually thin-walled, but with occasional mural nodules and papillary infoldings (Fig. 3.50).[84] Unilocular cystadenomas are also encountered occasionally (Fig. 3.51) and peripheral rim-like calcification can also be seen. On CT, multiloculated cystic mass is again usually seen although the septations are better demonstrated by ultrasonography. The CT density is variable depending on the composition of fluid which may be serous, mucinous, or purulent and may also contain hemosiderin or cholesterol crystals. The presence of crystalline or necrotic material may also result in echogenic fluid on sonographic examination. Cystadenomas are also hypovascular by angiography. Carcinomatous degeneration may occur rarely, and usually is not reliably predicted preoperatively unless neovascularity is recognized on angiography. The vast majority of these lesions are benign and usually do not communicate with the biliary tree, although the lesions originate from ductal epithelium. Rarely there may be communication with the bile ducts.

Differential diagnosis for biliary cystadenomas might include echinococcal cysts, which usually have smaller locules and daughter cysts, cystic metastatic disease, or cystic necrosis of primary or secondary malignancies. Abscesses

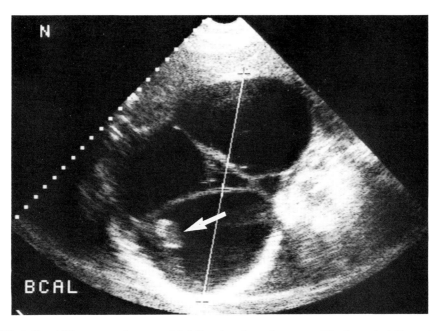

FIG. 3.49.   Biliary cystadenoma. Multiloculated cystic mass with characteristic septations as well as mural thickening and nodularity posteriorly (arrow).

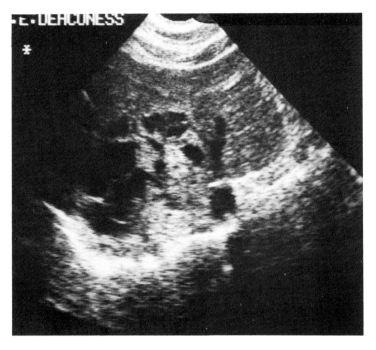

FIG. 3.50. Biliary cystadenoma with marked mural thickening but no malignant degeneration.

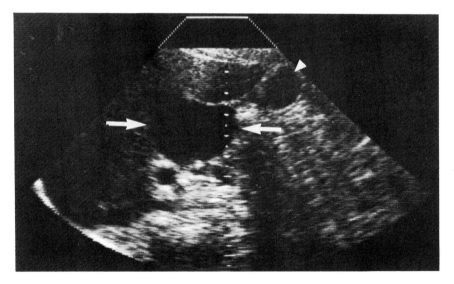

FIG. 3.51. Unilocular biliary cystadenoma (arrows) in the porta hepatis. The gallbladder is seen distally (arrowhead).

and partially liquified hematomas may also be in the differential diagnosis. An extrahepatic unilocular choledochal cyst could rarely have this appearance.

PRIMARY MALIGNANT DISEASE

This category should probably include both ampullary carcinoma and cholangiocarcinoma. Most ampullary tumors present early because of their strategic location causing biliary obstruction, and frequently the only sonographic finding is that of distal bile duct obstruction (Fig. 3.52). The mass may not be recognized but, if successfully imaged, has an appearance indistinguishable from that of pancreatic carcinoma (Fig. 3.53), which presents as a hypoechoic solid mass surrounding the periampullary portion of the distal common duct. Similarly, most patients with cholangiocarcinoma again present early when the masses are fairly small because of the abrupt onset of obstruction. While some authors have claimed success in visualizing this neoplasm in approximately 75 percent of cases,[85] our experience has been decidedly different. In the majority of our cases both involving the distal common duct as well as the bifurcation (Klatskin tumor), we have merely seen the effects of the obstruction with proximal ductal dilatation and narrowing at the site of tumor. Frequently the cholangiocarcinoma will grow submucosally along the ducts and may be difficult or impossible to detect even by the

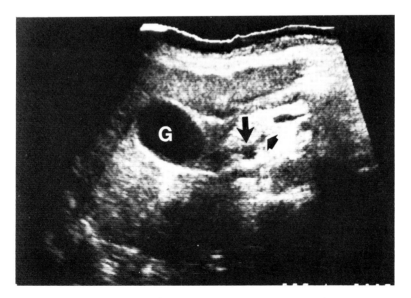

FIG. 3.52.   Ampullary carcinoma. Ultrasound through the low head of the pancreas shows common bile duct dilatation (arrow) and slight dilatation of the adjoining pancreatic duct (arrowhead) but the tumor was below resolution limits and could not be imaged. G = gallbladder.

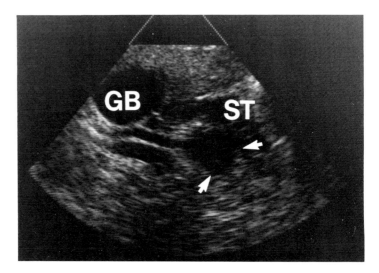

FIG. 3.53. Pancreatic carcinoma. The minimally dilated common duct terminates abruptly in a rounded hypoechoic mass (arrows). Note the somewhat dilated gallbladder, *GB*, and the stomach, *ST*, draped across the pancreatic tumor.

surgeon directly palpating the ducts. A smaller subset of patients will present with a definable mass either fungating within the duct lumen or, in the case of Klatskin tumor, extending for a variable distance into the surrounding hepatic parenchyma near the porta hepatis (Fig. 3.54). Metastases to the periportal lymph nodes and hepatic parenchyma may be seen.[86]

Despite the fact that these tumors present early and at times grow fairly slowly, the prognosis is still rather poor, probably in part because of the inadequate ability to define the full extent of the tumor even intraoperatively. We have noted a rather striking appearance of a cholangiocarcinoma at the bifurcation during intraoperative sonography (Fig. 3.55) where a large infiltrating tumor was demonstrated that was not well recognized by preoperative CT, ultrasound or angiography.

Metastatic Tumors

The most common nonprimary malignancy to result in bile duct dilatation is, of course, cancer of the head of the pancreas, where the obstruction is caused by direct invasion around the intrapancreatic segment of the distal common duct (Fig. 3.53). Occasionally, the metastatic spread of cancer of the pancreas may invade up the hepatoduodenal ligament and obstruct the common duct more proximally in its suprapancreatic portion. Similarly, metastatic disease to the periportal lymph nodes will often lead to proximal ductal obstruction, giving an appearance of dilated intrahepatic ducts in the left and right lobes but a normal or small extrahepatic common duct. Carcino-

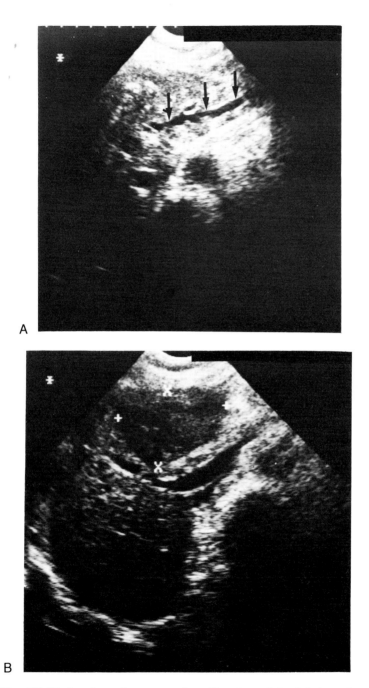

FIG. 3.54. (A) Cholangiocarcinoma causing dilatation of the left lateral segmental bile duct (arrows). (B) Large hypoechoic tumor in the medial segment of the left lobe extending to the porta and obstructing the left hepatic duct.

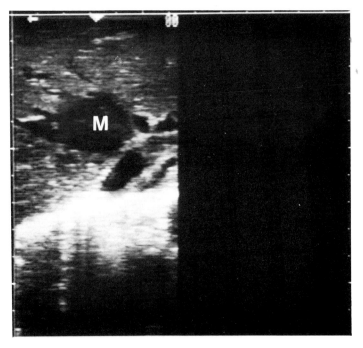

FIG. 3.55. Klatskin tumor seen on intraoperative sonography at the bifurcation of right and left ducts. This 2.5 cm mass, *M,* could not be visualized preoperatively.

mas of the colon, stomach, pancreas and breast are the most common primary malignancies to cause periportal bile duct obstruction (Fig. 3.56). Lymphoma can also involve the periportal nodes and can cause biliary obstruction as well, although since this tumor is somewhat softer than the carcinomas, one may see fairly extensive periportal lymphadenopathy without obstruction, and in fact this may be a clue to the diagnosis of lymphoma. Direct lymphomatous involvement of the pancreas or peripancreatic lymph nodes can also lead to obstruction of the distal common duct (Fig. 3.57).

Finally, one may see isolated obstruction of lobar or segmental intrahepatic ducts with the remainder of the system being normal in caliber. This can occur as a result of isolated cholangiocarcinoma but is more often seen due to hepatic parenchymal metastatic disease, where one of the metastatic lesions directly invades and obstructs a segmental ductal system. Generally the metastatic disease is readily appreciated, allowing one to distinguish this appearance from the segmental dilatation sometimes seen with sclerosing cholangitis.

CONGENITAL ABNORMALITIES

Choledochocele

Choledochocele refers to focal cystic dilatation of the intraduodenal portion of the common duct near the ampulla. This cystic area communicates with the duodenum and represents the terminus of the pancreatic duct. Choledo-

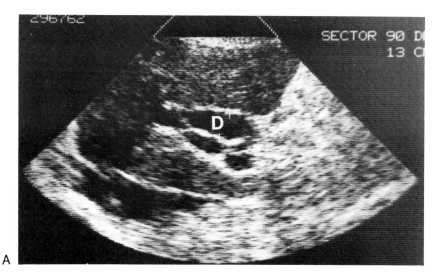

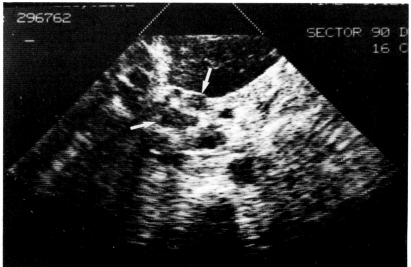

FIG. 3.56. Metastatic colon carcinoma. (A) Marked dilatation of the right main and common hepatic duct, *D*. (B) Periportal metastatic lymphadenopathy (arrows) causing the biliary obstruction.

choceles are typically small and usually not visualized sonographically due to surrounding gas in the duodenum.

Choledochal Cysts

Choledochal cysts are more common and are readily recognizable by ultrasound.[87] This anomaly occurs much more often in females and often presents in children or young adults. Symptoms include jaundice, which

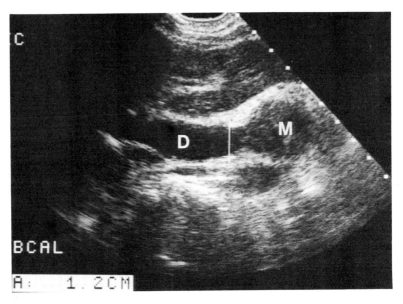

FIG. 3.57. Peripancreatic lymphoma presenting as a hypoechoic solid mass, *M*, obstructing the distal common duct, *D*.

occurs in 70 percent of cases, and pain from associated cholangitis as well as a palpable right upper quadrant mass. Typically a choledochal cyst presents with massive dilatation of the common bile duct, common hepatic duct, and cystic duct. Usually there is a very short localized stricture at the distal end of the common duct. The intrahepatic ducts are usually normal in caliber, although occasionally there may be central intrahepatic ductal dilatation as well. The lesion may be a result of abnormal insertion of the common duct into the distal pancreatic duct, resulting in reflux of pancreatic secretions into the common duct and resultant stricture and fibrosis. Complications of this disease include recurrent cholangitis and stone formation with occasional progression to biliary cirrhosis, and portal hypertension. There is also an increased incidence of cholangiocarcinoma developing in a choledochal cyst, and these tumors tend to be very aggressive with early metastases.

The typical ultrasonographic appearance of a choledochal cyst is that of massive dilatation of the extrahepatic biliary tree with little or no intrahepatic ductal dilatation (Fig. 3.58). This serves to distinguish, in most cases, this entity from Caroli's disease, as well as from other causes of distal common duct obstruction such as pancreatic carcinoma and stricture, where one would expect proportionate dilatation of the intrahepatic ducts.

Caroli's Disease

Caroli's disease is also a congenital autosomal recessive disorder in which there is segmental saccular dilatation of the intrahepatic ducts. While in most cases the common duct is not dilated, occasional involvement of the extrahe-

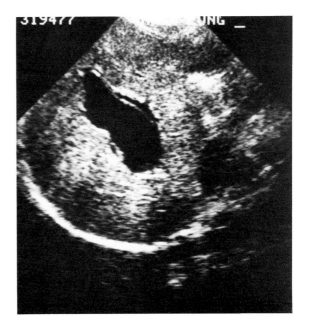

FIG. 3.58.   Choledochal cyst manifesting as massive tubular dilatation of the common hepatic duct. Note the absence of intrahepatic peripheral ductal dilatation.

patic ductal system can be seen. This results in an appearance of multiple cyst-like areas within the liver which communicate with the dilated biliary tree giving a so-called lollipop appearance on cholangiography. The sonographic appearance thus is that of intrahepatic ductal dilatation and cyst formation (Fig. 3.59) with usually a normal common duct.[88] Stones may be seen within the cyst or ducts and cholangitis is a frequent complication which may ultimately result in the formation of parenchymal liver abscesses. This disease also usually presents in young adults and has no major predilection for either sex. Approximately 80 percent of patients have associated medullary sponge kidney. Increased echogenicity and actual stone formation in the kidneys can be seen sonographically. There is also a speculative relationship with congenital hepatic fibrosis in which there is bile duct proliferation and multiple strictures with proximal cystic dilatation. The degree of dilatation is less than seen in Caroli's disease and the fibrosis predominates, resulting in early cirrhosis, portal hypertension, and liver failure. This disease is usually lethal in childhood. Probably congenital hepatic fibrosis and Caroli's disease represent opposite ends of a spectrum.

INFECTIOUS/INFLAMMATORY DISEASES

Oriental Cholangiohepatitis

Oriental cholangiohepatitis is an uncommon disease in the United States but is not unusual in the Far East and in Southeast Asia. Patients with this disorder have repetitive bouts of cholangitis and biliary obstruction secondary to stone formation, and present with colic, fever, and jaundice. The precise etiology of this disease is not clear. It occurs predominately in areas where

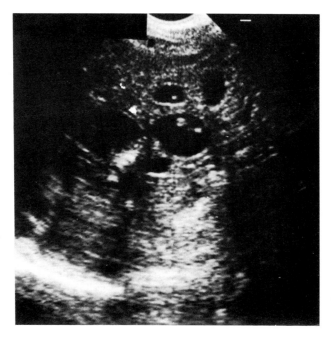

FIG. 3.59. Caroli's disease with multiple dilated intrahepatic ducts and periductal abscesses. Note the small stones floating within several dilated ducts.

infestation with the liver fluke, *Clonorchis sinensis* is endemic. However, many patients with oriental pyogenic cholangitis do not show evidence of *Clonorchis* infestation. The vast majority of patients have biliary infection, most often with *E. coli,* which can elaborate an enzyme (beta-glucuronidase) that deconjugates bilirubin and may result in calcium bilirubinate stone formation. The *E. coli* infection, however, may be present only because of the presence of biliary obstruction and multiple strictures.

The sonographic findings include variable dilatation of the common duct and intrahepatic ducts, often with areas of segmental dilatation interspersed with nondilated ducts.[89] Intrahepatic and extrahepatic biliary stones are often seen (Fig. 3.60). At times the stones are soft and sludge-like and may be difficult to recognize sonographically, being virtually isoechoic to the surrounding hepatic parenchyma.[90] Soft, sludge-like stone material in the common duct may be confused with an extrahepatic soft tissue mass. However, a lack of ability to demonstrate the normal common duct serves as a clue to the true etiology. Air within the biliary tree may also be seen in the presence of a gas-forming bacterial infection. There is an increased incidence of cholangiocarcinoma developing in patients with oriental cholangiohepatitis, presumably as a result of chronic irritation leading to dysplasia and subsequently neoplasia.

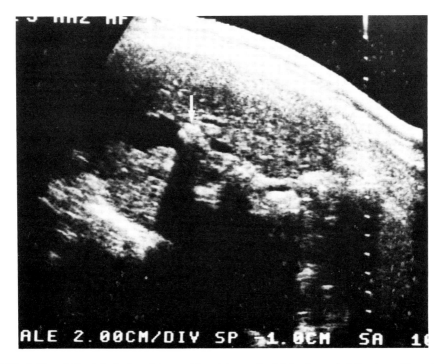

ALE 2.00CM/DIV SP -1.0CM SA 1(

FIG. 3.60. Oriental cholangiohepatitis with marked intrahepatic bile duct dilatation and extensive stone formation (one denoted by arrow).

Ascariasis

Ascariasis is a common infestational disease in the Far East, Russia, Africa and Latin America, and there are some endemic areas in the Southeastern United States, as well. The roundworm *Ascaris lumbricoides* usually infests the small bowel, most commonly the jejunum, but worms frequently enter the common bile duct as well as the gallbladder and intrahepatic ducts. The clinical presentation is of biliary colic, occasionally with fever, and elevation of liver enzymes. Jaundice occurs only occasionally as does acute cholecystitis. Parasitic liver abscesses and ascending cholangitis are infrequent complications. Infestation in endemic areas is especially common in children.

The sonographic appearance of biliary ascariasis is variable.[91, 92] The worm may appear as a moderately echogenic, nonshadowing, linear filling defect within the lumen of the common duct (Fig. 3.61), and occasionally multiple linear structures are seen in a spaghetti-like appearance when multiple worms are present in the duct. Occasionally the digestive tract of the worm may be visualized as an anechoic tubular structure within the outer walls of the worm. This may produce a bull's-eye appearance in short axis. When the worm is coiled, multiple rounded, tortuous, or tubular structures can be

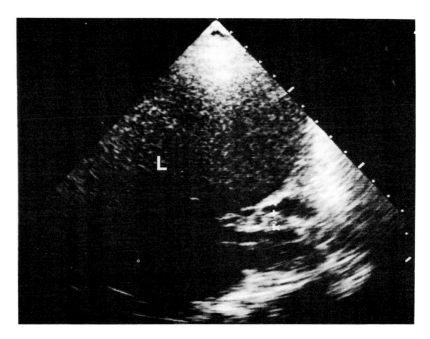

FIG. 3.61. Biliary ascariasis (denoted by *xs*) presenting as a moderately echogenic intraluminal mass within the common duct. *L*= liver. (Courtesy of Dr. Waraporn Issarapanichkit, Bankok, Thailand).

seen either within the gallbladder or the common duct. If any of these appearances is encountered and biliary ascariasis is clinically suspect, examination of the stool for worms or eggs should be undertaken to confirm the diagnosis. Treatment with mebendazole is usually successful in eradicating the infestation, although biliary and bowel obstruction may occur.

Sclerosing Cholangitis

Sclerosing cholangitis usually has no sonographic manifestations, although occasionally one may see segmental or subsegmental dilatation of the intrahepatic ducts proximal to an area of stricture.[93] This appearance can also be seen due to obstruction from intrahepatic parenchymal tumors, including primary cholangiocarcinoma, hepatoma, and metastases. The degree of dilatation seen in sclerosing cholangitis is usually minimal, however. Thickening of the wall of the common duct has been reported[94] (Fig. 3.62), presumably due to the desmoplastic inflammatory reaction commonly seen in this entity. The appearance is not specific, however, and could potentially be seen in other conditions such cholangiocarcinoma and possibly in suppurative cholangitis. Bile duct wall thickening may be simulated by redundant duct mucosa

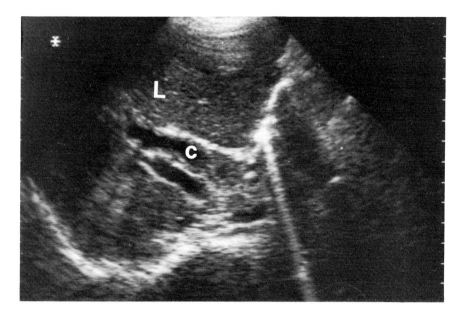

FIG. 3.62.   Sclerosing cholangitis. Note the dilated common hepatic duct, C, with thickened echogenic walls as a result of a fibrous stricture more distally in the common bile duct. L = liver.

after relief of a distal obstruction and collapse of a previously dilated duct. Changes of cirrhosis and portal hypertension may be seen in longstanding cases of sclerosing cholangitis.

CONCLUSION

Ultrasonographic imaging has revolutionized the work-up of biliary abnormalities. Continued improvements in the technique and especially the use of real time instrumentation make ultrasonography the primary imaging method of choice in the initial evaluation of diseases of the gallbladder and biliary tree. Other imaging modalities, such as CT scanning, radionuclide cholescintigraphy, ERCP, and transhepatic cholangiography can be rationally utilized as supplementary imaging techniques to confirm the ultrasonographic findings when necessary or to provide further, more specific evaluation of the disease process. In many instances, however, the ultrasonographic evaluation is complete and sufficient for accurate diagnosis, thus providing an extremely cost-effective and accurate test for evaluating biliary pathology.

REFERENCES

1. Kane RA: Ultrasonographic anatomy of the liver and biliary tree. Semin Ultrasound 1:87, 1980
2. Kane RA: Ultrasonographic evaluation of the gallbladder. CRC Crit Rev Diagn Imaging 17:107, 1982

3. Braverman DZ, Johnson ML, Kern F Jr: Effects of pregnancy and contraceptive steroids on gallbladder function. N Engl J Med 302:362, 1980

4. Taylor KJW, Rosenfeld AT, Graaff CS: Anatomy and Pathology of the Biliary Tree as Demonstrated by Ultrasound. p. 109. In Vol. 1. Diagnostic Ultrasound in Gastrointestinal Disease. Churchill Livingstone, New York, 1979

5. Edell S: A comparison of the "Phrygian cap" deformity with bistable and gray scale ultrasound. J Comput Ultra 6:34, 1978

6. Marchal G, Van de Voorde P, Van Dooren W, et al: Ultrasound appearance of the filled and contracted normal gallbladder. JCU 8:439, 1980

7. Callen PW, Filly RA: Ultrasonographic localization of the gallbladder. Radiology 133:687, 1979

8. Sukov RJ, Sample WF, Sarti DA, Whitcomb MJ: Cholecystosonography—the junctional fold. Radiology 133:435, 1979

9. Taylor KJW, Carpenter DA: The anatomy and pathology of the porta hepatis demonstrated by gray scale ultrasonography. JCU 3:117, 1975

10. Sommer FG, Filly RA, Minton MJ: Acoustic shadowing due to refractive and reflective effects. Am J Roentgenol 132:973, 1979

11. Crade M, Taylor KJW, Rosenfield AT, et al: Surgical and pathologic correlation of cholecystosonography and cholecystography. Am J Roentgenol 131:227, 1978

12. McCune BR, Weeks LE, O'Brien TF, Martin JF: "Pseudostone" of the gallbladder. Gastroenterology 73:1149, 1977

13. Sommer FG, Taylor KJW: Differentiation of acoustic shadowing due to calculi and gas collections. Radiology 135:399, 1980

14. Carroll BA: Gallstones: in vitro comparison of physical, radiographic, and ultrasonic characteristics. Am J Roentgenol 131:223, 1978

15. Filly RA, Moss AA, Way LW: In vitro investigation of gallstone shadowing with ultrasonic tomography. JCU 7:255, 1979

16. Jaffee CC, Taylor KJW: The clinical impact of ultrasonic beam focusing patterns. Radiology 131:469, 1979

17. Sigel B: Ultrasonography during biliary tract surgery. p. 53. In Sigel B (ed): Operative Ultrasonography. Philadelphia, Lea & Febiger, 1982

18. Crow HC, Bartrum RJ, Foote SR: Expanded criteria for the ultrasound diagnosis of gallstones. JCU 4:289, 1976

19. Carroll B, Sommer FG: Letters to the editor, JCU 9:A-30, 1981

20. Scheske GA, Cooperberg PL, Cohen MM, Burhenne HJ: Floating gallstones: the role of contrast material. JCU 8:227, 1980

21. Fakhry J: Sonography of tumefactive biliary sludge. AJR 139:717, 1982

22. MacDonald FR, Cooperberg PL, Cohen MM: The WES triad—A specific sonographic sign of gallstones in the contracted gallbladder. Gastrointest Radiol 6:39, 1981

23. Raptopoulos V, D'Orsi C, Smith E et al: Dynamic cholecystosonography of the contracted gallbladder: the double-arc-shadow sign. AJR 138:275, 1982

24. Chun GH, Deutsch AL, Scheible W: Sonographic findings in milk of calcium bile. Gastrointest Radiol 7:371, 1982

25. Love MB: Sonographic features of milk of calcium bile. J Ultrasound Med 1:325, 1982

26. Kane RA, Jacobs R, Katz J, Costello P: Porcelain gallbladder: ultrasound and CT appearance. Radiology 152:137, 1984

27. Filly RA, Allen B, Minton MJ, et al: In vitro investigation of the origin of echoes within biliary sludge. JCU 8:193, 1980

28. Simeone JF, Mueller PR, Ferrucci JT, et al: Significance of nonshadowing focal opacities at cholecystosonography. Radiology 137:181, 1980

29. Fiske CE, Laing FC, Brown TW: Ultrasonographic evidence of gallbladder wall thickening in association with hypoalbuminemia. Radiology 135:713, 1980

30. Sanders RC: The significance of sonographic gallbladder wall thickening. JCU 8:143, 1980

31. Lewandowski BJ, Winsberg F: Gallbladder wall thickness distortion by ascites. AJR 137:519, 1981

32. Carroll BA: Gallbladder wall thickening secondary to focal lymphatic obstruction. J Ultrasound Med 2:89, 1983

33. Juttner H-U, Ralls PW, Quinn MF, et al: Thickening of the gallbladder wall in acute hepatitis: ultrasound demonstration. Radiology 142:465, 1982

34. Handler SJ: Ultrasound of gallbladder wall thickening and its relation to cholecystitis. Am J Roentgenol 132:581, 1979

35. Marchal GJF, Casaer M, Baert AL, et al: Gallbladder wall sonolucency in acute cholecystitis. Radiology 133:429, 1979

36. Finberg HJ, Birnholz JC: Ultrasound evaluation of the gallbladder wall. Radiology 133:693, 1979

37. Ralls PW, Colletti PM, Lapin SA, et al: Real-time sonography in suspected acute cholecystitis. Radiology 155:767, 1985

38. Herlin P, Jonsson P-E, Karp W: Postoperative acute acalculous cholecystitis—an assessment of diagnostic procedures. Gastrointest Radiol 5:147, 1980

39. Deitch EA, Engel JM: Acute acalculous cholecystitis: ultrasonic diagnosis. Am J Surg 142:290, 1981

40. Hunter ND, Macintosh PK: Acute emphysematous cholecystitis: an ultrasonic diagnosis. Am J Roentgenol 134:592, 1980

41. Parulekar SG: Sonographic findings in acute emphysematous cholecystitis. Radiology 145:117, 1982

42. Mentzer RM, Golden GT, Chandler JG, et al: A comparative appraisal of emphysematous cholecystitis. Am J Surg 129:10, 1975

43. Graif M, Horovitz A, Itzchak Y, Strauss S: Hyperechoic foci in the gallbladder wall as a sign of microabscess formation or diverticula. Radiology 152:781, 1984

44. Kane RA: Complications of acute cholecystitis—ultrasonographic evaluation. Proc 24 Annu Meet Am Inst Ultrasound Med 1:170, 1979

45. Jenkins M, Golding RH, Cooperberg PL: Sonography and computed tomography of hemorrhagic cholecystitis. AJR 140:1197, 1983

46. Kane RA: Ultrasonographic diagnosis of gangrenous cholecystitis and empyema of the gallbladder. Radiology 134:191, 1980

47. Jeffrey RB, Laing FC, Wong W, et al: Gangrenous cholecystitis: diagnosis by ultrasound. Radiology 148:219, 1983

48. Wales LR: Desquamated gallbladder mucosa: unusual sign of cholecystitis. AJR 139:810, 1982

49. Madrazo BL, Francis I, Hricak H, et al: Sonographic findings in perforation of the gallbladder. AJR 139:491, 1982

50. Bergman AB, Neiman HL, Kraut B: Ultrasonographic evaluation of pericholecystic abscesses. AJR 132:201, 1979

51. Berk RN, van der Vegt JH, Lichtenstein JE: The hyperplastic cholecystoses: cholesterolosis and adenomyomatosis. Radiology 146:595, 1983

52. Price RJ, Stewart ET, Foley WD, et al: Sonography of polypoid cholesterolosis. AJR 139:1197, 1982

53. Carter SJ, Rutledge J, Hirsch JH, et al: Papillary adenoma of the gallbladder: ultrasonic demonstration. JCU 6:433, 1978

54. Detweiler DG, Biddinger P, Staab EV, et al: The appearance of adenomyomatosis with the newer imaging modalities: a case with pathologic correlation. J Ultrasound Med 1:295, 1982

55. Raghavendra BN, Subramanyam BR, Balthazar EJ, et al: Sonography of adenomyomatosis of the gallbladder: radiologic-pathologic correlation. Radiology 146:747, 1983

56. Rice J, Sauerbrei EE, Semogas P, et al: Sonographic appearance of adenomyomatosis of the gallbladder. JCU 9:336, 1981

57. Yeh HC: Ultrasonography and computed tomography of carcinoma of the gallbladder. Radiology 133:167, 1979

58. Yun HY, Fink AH: Sonographic findings in primary carcinoma of the gallbladder. Radiology 134:693, 1980

59. Ruiz R, Teyssou H, Fernandez N, et al: Ultrasonic diagnosis of primary carcinoma of the gallbladder: a review of 16 cases. JCU 8:489, 1980

60. Bluth EI, Katz MM, Merritt CRB, et al: Echographic findings in xanthogranulomatous cholecystitis. JCU 7:213, 1979

61. Bundy AI, Richie WGM: Ultrasonic diagnosis of metastatic melanoma presenting as acute cholecystitis. JCU 10:285, 1982

62. Phillips G. Pochaczevsky R, Goodman J, et al: Ultrasound patterns of metastatic tumors in the gallbladder. JCU 10:379, 1982

63. Kane RA: Ultrasonographic anatomy of the liver and biliary tree. Semin Ultrasound 1:87, 1980

64. Behan M, Kazam E: Sonography of the common bile duct: value of the right anterior oblique view. AJR 130:701, 1978

65. Laing FC, Jeffrey RB, Wing VW: Improved visualization of choledocholithiasis by sonography. AJR 143:949, 1984

66. Cooperberg PL: High-resolution real-time ultrasound in the evaluation of the normal and obstructed biliary tract. Radiology 129:477, 1978

67. Parulekar SG: Ultrasound evaluation of common bile duct size. Radiology 133:703, 1979

68. Wu C-C, Ho Y-H, Chen C-Y: Effect of aging on common bile duct diameter: a real-time ultrasonographic study. JCU 12:473, 1984

69. Graham MF, Cooperberg PL, Cohen MM, et al: The size of the normal common hepatic duct following cholecystectomy: an ultrasonographic study. Radiology 135:137, 1980

70. Mueller PR, Ferrucci JT Jr, Simeone JF, et al: Postcholecystectomy bile duct dilatation: myth or reality? AJR 136:355, 1981

71. Simeone JF, Mueller PR, Ferrucci JT Jr, et al: Sonography of the bile ducts after a fatty meal: an aid in detection of obstruction. Radiology 143:211, 1982

72. Hopman WPM, Rosenbusch G, Jansen JBMJ, et al: Gallbladder contraction: effects of fatty meals and cholecystokinin. Radiology 157:37, 1985

73. Weill F, Eisencher A, Zeltner F: Ultrasonic study of the normal and dilated biliary tree. Radiology 127:221, 1978

74. Conrad MR, Landay MJ, Janes JO: Sonographic "parallel channel" sign of biliary tree enlargement in mild to moderate obstructive jaundice. AJR 130:279, 1978

75. Laing FC, London LA, Filly BA, Filly RA: Ultrasonographic identification of dilated intrahepatic bile ducts and their differentiation from portal venous structures. JCU 6:90, 1978

76. Muhletaler CA, Gerlock AJ Jr, Fleischer AC, et al: Diagnosis of obstructive jaundice with nondilated bile ducts. AJR 134:1149, 1980

77. Cronan JJ, Mueller PR, Simeone JF, et al: Prospective diagnosis of choledocholithiasis. Radiology 146:467, 1983

78. Laing FC, Jeffrey RB Jr: Choledocholithiasis and cystic duct obstruction: difficult ultrasonographic diagnosis. Radiology 1446:475, 1983

79. Zeman R, Taylor KJW, Burrell MI, et al: Ultrasound demonstration of anicteric dilatation of the biliary tree. Radiology 134:689, 1980

80. Weinstein BJ, Weinstein DP: Biliary tract dilatation in the nonjaundiced patient. AJR 134:899, 1980

81. Glazer GM, Filly RA, Laing FC: Rapid change in caliber of the nonobstructed common duct. Radiology 140:161, 1981

82. Menu Y, Lorphelin JM, Scherrer A, et al: Sonographic and computed tomographic evaluation of intrahepatic calculi. AJR 145:579, 1985

83. Marchal G, Gelin J, Van Steenbergen WV, et al: Sonographic diagnosis of intraluminal bile duct neoplasm; a report of 3 cases. Gastrointest Radiol 9:329, 1984

84. Stanley J, et al: Evaluation of biliary cystadenoma and cystadenocarcinoma. GI Radiol 8:245, 1983

85. Subramanyam BR, Raghavendra BN, Balthazar EJ, et al: Ultrasonic features of cholangiocarcinoma. J Ultrasound Med 3:405, 1984

86. Machan L, Muller NL, Cooperberg PL: Sonographic diagnosis of Klatskin tumors. AJR 147:509, 1986

87. Kangarloo H, Sarti DA, Sample WF, et al: Ultrasonographic spectrum of choledochal cysts in children. Pediatric Radiol 9:15, 1980

88. Mittelstaedt CA, Volberg FM, Fischer GJ, et al: Caroli's disease: sonographic findings. AJR 134:585, 1980

89. Ralls PW, Colletti PM, Quinn MF, et al: Sonography in recurrent oriental pyogenic cholangitis. AJR 136:1010, 1981

90. Federle MP, Cello JP, Laing FC, Jeffrey RB Jr: Recurrent pyogenic cholangitis in Asian immigrants. Radiology 143:151, 1982

91. Cerri GC, Leite GJ, Simoes JB, et al: Ultrasonographic evaluation of ascaris in the biliary tract. Radiology 146:753, 1983

92. Schulman A, Loxton AJ, Heydenrych JJ, Abdurahman KE: Sonographic diagnosis of biliary ascariasis. AJR 139:485, 1982

93. Doyle TCA, Roberts-Thomson IC: Radiological features of sclerosing cholangitis. Australas Radiol 27:163, 1983

94. Carroll BA, Oppenheimer DA: Sclerosing cholangitis: sonographic demonstration of bile duct wall thickening. AJR 139:1016, 1982

4 The Spleen

ALFRED B. KURTZ

NORMAL ANATOMY

General Characteristics

The spleen is an intraperitoneal organ situated in the left upper quadrant (Fig. 4.1). It is the largest lymphoid structure in the body and is an important part of both the immunologic and reticuloendothelial systems.[1] The interior of the spleen is filled with red and white pulp. The white pulp is composed of tiny aggregates of lymphoid tissue surrounded by the red pulp of long irregular channels of red blood cells.

The spleen has a diaphragmatic and visceral surface[2] (Fig. 4.2). The diaphragmatic surface is convex and smooth. It is apposed to the caudal surface of the left hemidiaphragm which separates it from the caudal border of the left lung, left pleura, and left 9th through 11th ribs. The diaphragmatic surface is directed to the left, cranially and posteriorly, with its cranial margin extending medially toward the epigastrium. The visceral surface is concave and divided by a middle ridge into three flattened regions, the gastric, renal, and colic surfaces. The gastric surface, the largest of the three, is angled superiorly, medially and posteriorly and is in contact with the posterior wall of the stomach. The renal surface is directed posteriorly and medially and is adjacent to the cranial anterior surface of the left kidney and occasionally the left adrenal gland. The colic surface, the smallest of the three, is angled anteriorly and inferiorly and is in contact with the colon at the splenic flexure and the phrenicocolic ligament. Additionally, both the gastric and colic surfaces are closely related to the pancreatic tail.

The spleen is contained within a fibrous capsule. The visceral peritoneum adheres closely to this capsule except on its visceral gastric surface where the splenic hilum is located (Fig. 4.2). In this region, the capsule is reflected over splenic ligaments that attach to the left hemidiaphragm, left kidney, and stomach. These form the left border of the lesser sac (omental bursa) and convey the splenic artery and vein (Fig. 4.1). The splenic artery courses along the superior pancreatic border, divides into six or more branches before entering the hilum, and further subdivides into arterioles within the splenic

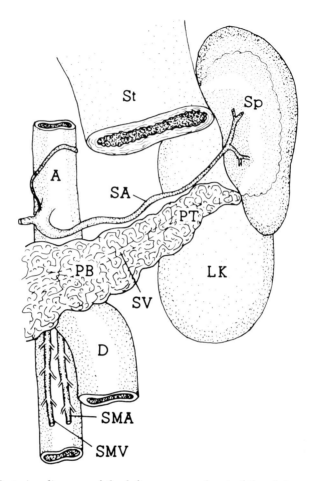

FIG. 4.1. Anterior diagram of the left upper quadrant of the abdomen. The spleen, *Sp*, is closely related to the left kidney, *LK*, pancreatic tail, *PT*, and stomach, *St*. The distal branches of the splenic artery, *SA*, and proximal branches of the splenic vein, *SV*, enter the splenic hilum. Most of the splenic vein courses posterior to the pancreatic tail and body, *PB*. *A* = aorta; *D* = duodenum; *SMA* = superior mesenteric artery; *SMU* = superior mesenteric vein.

red pulp. The smaller venules, not accompanying the arterioles, unite to form six or more branches that emerge from the hilum, combining to form the splenic vein.

Normal Variations

The spleen varies in position, size, shape, and number.

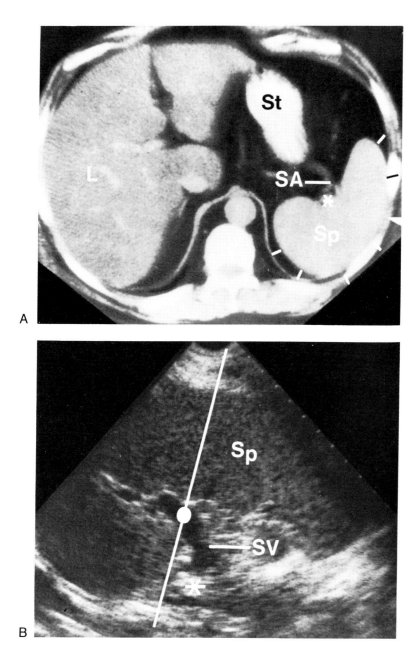

FIG. 4.2. (A) Contrast enhanced computed tomogram of the upper abdomen showing the normal spleen, *Sp,* and its standard position in the left upper quadrant.
Arrowhead denotes intercostal space through which (B), the oblique ultrasound image
of the normal spleen, was obtained. Pulsed range-gated Doppler is positioned within
the normal splenic vein, *SV.* * = splenic hilum on the concave visceral surface; dashes
denote convex diaphragmatic splenic surface; *SA* = splenic artery; *L* = liver.

Position

Due to its ligamentous attachments, the splenic position is fairly constant. If these attachments are lax, however, a finding that occurs in approximately 0.2 percent of cases, the spleen may lie in unusual positions and is then termed the "wandering spleen." The most common locations of the "wandering spleen" are the mid abdomen or left lower quadrant.[3] Unusual splenic positions may also occur following surgical removal of an adjacent organ, particularly the left kidney, or displacement by an adjacent mass. Clinically and radiographically, aberrant locations may cause considerable confusion. When ultrasound fails to image the spleen in its normal position, and a mass is detected elsewhere, the echogenicity and shape should be analyzed to determine if it is similar to that normally imaged for a spleen. If there is uncertainty as to whether the mass is the spleen, however, functional imaging tests such as Technitium 99m sulfur colloid radionuclide or contrast enhanced CT scans may be needed to confirm the diagnosis. Occasionally, while the spleen may still occupy the left upper quadrant, ligamentous laxity may permit it to rotate. The spleen can then assume an upside-down position with the concave visceral surface including the hilum located cephalad, adjacent to the hemidiaphragm, and the convex diaphragmatic surface situated medially and adjacent to the left kidney.

Size

The size, and therefore the weight, of the spleen is extremely variable. The spleen increases in weight from an average of 17 grams during the first year of extrauterine life to 170 grams by age 20.[2] The spleen then slowly involutes to an average of 122 grams by age 76 to 80 years of age. No linear measurements are available in children. In adults, the size and shape approximates that of a clenched fist with the average spleen measuring 12 cm in length, 7 cm in anteroposterior diameter, and 4 cm in width, and weighing 100 to 150 grams.[2]

Shape

In addition to the concave visceral and convex diaphragmatic surfaces, the spleen is a soft organ and frequently conforms to adjacent structures. There are also intrasplenic bulges termed "lobulations" that further alter the splenic contour. These lobulations may extend superiorly and medially to lie anterior to the left upper pole of the kidney, simulating an adjacent left adrenal or renal mass, or may extend partially behind the left kidney displacing it anteriorly.[4,5] Rarely, clefts between these lobulations can be deep and appear as focal abnormalities.

Number

In 10 to 30 percent of the population, accessory spleens, termed *splenules,* are present.[4] These vary in size from microscopic foci to 3 cm. When large, they may be detected sonographically as round or ovoid masses with hyperechoic rims and an internal echogenicity identical to that of the primary spleen.[6] Using ultrasound, a splenule can only be definitely diagnosed if its tortuous artery or straight vein can be identified and shown to originate from the main splenic artery and vein respectively.[6]

NORMAL ULTRASOUND EVALUATION

Technique

The spleen can be imaged with the patient in one of four positions: prone, supine, right-side-down posterior oblique, or true right lateral (right lateral decubitus). The prone position, while previously popular, is now the least used. This type of scanning frequently causes poor quality images and less splenic visualization due to interposed aerated lung in the left posterior costo-phrenic angle and sound attenuation from the back muscles.[7] The supine view is more commonly used but on occasion it too fails to permit full splenic visualization because of gas in the overlying stomach anteriorly or air in the left lung base laterally.[7,8] The right side down positions, posterior oblique and decubitus, are therefore preferable, since the spleen can be imaged closer to the transducer and through less muscle, thus permitting better intrasplenic detail and less chance of interposed gas or air.[7–11]

The type of ultrasound machine is also important. Static scanners permit visualization of overall splenic size and its internal architecture. Not uncommonly, however, these scanners fail to fully evaluate splenic echogenicity due to rib shadowing, a problem that can be at least partially overcome by scanning intercostally. Real-time imaging is comparable in resolution to static scanners and easier to maneuver between the ribs, particularly with small headed sector probes. As a result, although the entire spleen may not be routinely evaluated on a single image, real-time scanning can accurately analyze splenic echogenicity. In addition, since the spleen and left hemidiaphragm move with respiration, real-time ultrasound can determine if diaphragmatic movement is present and normal and can clearly visualize small splenic structures without the problem of image blurring caused by respiratory motion.

Since the spleen has variable positions and shapes, scanning maneuvers must be varied from patient to patient. One commonly used technique involves imaging the left upper quadrant in straight long and transaxial planes, with the long axis images obtained either anteroposteriorly or coronally[8] (Figs. 4.3, 4.4). While these views allow overall visualization of the contour of the spleen, rib shadowing frequently obscures its internal architecture. To overcome rib shadowing, two techniques may be employed: the transducer can be moved obliquely from the left shoulder toward the umbilicus along the intercostal spaces between the left 8th and 9th, 9th and 10th, or 10th and 11th ribs[10] (Fig. 4.4B) or if a static scanner is used, the transducer can be moved in a compound sector motion at each intercostal space (Fig. 4.4C). When the intercostal spaces are too narrow, these spaces can be widened by having the patient lie in one of the two right-side-down positions, stretching the left arm over the head and placing towels under the right

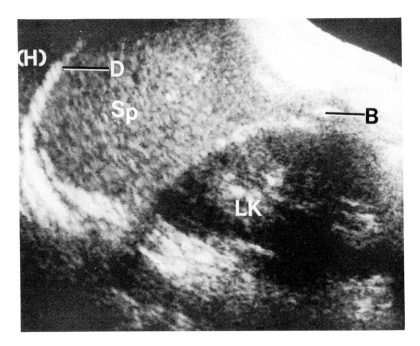

FIG. 4.3. Subcostal long axis ultrasound image of the normal spleen, *Sp,* and left kidney, *LK.* The spleen is more completely imaged than by the intercostal approach. Note the convex diaghragmatic surface, and the concave visceral surface adjacent to the left kidney. Also note that the splenic echogenicity is greater than that of the renal cortex. *D* = diaphragm; *B* = bowel with gas, causing shadowing; *(H)* = toward patient's head.

lower rib cage. Lastly, scanning can be performed subcostally, angling the transducer superiorly from the umbilicus toward the left shoulder (Fig. 4.3). Since this maneuver avoids the ribs, more complete visualization of the spleen, especially the superior margin, can commonly be obtained.

When imaging the spleen, the only anatomic landmark that can be consistently used as a reference point is the splenic hilum. The best method to image the hilum is with the patient either in a supine or one of the right-side-down positions. The images are performed intercostally or subcostally with the scan plane angled moderately cephalad. The patient is instructed to take progressively deeper breaths until the hilum is visualized (Fig. 4.2B). Then with respiration suspended, the transducer is swept superiorly and inferiorly to exam the entire spleen. This technique allows for imaging of the splenic hilum, parenchyma, contours, particularly the convex diaphragmatic surface, and the capsule.

The splenic hilum is evaluated for the normal artery and vein, abnormal vessels in the perihilar region (varices or collateral circulation), and perihilar adenopathy (Figs. 4.2B, 4.5A and 4.5B). The splenic vein can be visualized

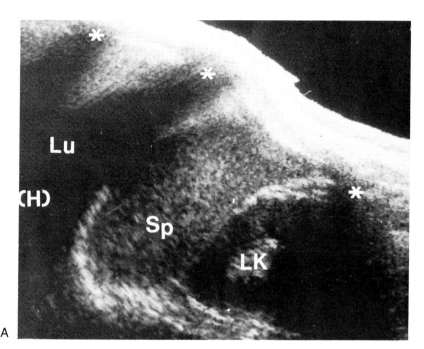

A

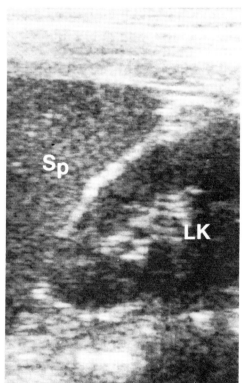

FIG. 4.4. Long axis ultrasound images of the normal spleen, *Sp,* and left kidney, *LK.* Note the echogenicity of the spleen is greater than that of the renal cortex. (A) Static scan obtained anteroposteriorly showing rib shadowing artifact (*) that obscures parts of the two organs. *Lu* = lung. (B) Real-time linear array scan obtained intercostally. Although the image shows less of the two organs, neither is obscured by the rib shadowing artifact. This same technique can be used with static scanning. (*Figure continues.*)

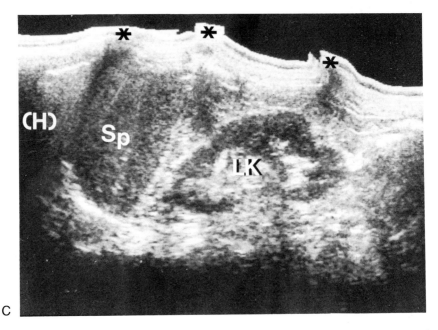

C

FIG. 4.4 (*Continued*). (C) Static scan obtained anteroposteriorly with a compounding sector motion at each intercostal space, *. Note that more of the two organs are imaged than in Figure 4.4A. (*H*) = toward patient's head.

from two approaches. The largest portion of the vein can be imaged from the anterior abdominal wall, where the vein is immediately posterior to the pancreatic body and tail. The proximal splenic vein, however, is best imaged at the splenic hilum with scans performed intercostally from the left flank through the splenic tissue (Fig. 4.2B). Although the normal range for splenic vein measurements has not been fully studied, it has been reported that a diameter up to 1.0 cm is normal in 87 percent of cases, while a diameter greater than 1.3 cm is present in 50 percent of cases of portal hypertension.[12] It has also been observed that the splenic vein varies in caliber with deep respiration in all normal subjects but only in 10 percent of cases of portal hypertension.[12] Therefore, a splenic vein that is larger than 1.3 cm in diameter and does not vary with respiration is suggestive of portal hypertension. If a duplex ultrasound system with pulsed range-gated Doppler is available, this too can be used to analyze the splenic vein by evaluating the direction of its blood flow. Normally, blood in the portal venous system flows from the spleen toward the liver. In cases of severe portal hypertension, this flow can become bidirectional or reversed. When scanning the vein intercostally or subcostally through the splenic parenchyma, the velocity tracing is normal if it is negative (away from the transducer). If the tracing is bidirectional or positive (toward the transducer), portal hypertension is present. The pulse range-gated Doppler can also be used to evaluate tubular or serpiginous

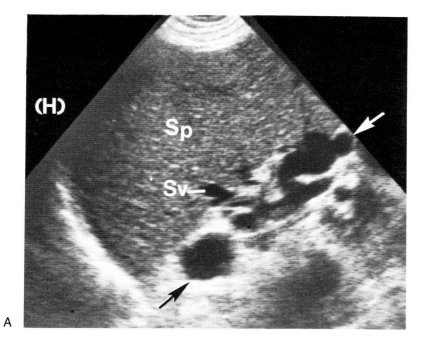

A

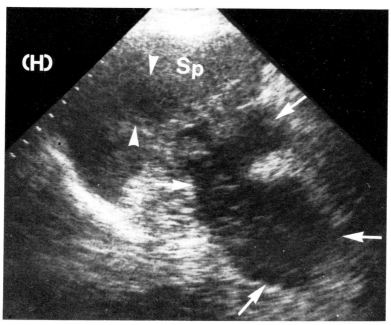

B

FIG. 4.5. Intercostal long axis real-time ultrasound sector images of the spleen, *Sp*, splenic hilum and perihilar region. (A) Perihilar varices, secondary to portal hypertension: Large tubular anechoic structures (denoted by arrows) in the perihilar region, adjacent to the splenic vein, *SV*. (B) Perihilar adenopathy, secondary to Hodkin's lymphoma. Large hypoechoic solid masses (denoted by arrows). Note a similar hypoechoic solid mass (denoted by arrowheads) within the spleen. (*H*) = toward patient's head.

structures in the splenic hilum. If a velocity tracing can be detected, these structures are vascular and represent either collateral channels or varices.

In summary, technique is very important when evaluating the spleen. It is recommended that real-time scanning be performed, either intercostally or subcostally, and that the patient be positioned right-side-down or supine. The splenic hilum is located by progressively deeper breaths and scanning then performed superiorly and inferiorly to image the entire spleen. When available, pulsed range-gated Doppler should be performed if splenic vein abnormality is suspected or if unusual tubular structures are identified in the perihilar region.

Splenic Echogenicity

The splenic parenchyma gives rise to uniformly moderate amplitude echoes. These are the result of small interfaces (back scatter or diffuse reflectors) that are angle independent so that the angle of the transducer does not influence their echogenicity. The splenic capsule, however, is a large bright interface (specular reflector) that is angle dependent.[8] This reflector can only be demonstrated when the angle of the ultrasound beam is perpendicular or nearly perpendicular to the capsule.

The spleen has been described as ranging in echogenicity from primarily hypoechoic[8] to hyperechoic.[11] With the patient supine, the normal spleen appears isoechoic[13] or slightly hypoechoic. In the prone position or when scanned transaxially over the ribs, the beam is more attenuated and the spleen appears to be more hypoechoic than the liver. When scanned in the right lateral decubitus or posterior oblique positions, however, observers have described the spleen as both hypoechoic[10] and hyperechoic.[11]

The reasons for these inconsistencies are puzzling and cannot be ascertained from these articles. It is possible that the differences are multifactorial, related to the echo patterns of the liver and spleen, how these organs are analyzed, or the amplification settings used. Both the liver and spleen have small backscatter reflectors (Fig. 4.6). Within the spleen the backscatter reflectors are more densely packed while those within the liver are disrupted by blood vessels with their strongly reflective larger specular walls (Fig. 4.6). At low amplifications settings, the specular reflectors of the liver stand out. At high amplication settings, however, the backscatter reflectors are more prominent. If the backscatter reflectors of the liver and spleen are compared, with the specular reflectors of the liver ignored, the echogenicities are approximately equal at normal amplification, with the spleen more hyperechoic at higher settings (Fig. 4.6). If, instead, the specular reflectors of the liver are compared with the backscatter reflectors of the spleen, the liver is more hyperechoic especially at lower amplifications settings.

While these descriptions of comparative echogenicity are constant when the liver and the spleen are scanned separately and the images compared,

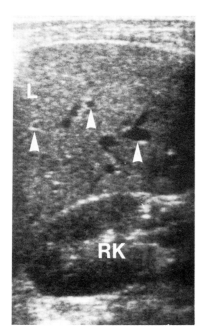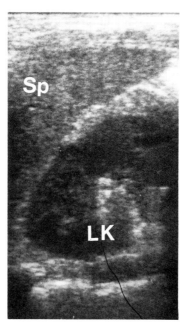

FIG. 4.6.   Comparative echogenicities of normal liver, *L*, and normal spleen, *Sp*, in the same patient. Both were scanned in the supine position, subcostally with moderate amplification settings used. Note the parenchyma of both organs (back-scatter reflectors) are equal in brightness. Arrowheads denote normal blood vessels, some with highly reflective walls, within the liver. *LK* = left kidney; *RK* = right kidney.

recently there has been a direct comparison of the two organs. When the left lobe of the liver extended into the left upper quadrant to abut on the superior and lateral splenic surface, the liver and spleen can be simultaneously scanned. It was shown that at the same depth from the transducer the liver echogenicity was less than that of the adjacent spleen.[14,15] In fact, the liver echogenicity was so decreased that the left lobe was initially misdiagnosed as a perisplenic fluid collection.

The spleen can also be evaluated relative to the left kidney.[16] Intercostal and subcostal long axis images in either the supine or right-side down positions will frequently image both organs. The splenic echogenicity is slightly greater than that of the renal parenchyma (Figs. 4.3 and 4.4). The renal parenchymal echoes can be made to falsely approximate the spleen if the amplification settings are kept too high.

In summary, at moderate to high amplification settings, when the liver is used as the standard, the spleen has approximately the same echogenicity as the liver and is greater in echogenicity than the left kidney. To obtain this comparative echogenicity, it is suggested that the liver and the spleen be scanned in one of two projections, keeping all other parameters constant. (1) The liver is imaged in the left-side-down posterior oblique or lateral decubitus position compared with the spleen imaged in the right-side-down posterior oblique or lateral decubitus position, both scanned either intercostally or subcostally or (2) both the liver and spleen are imaged with the patient supine, using the coronal long axis views scanned intercostally, the liver imaged through the right ribs and the spleen imaged through the left ribs (Fig. 4.6). If there is a prominent left lobe of the liver, however, the direct comparison of the left lobe to the adjacent spleen has shown the spleen to be more hyperechoic.

Splenic Size

The spleen is variable in shape and position so that its longest axis cannot always be identified. When it can be determined, however, the spleen should not be greater than 14 cm in cranial-caudal extent.[4] One observer, however, has stated that a normal spleen should not be more than 10 cm in long axis,[10] with its length obtained by scanning obliquely along the intercostal space between the 10th and 11th ribs[10]. This latter scan plane does not always give the longest cranial-caudal length, and a true subcostal coronal or longitudinal view is frequently better.

Because of the variabilities in splenic shapes, some observers have felt that a linear length is not an accurate representation of splenic size and have therefore attempted instead to refer to splenic areas and volumes. A cross-sectional splenic area has been calculated from images performed intercostally between the 8th and 9th ribs, following the longest axis of the spleen.[10,17,18] The splenic areas were evaluated both clinically and with follow up in vitro scans on 10 splenectomy specimens and were found to have a high correlation. Splenic volumes have been obtained, particularly in markedly enlarged spleens.[19] Transaxial images at right angles to the long axis of the spleen were performed at 2 cm intervals, with the areas of all the sections added together to equal a volume. Nine of these spleens were reexamined after splenectomy with a high correlation also obtained. Splenic volumes have additionally been calculated by multiplying the maximum splenic length, width, height, dividing by an arbitrary number 27, the lengths obtained from transaxial and long axis coronal scans.[20] While there was no comparison in this study to spleens following splenectomy, a high degree of accuracy was reported in separating normal from enlarged spleens.

The value of any of these methods lies in its ability to determine if the spleen is normal or mildly enlarged, since greatly enlarged spleens are clinically and sonographically obvious. Although it is not possible to determine which of these above methods is best, it is clear that none totally visualizes all of the curved splenic borders and therefore none truly represent splenic volumes. Any of these methods, however, would be of value in serial examinations to detect changes in splenic size with time.[10] Nuclear medicine studies have also been used to calculate splenic volumes[21,22] but are probably not more accurate than ultrasound volumes in detecting subtle splenic enlargement. Computed tomography would seem to offer the best method of calculating true volumes. In the supine position using rapid scanning to avoid respiratory movements, true transaxial sections can be obained without obscuring the splenic borders by air or bone. Areas of each section can be added together to equal a volume, with a high degree of accuracy found in true splenic volumes in both dogs and humans.[23]

The difficulties outlined above in obtaining an accurate splenic area or volume technique has led to "rough estimate" proposals. These estimates seem useful in quick analysis of splenic size. They may be as accurate as other methods in evaluating normal versus subtly enlarged spleens aside from the true volume technique of computed tomography. The estimates are as follows: (1) on transaxial scans the normal spleen should not project anterior to the anterior border of the aorta and on longitudinal images should not extend below the costal margins in 90 percent of cases,[8] and (2) an "eyeball" technique that states that if the spleen looks enlarged on ultrasound scans then it probably is.[9]

Splenic Contour

Splenic contour changes are usually easier to appreciate on CT scans or radioisotope images but can often be evaluated by ultrasound (Fig. 4.2). When there is generalized splenic enlargement, both the convex and concave surfaces usually become rounded with the spleen assuming a more globular shape.[4] Focal contour distortions from either normal lobulations or true pathology may also be analyzed. If the contour distortion is secondary to a pathologic abnormality, the echogenicity of the spleen should be altered, at least in the area of abnormality. On the other hand, contour changes with normal echogenicity most likely represent regions of normal lobulation. If after the ultrasound examination there is still uncertainty, a functional imaging study should be performed.

ABNORMAL ULTRASONOGRAPHIC FINDINGS
Criteria

Abnormalities of the spleen can be divided into (1) processes causing focal change, usually neoplasms, and (2) processes causing diffuse change, both benign and malignant and usually associated with splenomegaly. Ultrasound can detect these abnormalities using modifications of the criteria that were stated above for the evaluation of the normal spleen, i.e., echogenicity, size, and contour. Of these, echogenicity and size are the most important. Contour changes are less reliable since they are more difficult to appreciate and can occur in both normal and abnormal states.

The modified ultrasound criteria are as follows:

1. Echogenicity
   If focally abnormal—cystic versus solid, clarity of margins, through transmission.
   If diffusely abnormal—hypoechoic, isoechoic, or hyperechoic.
2. Size
   Normal or enlarged. If enlarged, localized or diffusely abnormal.
3. Contour changes
4. Additional features
   Can be suggestive of specific abnormalities, such as adenopathy.

Focal Splenic Enlargement

Splenic Cysts

The three types of splenic cysts are epidermoid, posttraumatic, and parasitic. Epidermoid cysts are usually solitary and have obtained a size of 15 cm or greater in diameter before detection. They are probably congenital in origin and are usually spherical, sharply circumscribed, and may calcify or contain peripheral trabeculations[24,25] (Fig. 4.7A). Posttraumatic cysts, usually encountered in older persons, are believed to be the final stage of a splenic hematoma.[4,25] These cysts are rarely totally anechoic and usually contain internal debris or fluid-debris levels (Fig 4.7B). Parasitic cysts, particularly hydatid, are rare in this country but, when detected, are indistinguishable from the other two types.

Other unusual benign lesions may occasionally mimic splenic cysts in size, shape, and ultrasound characteristics. These are dermoids, lymphangiomas, angiomas and cavernous hemangiomas.[26–28] Many have multiple septations. It is possible, although not previously described, that an angiomatous lesion could be diagnosed by detecting blood flow with Doppler evaluation. Migration of pancreatic fluid, a pseudocyst, may on occasion extend into the spleen and may even mimic a simple cyst[29] (Fig. 4.7C).

Splenic Abscesses

Splenic abscesses, while uncommon, are associated with high mortality rates of up to 60 percent.[30] They are relatively silent lesions and may go undetected until time of operation or autopsy. Patients commonly present with fever, nonspecific abdominal pain and tenderness, and occasionally with splenomegaly.[31] When a mass is imaged, it is frequently hypoechoic with ill-defined walls and moderately increased through transmission (Fig. 4.8). While gas may infrequently be detected within the abscess as a hyperechoic area, usually without shadowing, it is better appreciated with computed tomography.[32] If doubt exists as to whether a focal splenic mass is an abscess, nuclear medicine evaluation with Galium-67 citrate or, more specifically, Indium-111 labeled leukocytes is of value.

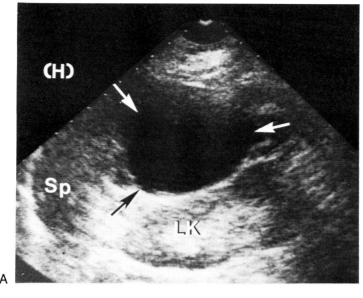

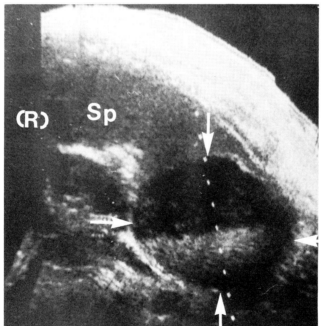

FIG. 4.7. Splenic cystic masses. Ultrasound long axis images in three different patients. (A) Epidermoid cyst (arrows). The cyst is anechoic with smooth walls and good through transmission. (B) Post traumatic cyst (arrows). Note internal echoes and fluid-debris level. (*Figure continues.*)

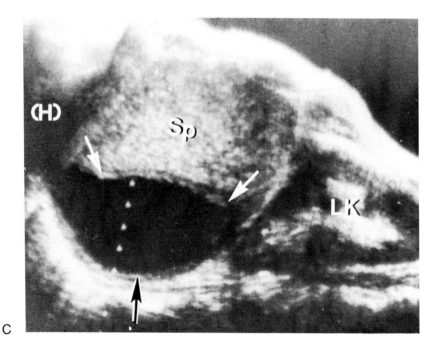

FIG. 4.7 (*Continued*). (C) Intrasplenic pseudocyst (arrows). This patient had a history of chronic relapsing pancreatitis. *Sp* = spleen; *LK* = left kidney; (*H*) = toward patient's head.

Splenic Malignancy

Primary splenic malignancies are extremely rare while metastatic disease and lymphoma are more common. Metastatic disease involves the spleen in up to 50 percent of patients with malignant melanoma and has also been detected in metastases from the lung, breast, and ovary.[33] The spleen is usually enlarged but on occasion may be normal in size. Metastases vary in echogenicity from hypo- to hyperechoic without a characteristic ultrasound pattern that can be ascribed to any type.[33]

The ability of ultrasound to detect lymphoma even when splenomegaly is present approaches only 50 percent, with higher accuracies reported in non-Hodgkin lymphoma.[34] When lymphomatous infiltration is imaged, it presents as either focal poorly marginated hypoechoic masses with decreased through transmission ranging in size from 3 mm to 3 cm (Fig. 4.9) or as a diffusely hypoechoic enlarged spleen. The diffusely abnormal spleen is felt to be the result of coalescence of these focal lesions.[11] Adenopathy in the splenic hilum may also be detected. Occasionally, lymphoma may present with the clinically and ultrasound findings suggestive of a splenic abscess.[34] To differentiate these two processes, a nuclear medicine study with Indium-111 labelled leukocyte is of value since it is positive only in inflammatory processes.

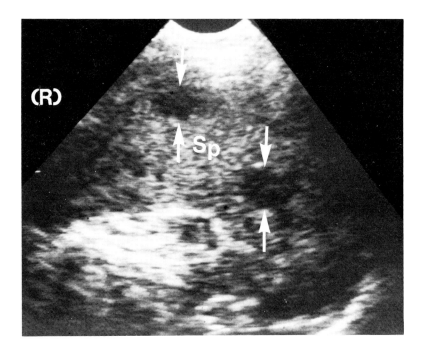

FIG. 4.8. Splenic abscesses in an immune-suppressed patient. Two of these masses (arrows) have low level internal echoes, smooth walls, and only moderate through transmission within the spleen, *Sp*. (*H*) = toward patient's head.

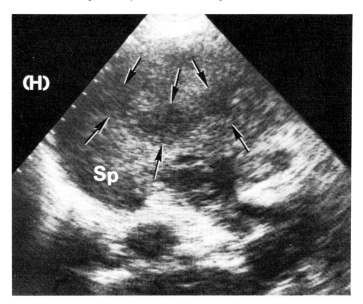

FIG. 4.9. Splenic lymphoma, Hodgkin type. Long axis ultrasound image showing hypoechoic solid masses (denoted by arrows) within the spleen, *Sp*. The masses have ill-defined margins and only moderate through transmission. Note the similarity of the ultrasound appearance of these to the abscesses of Fig. 4.8. (*H*) = toward patient's head.

Granulomatosis

Granulomatous disease, including sarcoidosis, tuberculosis, and histoplasmosis, can present as either focal or diffuse splenic abnormalities. When it presents as a focal abnormality, scattered hyperechoic punctate lesions are detected. These represent calcifications which have distal shadowing only when larger than 3 to 4 mm in size (Fig. 4.10). When there are questions as to whether calcifications are present, they can be more definitively detected by an abdominal radiograph or computed tomography. Less commonly, multiple focal hypoechoic areas with ill-defined walls and decreased through transmission may be encountered (Fig. 4.8). These lesions are granulomatous abscesses and can mimic other multiple hypoechoic abnormalities, including metastases and lymphoma.[35]

Trauma

Following acute trauma to the left upper quadrant, it may be technically difficult to scan the spleen due to pain, left rib fractures, open wounds, or bandages. Ultrasound can be used to evaluate splenic trauma once it has been shown that there is no significant vascular compromise to the spleen. Splenic lacerations and contusions (Fig. 4.11A), intrasplenic and subcapsular hematomas, and extrasplenic fluid collections (Fig. 4.11B) have all been suc-

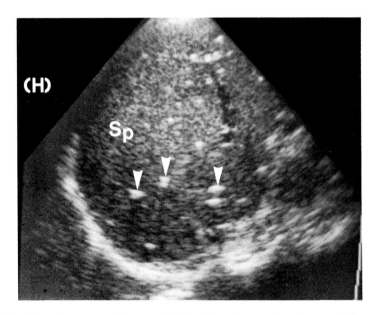

FIG. 4.10. Granulomatous disease. Calcifications. Long axis ultrasound image with multiple hyperechoic punctate lesions (denoted by arrowheads). No shadowing was seen, presumable due to their small size (all were less than 5mm). *Sp* = spleen; *(H)* = toward patient's head.

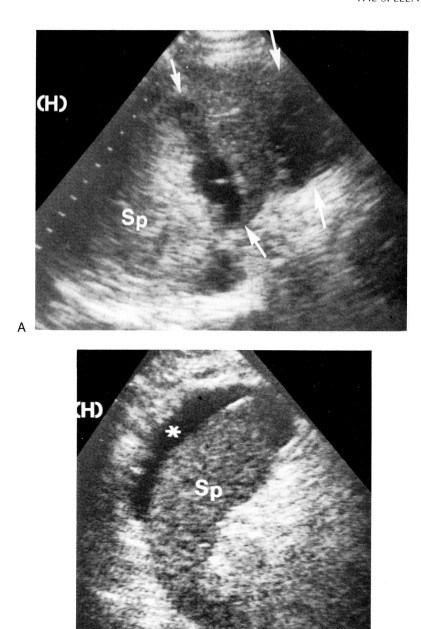

FIG. 4.11.   Splenic trauma in two different patients. (A) Splenic contusion. Long axis ultrasound image of spleen, *Sp*, 6 weeks after abdominal trauma showing two hypoechoic ill-defined linear defects (arrows). (B) Perisplenic fluid. Long axis ultrasound image of spleen (*Sp*) showing fluid (·) superior to its convex diaphragmatic surface 1 week after left upper quadrant abdominal trauma. (*H*) = toward patient's head.

cessfully imaged.[36] Following acute trauma, intraperitoneal and/or left pleural fluid frequently resorb within two to four weeks. Intrasplenic hematomas and contusions, however, while changing from hypo- to hyperechoic and then back to hypoechoic as the hematoma ages, may not fully resorb for as long as one year after injury.[36] Chronically, the spleen may be left with a residual small hyperechoic foci, presumably representing scar issue, or may revert back to normal.

Diffuse Splenic Enlargement

When splenomegaly occurs, the spleen extends below the left costal margin, and the technical difficulties encountered with scanning a normal-sized spleen intercostally and subcostally are therefore not a problem. Instead, long axis and transaxial images can be obtained below the costal margin through the soft tissues of the flank or anterior abdominal wall. The patient can be scanned in either the supine or right-side-down positions, with comparable images of the liver obtained in supine or left-side-down positions respectively.

While imaging an enlarged spleen is therefore easy, there have been discrepancies in the types of splenic echogenicities of different pathologic processes. The spleen has been found to be either hypo- or isoechoic, with one group suggesting that splenic echogenicity can also be hyperechoic.[37] Part of these discrepancies may be related to how the studies were performed, since some articles analyzed the splenic echogenicity without comparison to an adjacent organ[37,38] while others evaluated the echogenicity in comparison to the liver.[13] In these comparisons, untreated cases of lymphoma and leukemia were initially observed to decrease the splenic echogenicity, with an increase following treatment[13] (Fig. 4.12A and B). More recently, some untreated cases have been found to be hyperechoic and indistinguishable from treated cases.[38] Congestion of the spleen, usually secondary to cirrhosis, has been described as being of medium level echogenicity[37] and isoechoic in relation to the liver.[13] Erythropoietic diseases, myeloproliferative diseases, and reticuloendothelial hyperactivity have been reported to be medium-level in echogenicity and isoechoic in relation to the liver[11,13,37] (Fig. 4.12C). Chronic inflammatory diseases and granulocytopoietic abnormalities (such as tuberculosis, sarcoidosis, and malaria), have been described as both iso- and hyperechoic.[11,37,38]

The reasons for these discrepancies cannot be fully analyzed. They may be due, in part, to the concomitant changes in liver echogenicity caused by many pathologic processes. Since there is no external reference standard, it may be difficult or impossible to compare the liver and spleen if changes occur in both. Nevertheless an attempt to explain the reasons for these different echogenicities has been made.[11] By analyzing the regions of the spleen affected, i.e., the red or white pulp, it was found that the spleen is hypoechoic when the white pulp (lymphoid tissue) is involved and iso- or hyperechoic when the red pulp (blood containing regions) is affected. Whatever the rea-

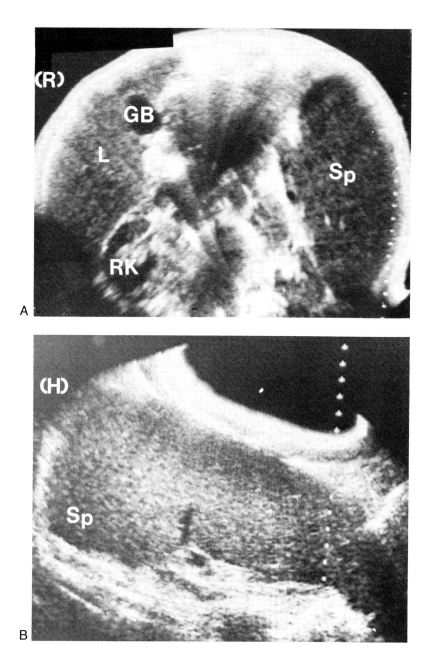

FIG. 4.12.   Splenomegaly with diffuse changes in echogenicity in 3 different patients.
(A) Acute lymphocytic leukemia. Transaxial ultrasound image showing an enlarged,
diffusely hypoechoic spleen, *Sp.* Compare echogenicity to normal liver, *L.* (B) Treated
lymphoma. Long axis ultrasound image showing uniform increased splenic, *Sp,* echogenicity. (*Figure continues.*)

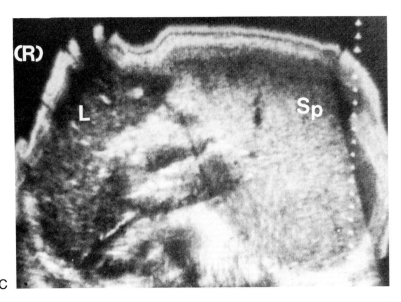

C

FIG. 4.12 (*Continued*). (C) Myeloid Metaplasia. Transaxial ultrasound image showing a massively enlarged uniformly hyperechoic spleen, *Sp*, when compared to the normal echogenicity of the liver, *L*. *GB* = gallbladder; *RK* = right kidney; (*H*) = Toward patient's head; (*R*) = toward patient's right side.

sons, though, the splenic echogenicity has limited value in predicting the type of pathologic process causing splenomegaly. If the spleen is hypoechoic it is almost certainly caused by diffuse lymphoma or leukemia. If the spleen is iso- or hyperechoic, however, it may be caused by any pathologic process.

In the past, ultrasound has been limited solely to the imaging of the splenic pathologic processes. Reluctance to perform biopsy and drainage procedures was based on the prominent splenic vascularity and difficulty of access secondary to the adjacent ribs, lung, and splenic flexure of the colon. Nevertheless, recently biopsies using 20 and 22 gauge needles and drainages using larger bore catheters have been performed without significant morbidity and mortality.[39] It is recommended, however, that a computed tomogram be obtained prior to the procedure to accurately assess adjacent bowel and lung and to obtain the best route for the biopsy or aspiration.

COMPARISON OF DIFFERENT IMAGING MODALITIES IN THE DETECTION OF SPLENIC ANOMALIES

The three primary noninvasive imaging modalities available to image the spleen are ultrasound, computed tomography (CT), and nuclear medicine. They are complimentary tests since all use different types of transmitted energy. In general, ultrasound and CT offer better anatomic analysis, while contrast-enhanced CT and Technetium-99m sulfur colloid nuclear medicine scans give functional information. To date, there have not been large studies analyzing these three modalities in the evaluation of splenic processes.

In acute trauma, contrast-enhanced CT is the procedure of choice, permitting evaluation of the splenic structure and function, and also the adjacent abdominal organs and intraperitoneal cavity.[4,40,41] Although ultrasound may give similar structural and anatomic information about the spleen, ultrasound cannot accurately evaluate its vascular integrity. Also, trauma frequently limits the ultrasound examination since neither the patient nor the transducer can be moved into all the appropriate positions. Although nuclear medicine can evaluate the anatomic and vascular integrity of the spleen, it is unable to image the surrounding structures. As a result, contrast-enhanced CT is considered the procedure of choice, with angiography available as a second test if splenic integrity is still in question (Fig. 4.13). Following the acute phase, particularly when conservative management of the spleen is warranted, ultrasound may be used to follow splenic and perisplenic trauma.

In the splenic evaluation for nontraumatic focal or diffuse disease, either ultrasound or Technetium-99m sulfur colloid nuclear medicine scans could be the first study (Fig. 4.13). There are shortcomings to both; nuclear medicine is chosen as the initial modality since it allows assessment of splenic function.[42] In the evaluation of splenic size, nuclear medicine images are usually sufficient, especially to differentiate a normal from a moderate to

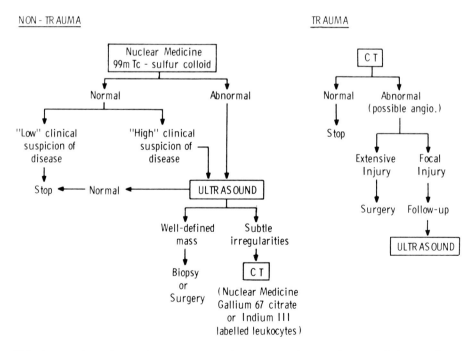

FIG. 4.13.   Flow charts of nontrauma and trauma work-ups of potential abnormalities of the spleen.

markedly enlarged spleen. In cases of minimal and mild enlargement or for the detection of changes of splenic size over time, nuclear medicine scan is frequently inaccurate due to variations in patient position, even when multiple projections are used. As a result, since ultrasound may be more tailored to the patient, it is recommended as a second study when subtle splenic enlargement is suspected and for follow up of serial size changes. In addition, when the spleen is enlarged on nuclear medicine images, ultrasound should be performed to evaluate the type of echogenicity associated with the splenomegaly.

Focal lesions are accurately detected by all three modalities, provided the abnormality is greater than 1 to 2 cm in size. Nuclear medicine, however, is nonspecific, showing predominantly photon poor areas. Ultrasound and CT are able to evaluate abnormal areas for cystic and solid components. While both can detect bright reflectors of calcium or gas, CT is frequently needed to differentiate the two. Nuclear medicine may miss subcapsular fluid collections that are easily appreciated by ultrasound and CT.

REFERENCES

1. Ham AW, Cormack DH: Lymphatic tissue. p. 355. In Histology. J.B. Lippincott Company, Philadelphia, 1979
2. Gray H: The spleen. p. 772. In Goss CM (ed): Gray's anatomy. Lea & Febiger, Philadelphia, 1966
3. Gordon DH, Burrell MI, Levin DC, et al: Wandering spleen—the radiological and clinical spectrum. Radiology 125:39, 1977
4. Koehler RE: Spleen. p. 243. In Lee JKT, Sagel SS, Stanley RJ (eds): Computed body tomography. Raven Press, New York 1983
5. Gooding GAW: The ultrasonic and computed tomographic appearance of splenic lobulations: a consideration in the ultrasonic differential of masses adjacent to the left kidney. Radiology 126:719, 1978
6. Subramanyam BR, Balthazar EJ, Horii SC: Sonography of the accessory spleen. AJR 143:47, 1984
7. Carlsen EN: Liver, gallbladder, and spleen. Radiol Clin North Am 8:543, 1975
8. Leopold GR, Asher WM: Spleen. p. 76. In Leopold GR, Asher WM (eds): Fundamentals of abdominal and pelvic ultrasonography. WB Saunders, Philadelphia 1975
9 Cooperberg P: Ultrasonography of the spleen. p. 244. In Sarti DA, Sample WF (eds): Diagnostic Ultrasound Text and Cases. G.K. Hall & Company, Boston, 1980
10. Taylor KJW: Reticuloendothelial system. p. 225. In Goldberg BB, (ed): Abdominal Gray Scale Ultrasonography. John Wiley & Sons, New York, 1977
11. Mittelstaedt CA: Ultrasound of the spleen. Semin Ultrasound 2:233, 1981
12. Bolondi L, Gandolfi L, Arienti V, et al: Ultrasonography in the diagnosis of portal hypertension: diminished response of portal vessels to respiration. Radiology 142:167, 1982
13. Mittelstaedt CA, Partain CL: Ultrasonic-pathologic classification of splenic abnormalities: gray-scale patterns. Radiology 134:697, 1980
14. Li DKB, Cooperberg PL, Graham MF, Callen P: Pseudoperisplenic "fluid collections": a clue to normal liver and spleen echogenic texture. J Ultrasound Med 5:397, 1986
15. Crivello MS, Peterson IM, Austin RM: Left lobe of the liver mimicking perisplenic collections. J Clin Ultrasound 14:697, 1986

16. Rosenfield AT, Taylor KJW, Jaffee CC: Clinical applications of ultrasound tissue characterization. p. 31. In James AE, Jr. (ed) The Radiologic Clinics of North America Symposium on Advances in Ultrasonography. W.B. Saunders Company, Philadelphia, 1980

17. Koga T: Correlation between sectional area of the spleen by ultrasonic tomography and actual volume of the removed spleen. J Clin Ultrasound 7:119, 1979

18. Koga T, Morikawa Y: Ultrasonographic determination of the splenic size and its clinical usefulness in various liver diseases. Radiology 115:157, 1975

19. Kardel T, Holm HH, Rasmussen SN, Mortensen T: Ultrasonic determination of liver and spleen volumes. Scand J Clin Lab Invest 27:123, 1971

20. Pietri H, Boscaini M: Determination of a splenic volumetric index by ultrasonic scanning. J Ultrasound Med 3:19, 1984

21. Mattsson O: Scintigraphic spleen volume calculation. Acta Radiol(Diagn) 1982; 23:471–477

22. Ingeberg S, Stockel M, Sorensen PJ: Prediction of spleen size by routine radioisotope scintigraphy. Acta Haematol 69:243, 1983

23. Moss AA, Friedman MA, Brito AC: Determination of liver, kidney, and spleen volumes by computed tomography: an experimental study in dogs. J Comput Assist Tomogr 5:12, 1981

24. Bhimji SD, Cooperberg PL, et al: Ultrasound diagnosis of splenic cysts. Radiology 122:787, 1977

25. Dachman AH, Ros PR, Murari PJ, et al: Nonparasitic splenic cysts: a report of 52 cases with radiologic-pathologic correlation. AJR 147:537, 1986

26. McQuown DS, Fishbein MC, Moran ET, Hoffman RB: Abdominal cystic lymphangiomatosis: report of a case involving the liver and spleen and illustration of two cases with origin in the greater omentum and roof of the mesentary. J Clin Ultrasound 3:291, 1975

27. Kaufman RA, Silver TM, Wesley JR: Preoperative diagnosis of splenic cysts in children by gray scale ultrasonography. J Ped Surg 14:450, 1979

28. Ros PR, Moser RP Jr, Dachman AH, et al: Hemangioma of the spleen: radiologic-pathologic correlation in ten cases. Radiology 162:73, 1987

29. Weil F, Brun PH, Rohmer P, Belloir A: Migrations of fluid of pancreatic origin: ultrasonic and CT study of 28 cases. Ultrasound Med Biol 9:485, 1983

30. Chulay JD, Lankerani MR: Splenic abscess—report of 10 cases and review of the literature. AM J Med 61:513, 1976

31. Dubbins PA: Case reports—ultrasound in the diagnosis of splenic abscess. Br J Radiol 53:488, 1980

32. Sommer FG, Gonzalez R, Taylor KJW: Computed tomography and ultrasound findings of a gas-containing splenic abscess. Yale J Biol Med 53:161, 1980

33. Murphy JF, Bernardino ME: The sonographic findings of splenic metastases. J Clin Ultrasound 7:195, 1979

34. Carroll BA, Ta HN: The ultrasonic appearance of extranodal abdominal lymphoma. Radiology 136:419, 180

35. Cunningham JJ: Ultrasonic findings in isolated lymphoma of the spleen simulating splenic abscess. J Clin Ultrasound 6:412, 1978

36. Lupien C, Sauebrie EE: Healing in the traumatized spleen: sonographic investigation. Radiology 151:181, 1984

37. Taylor KJW, Milan J: Differential diagnosis of chronic splenomegaly by grey-scale ultrasonography: clinical observations and digital A-scan analysis. Br J Radiol 49:519, 1976

38. Siler J, Hunter TB, Weiss J, Haber K: Increased echogenicity of the spleen in benign and malignant disease. AJR 134:1011, 1980

39. Quinn SF, vanSonnenberg E, Casola G, et al: Intervention radiology in the spleen. Radiology 161:289, 1986

40. O'Shaughnessy LS, Gosink BB: Imaging of the spleen—CT, ultrasound and nuclear medicine. Applied Radiol 13(3):39, 1984

41. Federle MP, Griffiths B, Minagi H, Jeffrey RB Jr: Splenic trauma: evaluation with CT. Radiology 162:69, 1987

42. Shirkhoda A, McCartney WH, Staab EV, Mittelstaedt CA: Imaging of the spleen: a proposed algorithm. AJR 135:195, 1980

5 The Pancreas

BARRY B. GOLDBERG

Numerous chapters have been written relating to the usefulness and limitations of ultrasound in the evaluation of the pancreas.[1-3] Since this volume is intended to be part of an update of an earlier work, no attempt will be made to review in depth that which has already been published.[4] This chapter reviews our basic knowledge of the usefulness of ultrasound in the evaluation of the pancreas, as well as discusses the latest techniques that have been developed to improve our ability to delineate the various abnormalities that can be seen by ultrasound.

It is quite obvious to anyone who has performed a pancreatic ultrasound examination that it is one of the most difficult intra-abdominal organs to image. The pancreas is nonencapsulated and multilobulated, and is usually long and irregular in shape. It extends transversely across the upper abdomen with its tail being at a slightly higher level than its head. Its identification is based mainly on the delineation of vessels located posterior to it; i.e., the splenic vein and portal vein confluence (Fig. 5.1). The stomach, located anteriorly, is usually collapsed, but when filled can be used to better define the anterior borders of the pancreas and especially its body and tail. The region of the pancreatic head is defined laterally by the descending portion of the duodenum. On occasion, the gastroduodenal artery can be seen in the lateral superior aspect of the pancreatic head with the common bile duct just inferior to it (Fig. 5.2). An uncinate process extends from the medial inferior aspect of the head to the superior mesenteric vein, and can even extend as far as the superior mesenteric artery. The body of the pancreas is perhaps most easily visualized ultrasonically, being generally perpendicular to the ultrasound beam and the area where the pancreatic duct can be most easily delineated. The tail, extending as far as the splenic hilum, presents the most difficult portion of the pancreas to visualize. In fact, this can be considered the Achilles' heel of ultrasound, making CT in general a much more reliable method for imaging the entire pancreas.

There is significant variation in the position of the pancreas. In addition, movement of the pancreas with respiration has been documented using real-time ultrasound. It has been shown that the excursion between maximum

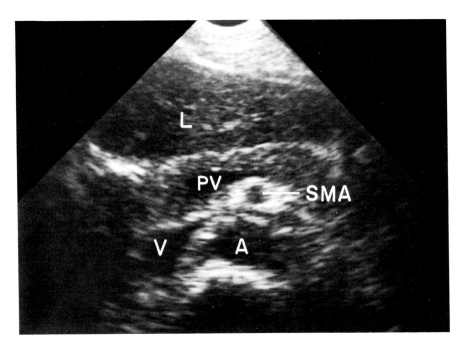

FIG. 5.1. Transverse ultrasonogram of the normal pancreas delineates the various vessels posteriorly (*PV* = portal vein confluence, *SMA* = superior mesenteric artery, *A* = aorta, *V* = vena cava and *L* = liver). (*D* = the area of acoustic shadowing due to air in the duodenum.)

inspiration and expiration may be as much as 3.5 cm with the average being 1.8 cm in the supine position, 1.9 when prone, and 2.2 in the lateral decubitus position.[5] Thus, when obtaining a frozen image, it is often best to ask the patient to hold his/her breath. There is also significant variation in the shape and size of the pancreas and, on rare occasions, even its location, i.e., a left-sided pancreas.[6]

ADVANCES IN ULTRASOUND TECHNIQUES

Throughout the years, the attempts at visualization of the pancreas by ultrasound have led to many diverse approaches, some of which have had little or no impact, and others of which have helped significantly. The key problem in the development of all the methods used has been the presence of bowel gas, particularly when it is obscuring portions of the tail of the pancreas. These techniques include scanning through the left lobe of the liver, particularly helpful in the evaluation of the pancreatic head and body.[7] When this is not possible in the supine position, having the patient sit or stand will often cause the large bowel to drop, air to enter the fundus of the stomach, and the liver to descend over the pancreas, displacing any bowel and thus improving the chance to image the pancreas. Of course, for an examination

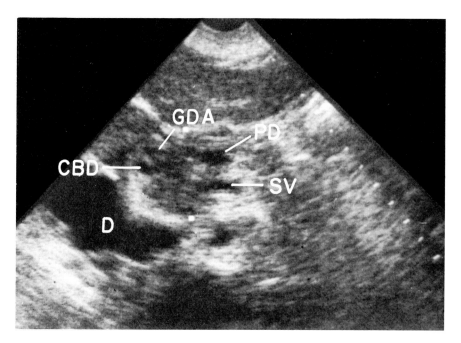

FIG. 5.2. Ultrasonic image of the head of the pancreas delineates the common bile duct, *CBD*, and gastroduodenal artery, *GDA*. Note the fluid-filled portion of the duodenum, *D*. (*PD* = prominent pancreatic duct, *SV* = portion of the splenic vein).

of the pancreas the patient should be fasting. In our facility, we routinely have the patient fast overnight and we perform the studies in the morning.

The head of the pancreas is usually seen by scanning through the liver with the patient supine, but with rotation to the left, with the right shoulder off the table. This is also the recommended view for obtaining images of the common bile duct. The most difficult problem has been, and still remains, the examination of the pancreatic tail. Various methods have been tried in an attempt to improve the ultrasonic visualization of this area, including the use of metoclopramide, with the object of increasing peristalsis, resulting in emptying of the stomach and thus of the gas that might obscure the pancreas. In fact, in one study, visualization of the pancreas was improved by 44 percent.[8] In another study, secretin was utilized to improve pancreatic imaging. It was found that within 4 to 5 minutes after this was administered, the pancreatic secretions flowed into the duodenum, producing a fluid-filled area around the head of the pancreas which improved its visualization, as well as the visualization of the pancreatic duct.[9] Several specific techniques have been utilized to evaluate the tail of the pancreas. When standard supine methods have failed, the patient can be turned prone to look at the tail through the kidney.[10] However, this technique has had limited success since one cannot be sure that the entire tail has been visualized. More recently, some limited success has been reported by using the spleen as an acoustic window with the patient supine. It is reported that there was good visualization of the pancreatic tail in 14 percent of cases and fair visualization in 22 percent.[11] It is also suggested that if this method fails, the fluid-filled stomach approach should be utilized. With this approach, a success rate of approximately 60 percent has been reported[12] (Fig. 5.3).

Various solutions, including a soup made from mince meat, have been used to fill the stomach.[13] The most common solution, however, is water. The amount that must be given varies from patient to patient, depending principally on the rate at which the liquid exits the stomach. In order to prevent this, it is often best to have the patient lie supine with his/her right side up and left side down, drinking water through a straw, allowing for the liquid to collect within the antrum and fundus of the stomach. Once there is an adequate amount present, which is determined by the ability to visualize the liquid within the stomach, the patient can be repositioned and the movement of the fluid followed with real-time ultrasound. Both supine and erect approaches can be attempted, with the success of visualizing the tail and other portions of the pancreas varying from individual to individual, but appearing to improve when the patient is erect and has a fluid-filled stomach (49 to 84 percent for the head, 52 to 92 percent for the body, and

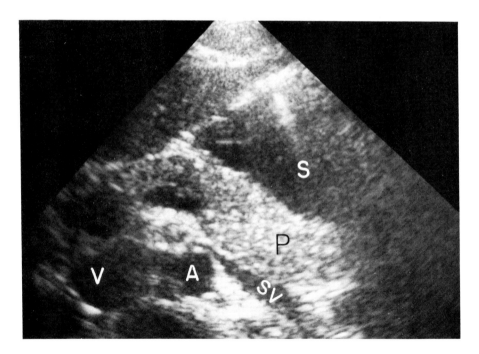

FIG. 5.3.   Transverse ultrasonogram demonstrates fluid within the stomach, *S*, allowing for visualization of the tail of the pancreas, *P* (*SV* = splenic vein, *A* =aorta, *V* = vena cava).

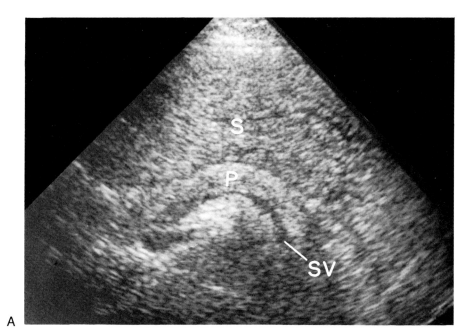

A

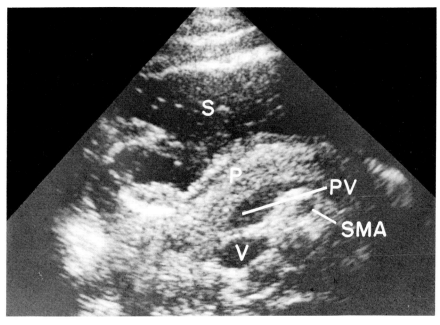

B

FIG. 5.4. (A) Transverse ultrasonogram delineates a portion of the pancreas, *P*, not well seen although significant fluid is seen within the stomach, *S*. The stomach is not well defined due to a marked increase in its echogenicity, the result of the presence of both macro- and micro-air bubbles (*SV* = splenic vein). (B) Ultrasonic images obtained several minutes later. During this interval the micro- and macro-air bubbles have dissipated, allowing for easy visualization of the stomach, *S*, and improved definition of the pancreas, *P* (*PV* = portal vein, *SMA* = superior mesenteric artery, and *V* = vena cava).

from 10 to 67 percent for the tail.[14] During the procedure, it may be necessary to ask the patient to drink additional liquid. It should be realized that, in general, when the patient is drinking, the liquid that first appears in the stomach is quite echogenic, so much so that it may be impossible to visualize the pancreas. Waiting at least several minutes will allow for both the macro and micro air bubbles that are within the swallowed liquid to thereafter dissipate (Figs. 5.4A and 5.4B). This will significantly increase the chances of success.

PANCREATIC MEASUREMENTS

While measurement of the pancreas is possible, due to its variation in shape, the usefulness of these measurements is sometimes in question. It is helpful in directing our attention to suspicious areas of enlargement. In fact, if an area of the pancreas is found to be larger than it should be, and no abnormality is detected by ultrasound, this is a definite indication for obtaining a CT examination. There are numerous articles about measuring the various portions of the pancreas. In general, it can be stated that on cross sectional imaging, when the pancreatic head is less than 30 mm and the body and tail less than 25, it is always within normal limits. However, it appears that the pancreatic head can be normal up to 35 mm and the tail to the same size.[15]

One must also remember that these measurements, taken from transverse ultrasound images, do not take into account the variable size of the pancreas in a cephalad-caudad dimension. This probably accounts for some of the variation in measurement in the various series that have been published. In fact, it has been reported that the cephalad-caudad length of the pancreas may be as much as 60 mm. In a recent article, the maximum anteroposterior diameter of the head of the pancreas was 2.2 ± 0.3 cm and the maximum diameter of the body of the pancreas 1.8 ± 0.3 cm. No attempt was made to measure the tail of the pancreas due to the difficulty of visualizing the entire tail in most cases. This particular population was much larger than other groups consisting of healthy subjects with correlation of organ size with sex, age, weight, height and body surface area.[16] In one study in which both ultrasound and CT were compared, there was significant variation in both the size and shape of the tail between the two. It was found that, in many cases, ultrasound demonstrated the tail to be going in a more dorsal direction, whereas with CT it was seen to be changing direction and curving toward the splenic hilum (Figs. 5.5A and 5.5B). It was felt that this was an artifact of ultrasound which seems to occur particularly in heavier patients and those with an excessive amount of bowel gas.[17]

While the importance of using measurements is to look for an abnormal increase in size, there are some instances in which the pancreas can be smaller than average. This appears to be particularly true in diabetes mellitus. A recent study shows that in those patients with insulin-dependent diabetes, the pancreas, on average, is smaller than in normals. In addition, the pancreas

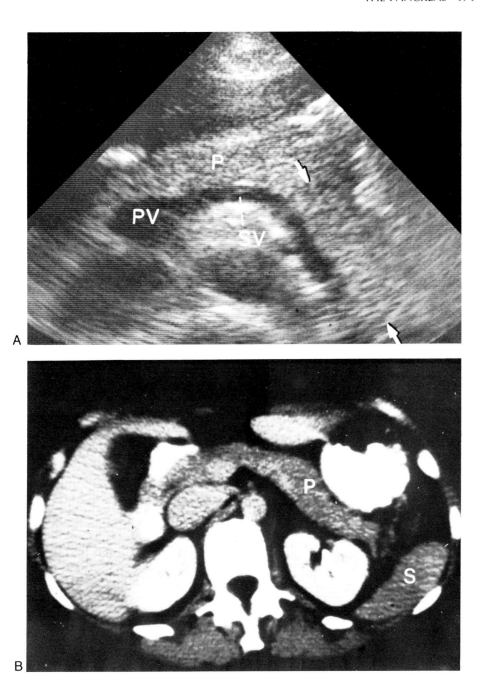

FIG. 5.5. (A) Transverse image of the pancreas demonstrates the tail to be projecting in a more dorsal direction (arrows). (*P* = pancreas, *PV* = portal vein, *SV* = splenic vein.) (B) Transverse CT section of the pancreas shows the tail to be actually extending up toward the region of the splenic hilum (*P* = pancreas, *S* = spleen).

is smaller in patients with insulin-dependent diabetes than with the non-insulin-dependent disease.[18]

PANCREATIC DUCT

In addition to measuring the pancreas, it is also possible to visualize and measure the diameter of the pancreatic duct. (Fig. 5.6) The duct is best seen in the body of the pancreas, but careful scanning may also demonstrate portions of it within the head and, to a lesser extent, the tail. It is important to demonstrate this tubular structure lying within the parenchyma of the pancreas, since it can sometimes be confused with minimal fluid in the antrum of the stomach or the splenic vein posteriorly[19] (Fig. 5.7). If there is confusion, placing fluid within the stomach eliminates this problem. Using Doppler to demonstrate fluid flow within the splenic vein is also possible but, in actuality, scanning the pancreas in both the longitudinal and transverse plane should clearly demonstrate the duct to be surrounded by pancreatic tissue. There has been some controversy as to what are the limits of normal for the diameter of the duct. While the generally accepted measurement of the inner luminal dimension is up to 2 mm, it has been shown that the mean diameter of the duct in the area of the head was 3 mm, in the body, 2.1 mm, and at the junction of the body and tail, 1.6 mm.[20] In cases where it becomes important

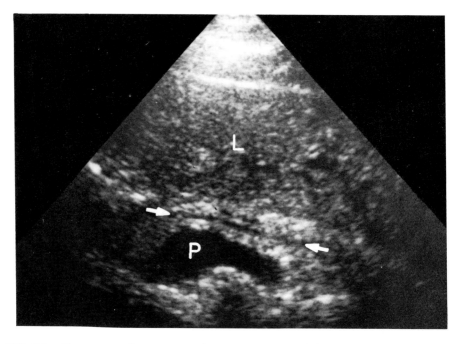

FIG. 5.6.   Transverse ultrasonogram images a portion of the normal pancreatic duct (arrows). (P = portal vein, L = liver.)

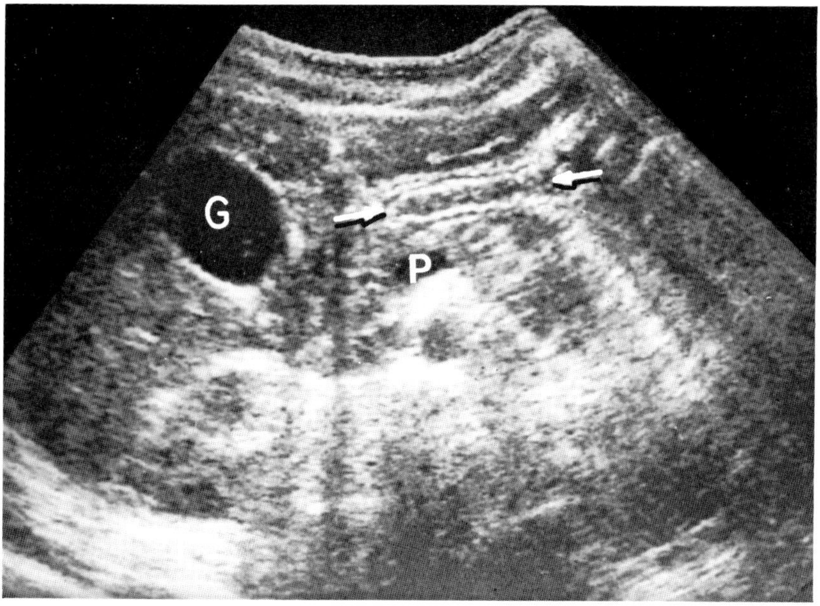

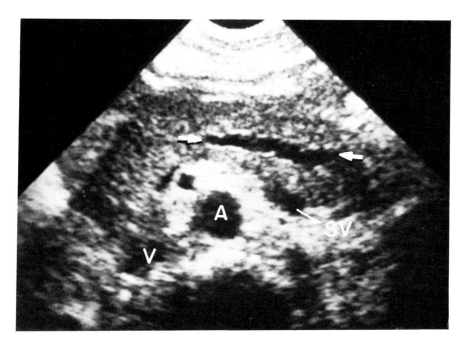

FIG. 5.7. Transverse image of the pancreas demonstrates the empty stomach (arrows) located just anterior to the body of the pancreas. It may sometimes be confused for a portion of the pancreatic duct (*P* = portal vein, *G* = gallbladder).

FIG. 5.8. Transverse ultrasonogram reveals a prominent pancreatic duct (arrows) after hormonal stimulation (*SV* = splenic vein, *V* = vena cava, *A* = aorta).

to visualize the duct, the use of secretin has shown positive results, i.e., an increase in the size of the pancreatic duct in a high percentage of cases within a few minutes after injection[9] (Fig. 5.8). In fact, this technique has been used to evaluate for ampullary stenosis. Using secretin stimulation, it was recently reported that a positive test result was associated with a 90 percent success rate in predicting recurrent pancreatitis and ameliorating pain.[21] These results have not been confirmed, and this should still be considered experimental. While the pancreatic duct generally is echo-free with reflections only from the walls, it has been reported that after transampullary septectomy, air can enter the pancreatic duct as it does the biliary system, resulting in its becoming echogenic. It generally appears as a noncontinuous echogenic line, varying in thickness, within the pancreatic duct.[22]

ECHOGENICITY OF THE PANCREAS

It has been recorded that the echogenicity of the normal pancreas is about equal to, or slightly greater than, that of the adjacent liver echotexture. In addition, it has been shown that with increasing age, particularly past 60, as well as with increasing body fat, the echogenicity of the pancreas increases (Fig. 5.9). An attempt has been made to even grade the echogenicity with grade 1 being a pancreas with echogenicity equal to that of the liver, grade

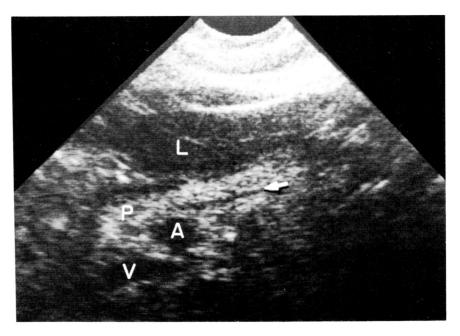

FIG. 5.9. Transverse ultrasonogram shows the increased echogenicity of the pancreas, *P*, relative to the liver, *L*. Note the normal pancreatic duct (arrow). (*A* = aorta, *V* = vena cava.)

2 slightly greater than the liver, grade 3 definitely greater, and grade 4 when the pancreas was as echogenic as the retroperitoneal fat.[23] The significance of these changes has not been established and, therefore, all may well be considered to be within the limits of normal variation. Comparing the echogenicity with CT showed that, generally, those pancreases with an increased echogenicity had a more nonhomogeneous CT scan, with evidence that one of the causes was fatty infiltration within the pancreas. It has also been seen that these pancreases with marked increased echogenicity, have thickness which appears to be greater than the CT measurements, probably due to the fact that ultrasound could not always distinguish between the surrounding echogenic retrojejunal fat and the outer limits of the pancreas, due to their similarity in echotexture.[24]

ABNORMALITIES OF THE PANCREAS

Abnormalities of the pancreas may be divided into either benign or malignant processes, focal or diffuse. As one might expect, there is significant overlap and, often, clinical findings and laboratory results must be utilized along with the ultrasound and other supportive imaging data to arrive at an appropriate differential diagnosis. In delineating abnormalities, ultrasound characteristics include evaluation of the size of the area of interest, its contour, and the disruption of the internal echogenicity. Secondary signs include dilation of the pancreatic duct and the common bile duct, as well as evidence of metastatic spread, if malignant, to adjacent lymph nodes, peritoneum, and such organs as the liver.

DIFFUSE PANCREATIC ABNORMALITIES

Under this category the most common is pancreatitis, both acute and chronic, although, in rare cases, one can have diffuse involvement of the pancreas by tumor. Mild acute pancreatitis may not show on ultrasound examination. However, when the pancreatitis is moderate to severe in nature, there is a decrease in its overall echogenicity relative to the liver. This comparison, of course, assumes that the liver itself is normal in echo texture (Fig. 5.10). The more severe the pancreatitis, the more likely the pancreas is to be enlarged. In mild cases of acute pancreatitis the initial ultrasound images are unlikely to demonstrate any recognizable change in the appearance of the pancreas. If there is an elevated serum amylase, it can be assumed that the patient has pancreatitis. This initial relatively normal baseline ultrasound study can be used to evaluate for any progressive changes that might occur. The more severe the process, usually, the more difficult it is to image the pancreas in its entirety due to resulting paralytic ileus and obscuring of major portions of the pancreas by overlying bowel gas. The greater the severity, the greater will be the increased sound transmission and decrease in overall internal echogenicity. With these severe cases, CT will also have a low attenuation number consistent with increase in fluid within the inflamed pancreas.

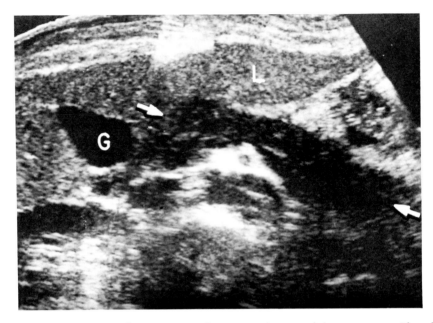

FIG. 5.10. Transverse ultrasonogram shows prominence of the pancreas with a decrease in its echogenicity (arrows) relative to the liver, L, consistent with a diagnosis of acute pancreatitis (G = gallbladder).

Fulminant pancreatic necrosis and hemorrhagic pancreatitis, in general, are not adequately evaluated by ultrasound due to overlying bowel gas, the result of associated paralytic ileus. Thus, in these cases, CT becomes the study of choice. Besides diffuse enlargement, it is possible for pancreatitis to occur focally, making differentiation between a tumor difficult just from the images alone (Fig. 5.11). If there is an elevated serum amylase, pancreatitis is considered as the primary diagnosis, although it is recognized that a tumor itself may cause pancreatitis, which can mask the tumor. Unfortunately, both pancreatic carcinomas and focal areas of pancreatitis often exhibit the same decreased echo texture relative to the rest of the pancreas. If the serum amylase is not elevated, pancreatic tumor becomes the most likely diagnosis. Serial examinations, as the patient responds to treatment, are often useful in making an appropriate differential diagnosis (Fig. 5.12A and 5.12B).

Phlegmons may also cause focal enlargement. This necrotic, focal pancreatitis may be confusing in terms of the ultrasound images, but is clarified by the clinical history and laboratory studies, which will usually indicate a severe pancreatitis. CT, in cases of focal masses, may also not be helpful since tumors or focal pancreatitis may produce a similar pattern. However, overall, CT has an advantage over ultrasound in the evaluation of severe, acute pancreatitis.[25] This also appears to be the case in the evaluation of acute pancreatic trauma, in which case CT is able to demonstrate the presence of acute pancreatic fractures, while ultrasound, despite technically adequate

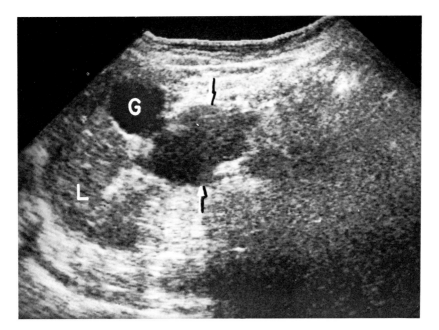

FIG. 5.11.   Transverse image of the pancreas demonstrates focal enlargement of the head of the pancreas (arrows). The overall echogenicity of this region is less than that of the adjacent liver in this patient with a history of pancreatitis (G = gallbladder, L = liver).

visualization of the pancreas, fails to demonstrate these changes.[26] It appears that in these cases, the echogenicity of the peripancreatic hemorrhage may obscure the plane of the fracture within the normally echogenic pancreatic parenchyma.

Ultrasound can be utilized in the serial evaluation of patients with proven acute pancreatitis. It has been shown that while the initial ultrasound appearance may be within normal limits, changes with time can often be documented. In addition, once an abnormal pancreas has been demonstrated, follow-up studies will show the progression of the inflammatory process. The changes can take several directions. In the more mild cases, it has been shown that the ultrasound pattern may return to normal, along with the size, if enlarged. In more moderate to severe cases, healing may occur with a resulting increase in the echogenicity of the pancreas. This increase may be fairly uniform in nature or may be irregular, presenting a mottled appearance. The cause of these changes is felt to be related principally to fibrosis and calcification in the parenchyma or along the duct, the result of healing of the acute process (Fig. 5.13A and 5.13B). These calcifications often present as scattered random highly reflective areas and, classically, if thick enough, produce acoustic shadowing (Fig. 5.14). Unfortunately, many of these calcifications are smaller than the beam width so that shadowing may not be

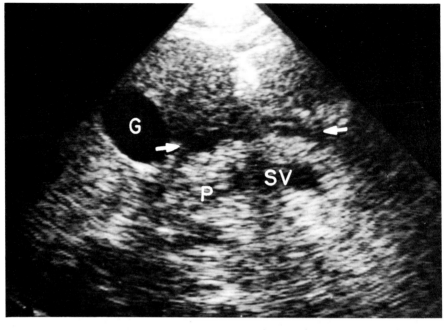

A

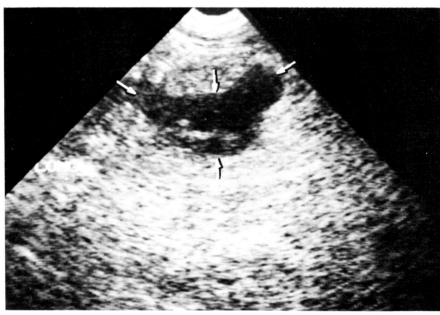

B

FIG. 5.12.   (A) Initial transverse ultrasonogram of a patient with a history of severe acute pancreatitis demonstrated the pancreas, P, to be increased in echogenicity, the result of a long history of previous bouts of pancreatitis. During this acute phase a small collection of fluid is seen outlining the upper surface of the pancreas (arrows). (SV = splenic vein, G = gallbladder.) (B) Follow-up ultrasound examination obtained 4 days later demonstrates the presence of a developing collection (arrows) located in the region where the pancreas had been previously well visualized, the result of severe pancreatitis.

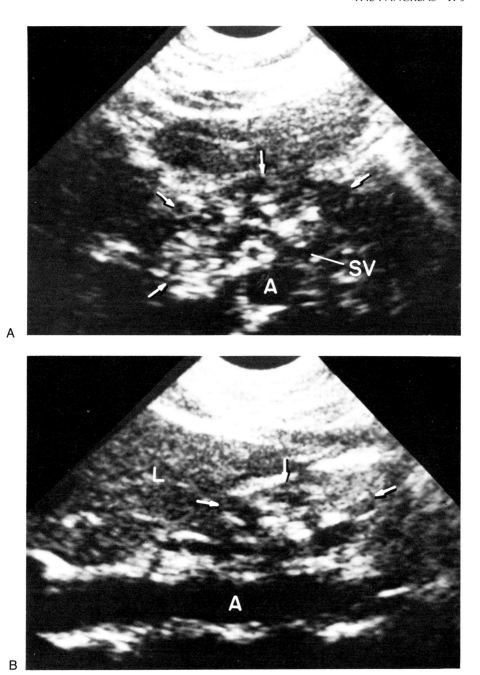

FIG. 5.13.   (A) Transverse image of the pancreas (arrows) showed it to be irregular
in echotexture presenting with a mottled appearance due to fibrosis and calcification.
(*SV* = splenic vein, *A* = aorta.) (B) Longitudinal image of the same pancreas (arrows)
demonstrating changes consistent with a diagnosis of chronic pancreatitis (*L* = liver,
A = aorta).

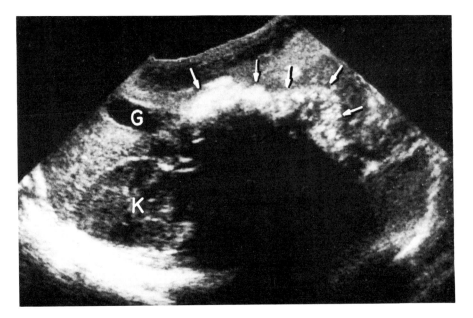

FIG. 5.14. Transverse image of a highly echogenic pancreas (arrows) producing marked acoustic shadowing the result of extensive calcification. (K = kidney, G = gallbladder.)

present, making a definite diagnosis of the presence of calcification impossible.

In cases of chronic pancreatitis, the size is most often within normal measurement limits. Obviously, in the transition from acute to chronic pancreatitis, the pancreas tends to decrease in size with time as the healing process continues. At the same time, there is usually an increase in parenchymal echogenicity.

Similar types of changes have been reported in cystic fibrosis.[27] The changes in this disorder are the result of similar changes that occur in chronic pancreatitis; that is, increase in tissue echogenicity felt to be the result of fibrosis.[28] In terms of diagnosing chronic pancreatitis, one study had a sensitivity of 93 percent. In addition, this same study has shown that the amount of pancreatic calcification decreased from head to tail in most patients, and that foci of calcification greater than 5 mm in diameter were almost always associated with pancreatic duct dilatation[29] (Fig. 5.15). While acute pancreatitis may heal with the changes previously described for chronic pancreatitis, another common pathway is the development of pseudocysts. This process is an attempt of the body to wall off the inflammatory process created by the destruction of tissues by the pancreatic enzymes. In fact, the patient may begin to feel better at the same time that the pseudocyst is forming, due to the walling off of the area of active inflammation. In their classical form, pseudocysts are well defined, smooth-walled, and the fluid within

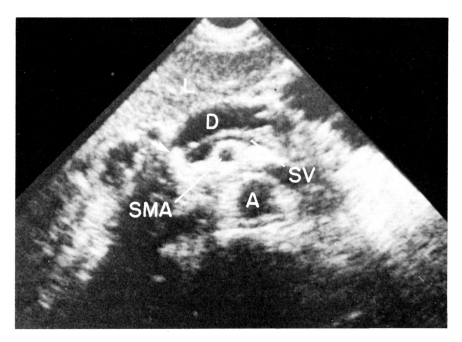

FIG. 5.15.   Transverse image of the pancreas demonstrates a dilated pancreatic duct, *D*, the apparent result of obstruction by a pancreatic stone (arrow) in this patient with a history of severe chronic pancreatitis (*SV* = splenic vein, *SMA* = superior mesenteric artery, *A* = aorta, *L* = liver).

them is echo-free (Fig. 5.16). However, if the ultrasound examination is performed during the process of the pseudocyst formation, it may appear mainly solid, or at least complex in nature. Serial evaluation will show gradual clearing of the internal echoes and better definition of the walls (Fig. 5.17A and 5.17B). Debris may be found within a pseudocyst either during its formation or as a complication after a pseudocyst has matured, due to infection or hemorrhage. Pseudocysts may also be loculated and have bright reflectors along the walls representing calcification. Pseudocysts can occur in patients with a history of chronic pancreatitis during episodes of reexacerbation; that is, the imposition of acute pancreatitis on chronic pancreatitis. In these cases, the echogenicity of the pancreas will decrease and the areas of calcification will be spread further apart due to swelling of the pancreas.

Without a history of pancreatitis, the possibility of mistaking a complicated pseudocyst for a cystadenoma or cystadenocarcinoma would be possible. However, with the appropriate history, such a mistake is unlikely. An abscess may also present as a complex mass, though the walls are usually more irregular and, if there is a gas-forming organism, the appearance is quite different than that of a pseudocyst. This can be easily confirmed with a CT examination. Other masses that can masquerade as pseudocysts include he-

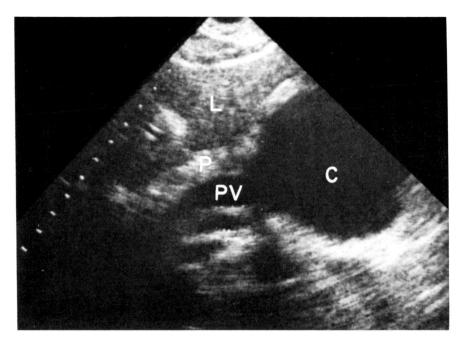

FIG. 5.16. Transverse ultrasonogram of the pancreas, *P*, in which a moderately large well-circumscribed cystic mass is seen within the tail, consistent with a diagnosis of pancreatic pseudocyst, *C*. (*PV* = portal vein, *L* = liver.)

matomas and loculated ascites although, here again, there is usually a history in the case of hematoma, or the presence of fluid elsewhere in the abdomen in the case of ascites.

Pseudocysts may develop quite rapidly after the onset of acute pancreatitis and may be single or multiple. In addition, while the majority form within or adjacent to the pancreas, they may extend far beyond these confines into the retroperitoneum, pelvis, and even the mediastinum.

Serial examinations are recommended in the following of patients with acute pancreatitis to evaluate for the development of pseudocysts and to follow their maturation process. It has been reported that pseudocysts may regress or disappear spontaneously. Most commonly, this is the result of drainage into the pancreatic duct or directly into the adjacent bowel. In addition, there can be rupture of a pseudocyst intraperitoneally, often resulting in peritonitis. While with severe pancreatitis the ultrasound examination may be limited due to overlying bowel gas, usually by the time the pseudocyst has developed the inflammation has cleared, so it is usually possible to delineate the peripancreatic regions in order to determine the presence of a pseudocyst. If, however, this area is still obscured by overlying bowel gas, then CT would be the study of choice. While uncommon, true cysts of the pancreas do occur, most often in association with polycystic renal disease.

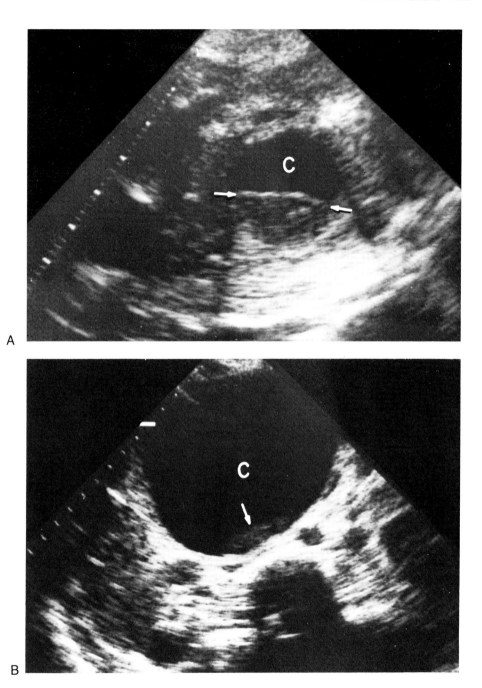

FIG. 5.17.   (A) Transverse image of a developing pseudocyst, C, with a debris level (arrows). (B) Follow-up examination 7 weeks later showed significant enlargement of the previously detected pancreatic pseudocyst, C. Only minimal debris remains (arrow).

In these cases there is, of course, usually no history of acute or chronic pancreatitis.[30]

PANCREATIC TUMORS

Ultrasound not only evaluates for diffuse processes of the pancreas, but also evaluates for focal masses, particularly tumors. It has the ability to determine the size and internal character of the mass. It can easily differentiate cystic from solid masses, as well as those that are more complex in nature. While primary adenocarcinoma is the most commonly seen solid mass, the differential would include focal pancreatitis, abscess, metastatic disease, and lymphoma. The vast majority of tumors are less echogenic than the pancreatic parenchyma. This is particularly so in the case of older patients in whom the pancreas is generally increased in echogenicity (Fig. 5.18). In fact, it is in these types of pancreases that small lesions, that is, lesions that do not

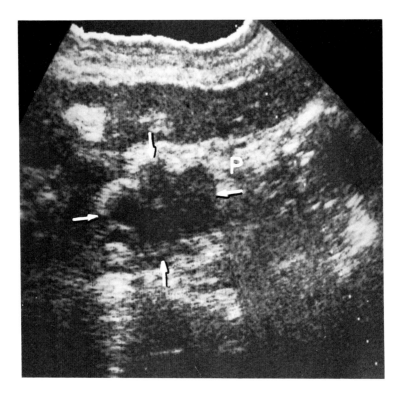

FIG. 5.18. Transverse ultrasonic image of an echogenic pancreas, *P*, reveals an irregular hypoechoic mass (arrows) easily differentiated from the adjacent portions of the pancreas which proved to be pancreatic cancer. (Goldberg BB, Kurtz AB (eds): Pancreas. In Goldberg AB (ed): Abdominal Ultrasonography. 2nd Ed. © Copyright 1984. Reprinted by permission of John Wiley & Sons, Inc.)

produce enlargement and are usually less than 3 cm in diameter, can be identified ultrasonically. A recent study has shown the usefulness of ultrasound combined with serum tumor markers in the diagnosis of pancreatic cancer less than 3 cm in diameter. By combining the two results, it was felt that there was an increased chance of detecting pancreatic cancer at an earlier stage of its development.[31]

Obviously, if the entire pancreas cannot be adequately visualized, CT becomes the study of choice for the evaluation of pancreatic carcinoma.[32] In terms of echogenic solid masses, 90 percent are malignant.[33] When a tumor undergoes necrosis, it presents as a complex mass. In these cases, the differential would include phlegmon, hematoma, abscess, or such cystic pancreatic tumors as cystadenomas or cystadenocarcinomas. Since the majority of tumors occur in the head of the pancreas, secondary signs often are present, such as dilatation of the pancreatic and/or common bile ducts (Fig. 5.19A and 5.19B). In some cases with duct dilatation, the tumor itself may not be seen. Besides pancreatic masses, tumors of the ampulla of Vater can also produce ductal dilatation. If no specific mass is seen, the differential must also include stricture or stone. Rarely, a heterotopic pancreas may mimic carcinoma. In one case ectopic tissue arising near the ampulla of Vater caused common bile duct obstruction, producing obstructive jaundice.[34]

Pancreatic tumors may invade or compress adjacent vessels. It is not uncommon to find obstruction of a portion of the portal venous system. When ultrasound was compared to angiography in terms of compression, displacement, or occlusion, there was a sensitivity of 90 percent and a specificity of 95 percent for the splenic vein and slightly lesser percentages for the main portal vein and superior mesenteric vein. It was concluded that ultrasound can make angiography prior to laparoscopy unnecessary in many cases.[35] When a solid mass is detected, not only should the pancreas, common bile, and pancreatic ducts be evaluated, but adjacent areas as well to evaluate for evidence of extension, either direct or at a distance. Lymphadenopathy is not uncommon, nor is venous obstruction. If the splenic or portal vein cannot be seen, this certainly is suggestive of vascular occlusion. Other signs of spread include compression of the vena cava, as well as the presence of ascites and liver metastasis.

While the vast majority of solid tumors are malignant, there are some benign tumors, in particular, islet cell tumors, and microcystic adenomas, which contain such small cysts that they often present as a solid mass. They have good sound transmission as a result of the multiple small cysts. These tumors are usually well circumscribed (Fig. 5.20). However this, in itself, does not allow for a definitive diagnosis of a benign lesion. In the case of islet cell tumors, they occur most commonly in Langerhans' islets located predominantly in the body and tail. They may also be quite small and are often undetectable by ultrasound. Metastatic and lymphomatous masses occur more commonly about the region of the head and body of the pancreas. When large, they may compress or displace the pancreas, making it difficult to distinguish from a pancreatic carcinoma. On occasion, differentiation may

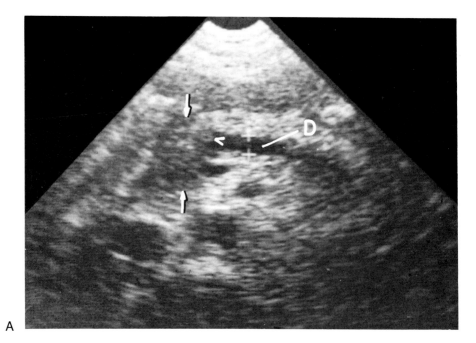

A

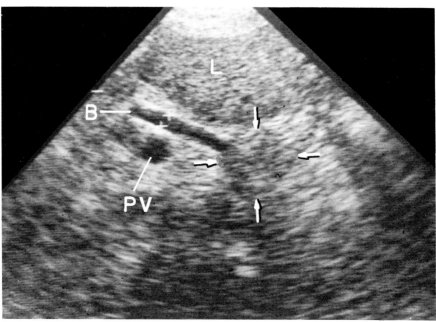

B

FIG. 5.19.   (A) A solid mass is seen within the head of the pancreas (arrows) producing dilatation of the pancreatic duct, *D,* which measured 8 mm in diameter. There is apparent extension of this pancreatic tumor into the pancreatic duct (arrowhead). (B) Longitudinal ultrasonic image showed associated dilatation of the common hepatic and bile ducts, *B,* extending down to the region of the tumor (arrows). (*PV* = portal vein, *L* = liver.)

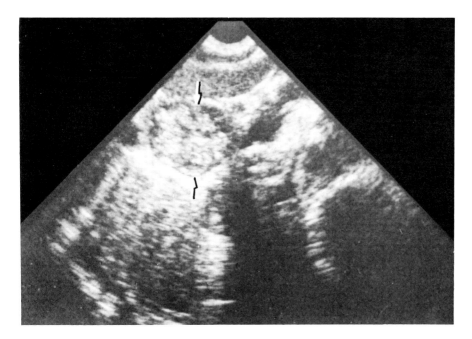

FIG. 5.20.   Transverse ultrasonogram reveals a well-circumscribed solid mass (arrows) within the head of the pancreas, which proved to be a pancreatic adenoma.

be possible since lymphomas tend to be relatively less echogenic and more irregular, with individually involved lymph nodes identified. In addition, lymphoma often projects posterior to the splenic and portal veins, which is usually not the case with pancreatic carcinoma (Fig. 5.21). However, even these findings are not specific since, on rare occasions, pancreatic carcinomas have been reported to extend posteriorly to the splenic vein.[36] While pancreatic cystadenomas and cystadenocarcinomas are relatively uncommon, they often present as complex, predominantly cystic masses, with septations and thick walls, although they may have a smooth outer contour[37] (Fig. 5.22). Calcification may be present along the periphery of the mass. Differentiation between cystadenoma and cystadenocarcinoma, i.e., benign versus malignant characteristics, is not possible. All such masses must be considered potentially malignant. These tumors tend to be hypervascular and may contain some central calcification.[38] In children, pancreatoblastomas are rare tumors usually presenting as complex cystic masses. This type of tumor is often called infantile carcinoma of the pancreas, but has a much better prognosis than adult pancreatic carcinoma. It occurs most commonly in the head of the pancreas and is believed to arise from the ventral pancreas. Usually the tumor may be totally excised and the prognosis is generally good. It can be associated with the Wiedmann-Beckwith syndrome.[39] Research is ongoing in our facility to evaluate the use of Doppler imaging in the evaluation of tumors to determine their degree of vascularity. While the vast majority of tumors examined have shown no increase in vascularity, that is, no signifi-

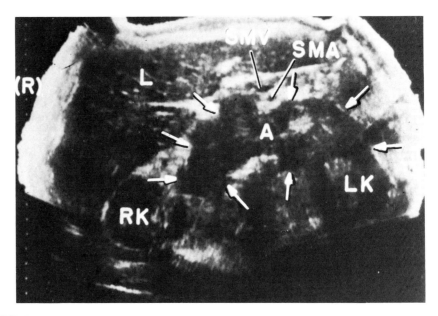

FIG. 5.21. Transverse image of the mid abdomen demonstrated the presence of a lobulated hypoechogenic solid mass (arrows) surrounding the aorta, *A*. The mass was located posterior to the superior mesenteric artery, *SMA*, and superior mesenteric vein, *SMV*. This proved to be a metastatic mass of nodes rather than a pancreatic carcinoma. (*L* = liver, *RK* = right kidney, *LK* = left kidney.) (Goldberg BB, Kurtz AB (eds): Pancreas. In Goldberg AB (ed) Abdominal Ultrasonography. 2nd Ed. © Copyright 1984. Reprinted by permission of John Wiley & Sons, Inc.)

cant Doppler signal could be detected, flow has been demonstrated in several pancreatic tumors. These were proven to be hypervascular tumors by angiography. In these cases, a distinctive ultrasound pattern was detected, felt to be arising from multiple tumor vessels (Fig. 5.23A and 5.23B).

ENDOSCOPIC ULTRASOUND

One of the newest approaches to imaging of the pancreas is through a specially developed flexible endoscope containing a high resolution ultrasound transducer. The endoscope is passed through the esophagus into the stomach, which is often fluid-filled to allow for easy transmission of the ultrasound beam through the stomach wall. While this technique has been used to evaluate the heart through the esophagus, of particular interest in this chapter is its usefulness in the evaluation of various aspects of the pancreas. It produces ultrasonic images superior to the conventional approach and it appears to be a valuable complement to conventional imaging, including ultrasound and CT.[40–42] It seems to be superior to conventional ultrasound in the diagnosis of ampullary abnormalities. However, the most promising use of endo-

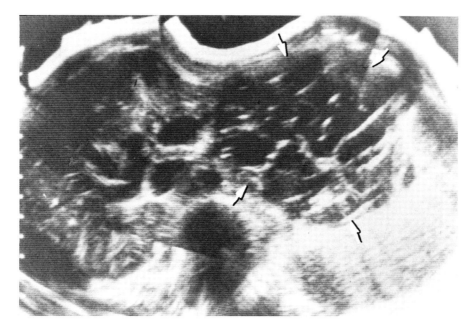

FIG. 5.22.   Transverse ultrasonogram of the pancreas delineates a septated cystic mass (arrows) which proved to be a cystadenocarcinoma. (Courtesy of Arnold C. Friedman, M.D., Department of Diagnostic Imaging, Temple University Hospital, Philadelphia, Pennsylvania.)

scopic ultrasound appears to be in the staging of local resectability of pancreatic and periampullary malignancies.[43] With this technique, it was possible to detect the presence of adjacent nodes and delineate the borders of the tumor, including its relationship to adjacent blood vessels. While this technique certainly will not replace the primary role of ultrasound and CT in the initial evaluation of pancreatic abnormalities, if these approaches are equivocal, endoscopic ultrasound appears to have an increasingly important role in helping to make a definitive diagnosis.

PANCREATIC BIOPSY

Ultrasound continues to be an important method of not only detecting the presence of tumors, but also of guiding needles percutaneously into an area of interest. In many cases, surgery is avoided once biopsy proof is obtained. With this information, radiation therapy or chemotherapy can be instituted.[44, 45] Most of the techniques utilized now involve a fine needle aspiration biopsy. In our facility, the cytologist is present at the time of the procedure and is able to immediately analyze the tissue, reducing the need for multiple biopsies. A recent study has shown that the accuracy of percutaneous versus operative biopsy is equivalent and, therefore, percutaneous aspiration should be given precedence since it obviates the need for explor-

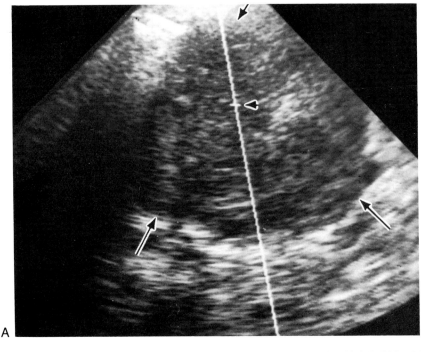

A

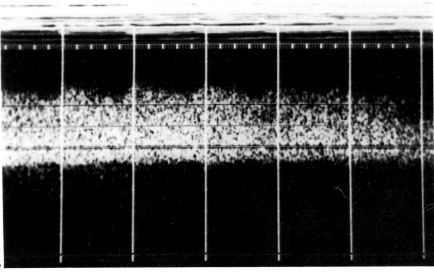

B

FIG. 5.23.   (A) Transverse ultrasonogram demonstrates the presence of a large solid mass (arrows) in the region of the body of the pancreas. Note line with marker (arrowhead) delineating the site of Doppler sample from within the tumor. (B) Doppler spectral analysis of this mass showed a marked increase in blood flow throughout both systole and diastole, which was felt to be the result of multiple arteriol-venous communications found within many tumors. Subsequent arteriography demonstrated a highly vascular pancreatic tumor.

atory laparoscopy.[46] Finally, should surgery be needed, ultrasound has proven useful during the procedure to localize lesions within the pancreas that cannot be easily palpated. This has been particularly true in instances such as small insulinomas, where the visual appearance of the surface of the pancreas, or palpation, may produce no lead as to the exact site of the area of abnormality. In addition, extension of tumors posteriorly may be better delineated using intraoperative ultrasound. Lymph node involvement, as well as extension of tumor beyond the confines of the pancreas, can also be demonstrated at the time of surgery, providing information that is often not appreciated by other noninvasive methods, including CT and conventional ultrasound.[47]

CONCLUSION

Ultrasound has, and will continue to play, an important role in the evaluation of various pancreatic abnormalities. While newer cross-sectional imaging procedures including CT and MR have limited some of its usefulness, it still has an important place. With the introduction of new approaches, including Doppler and endoscopic ultrasound, as well as its continued importance in the guiding of needles for aspiration biopsy and at surgery for localization, in many respects its usefulness may well increase.

REFERENCES

1. Taylor KJW, Pollock D, Crade M: Pancreatic ultrasonography: techniques, artifacts and clinical results. In Moss AA, Goldberg HI (eds): Computed Tomography, Ultrasound and X-ray. p. 81. University of California Press, San Francisco, 1980
2. Leopold GR: Ultrasonography. In Margulis AR, Burhenne HJ (eds): Alimentary Tract Radiology V.2; 3rd Ed. p. 1243. CV Mosby, St. Louis, 1983
3. Kurtz AB, Goldberg BB: Pancreas. In Goldberg BB (ed): Abdominal Ultrasonography. 2nd Ed. p. 163. John Wiley & Sons, New York, 1984
4. Sample WF, Sarti DA: Diagnosis of pancreatic disease by ultrasound and computed tomography. p. 85. In Taylor, KJW (ed): Diagnostic Ultrasound in Gastrointestinal Disease. Churchill Livingstone, Inc., New York, 1979
5. Bryan PJ, Custar S, Haaga JR, Balsara V: Respiratory movement of the pancreas: an ultrasonic study. J Ultrasound Med 3:317, 1984
6. Dunn DD, Gibson RN: The left-sided pancreas. Radiology 159:713, 1986
7. Lee JKT, Stanley RJ, Melson GL, Sagel SS: Pancreatic imaging by ultrasound and computed tomography. Radiology Clin North Am 16(1):105, 1979
8. duCret RP, Jackson VP, Rees C, et al: Pancreatic sonography: enhancement by metoclopramide. AJR 146:341, 1986
9. Bolondi L, Gaiani S, Casanova P, et al: Improvement of pancreatic ultrasound imaging after secretin administration. Ultrasound Med Biol 9:497, 1983
10. Goldstein HM, Katragadda CS: Prone view ultrasonography for pancreatic tail neoplasms. Am J Roentgenol 131:231, 1978
11. Paivansalo M, Suramo I: Ultrasonography of the pancreatic tail through spleen and through fluid-filled stomach. Europ J Radiol 6:113, 1986

12. Kolmannskog F, Swensen T, Vatn MH, Larsen S: Computed tomography and ultrasound of the normal pancreas. Acta Radiol (Diagn) 23:443, 1982

13. Vuoria P, Suramo I, Hyvarinen S: Transmission media for ultrasonography. Radiology 135:520, 1980

14. MacMahon H, Bowei JD, Beezhold C: Erect scanning of pancreas using a gastric window. AJR 132:587, 1979

15. Weill F, Schraub A, Eisenscher A, Bourgoin A: Ultrasonography of the normal pancreas. Radiology 123:417, 1977

16. Niederau C, Sonnenberg A, Muller JE, et al: Sonographic measurements of the normal liver, spleen, pancreas, and portal vein. Radiology 149:537, 1983

17. Suramo I, Lohela P, Lahde S, et al: The "ghost tail" of the pancreas in ultrasonography. Europ J Radiol 2:139, 1982

18. Gould IM, Newell S, Green SH, George RH: Size of pancreas in diabetes mellitus: a study based on ultrasound. Br Med J 291:6504, 1985

19. McGahan JP: The posterior gastric wall: a possible source of confusion in the identification of the pancreatic duct. J Clin Ultrasound 12:366, 1984

20. Hadidi A: Pancreatic duct diameter: sonographic measurement in normal subjects. J Clin Ultrasound 11:17, 1983

21. Warshaw AL, Simeone J, Schapiro RH, et al: Objective evaluation of ampullary stenosis with ultrasonography and pancreatic stimulation. Am J Surg 149:65, 1985

22. Braver JM, Jones TB, Brooks JR: The sonographic appearance of the pancreatic duct following transampullary septectomy. Ultrasound Med 5:459, 1986

23. Worthen NJ, Beabeau D: Normal pancreatic echogenicity: relation to age and body fat. AJR 139:1095, 1982

24. Paivansalo M: Normal pancreatic echogenicity: relation to structural unevenness and thickeness in CT. Annals of Clin Research 16:69, 1984

25. Block S, Maier W, Bittner R, et al: Identification of pancreas necrosis in severe acute pancreatitis: imaging procedures versus clinical staging. Gut 27:1035, 1986

26. Jeffrey RB, Laing FC, Wing VW: Ultrasound in acute pancreatic trauma. Gastrointest Radiol 11:44, 1986

27. Swobodnik W, Wolf A, Wechsler JG, et al: Ultrasound characteristics of the pancreas in children with cystic fibrosis. J Clin Ultrasound 13:469, 1985

28. Shawker TH, Linzer M, Hubbard VS: The diagnostic significance of pancreatic size and echo amplitude. J Ultrasound Med 3:267, 1984

29. Gilinsky NH, Leung JWC, Heron C, Cotton PB: Calcific pancreatitis: Calcification patterns and pancreatogram correlations. Clinical Radiology 35:401, 1984

30. Shirkoda A, Mittelstaedt C: Demonstration of pancreatic cysts in adult polycystic disease by computed tomography and ultrasound. AJR 131:1074, 1978

31. Iishi H, Yamamura H, Masahaur T, Okuda S, Kitamura T: Value of ultrasonographic examination combined with measurement of serum tumor markers in the diagnosis of pancreatic cancer of less than 3 cm in diameter. Cancer 57:1947, 1986

32. Ormson MJ, Charboneau JW, Stephens DH: Sonography in patients with a possible pancreatic mass shown on CT. AJR: 148:551, 1987

33. Katz RJ, Behan M, Herbstman C, et al: Sonography and CT of the pancreas. Seminars in Ultrasound 1(3):209, 1980

34. O'Reilly DJ, Craig RM, Lorenzo G, Yokoo H: Heterotopic pancreas mimicking carcinoma of the head of the pancreas: a rare cause of obstructive jaundice. J Clin Gastroenterol 5:165, 1983

35. Garra BS, Shawker TH, Doppman JL, Sindelar WF: Comparison of angiography and ultrasound in the evaluation of the portal venous system in pancreatic carcinoma. J Clin Ultrasound 15:83, 1987

36. Abiri MM, Kirpekar M: An unusual anatomic location of pancreatic masses. J Ultrasound Med 5:703, 1986

37. Wolson AH, Walls WJ: Ultrasonic characteristics of cystadenoma of the pancreas. Radiology 119:203, 1976

38. Friedman AC, Lichtenstein JE, Dachman AH: Cystic neoplasms of the pancreas. Radiology 149:45, 1983

39. Koh THHG, Cooper JE, Newman CL, et al: Pancreatoblastoma in a neonate with Wiedemann-Beckwith syndrome. Eur J Pediatr 145:435, 1986

40. Strohm WD, Kurtz W, Hagenmuller F, Classen M: Diagnostic efficacy of endoscopic ultrasound tomography in pancreatic cancer and cholestasis. Scand J Gastroenterol 19:18, 1984

41. Kukuda M, Nakano Y, Saito K, et al: Endoscopic ultrasonography in the diagnosis of pancreatic carcinoma. Scand J Gastroenterol 19:65, 1984

42. Classen M, Strohm WD, Kurtz W: Pancreatic pseudocysts and tumors in endosonography. Scand J Gastroenterol 19:77, 1984

43. Tio TL, Tytgat GNJ: Endoscopic ultrasonography in staging local resectability of pancreatic and periampullary malignancy. Scand J Gastroenterol 21:135, 1986

44. Tatsuta M, Yamamoto R, Yamamura H, et al: Cytologic examination and CEA measurement in aspirated pancreatic material collected by percutaneous fine-needle aspiration biopsy under ultrasonic guidance for the diagnosis of pancreatic carcinoma. Cancer 52:693, 1983

45. Hajdu EO, Kumari-Subaiya S, Phillips G: Ultrasonically guided percutaneous aspiration biopsy of the pancreas. Seminars in Diagnostic Pathology 3:166, 1986

46. Savarino V, Ceppa P, Biggi E, et al: Comparative study of percutaneous and preoperative fine-needle aspirations in the diagnosis of pancreatic cancer. Hepato-gastroenterol 33:75, 1986

47. Sigel B, Mach J, Ramos JR, et al: The role of imaging ultrasound during pancreatic surgery. Annals of Surgery 200:486, 1984

6 The Gastrointestinal Tract

PAUL A. DUBBINS

Fifteen years ago the title of this chapter would have been the role of the gastrointestinal tract in ultrasound imaging rather than the role of ultrasound imaging of the gastrointestinal tract. Early work had recognized the difficulties that bowel gas and other intestinal contents produced for adequate ultrasound imaging of the intra-abdominal organs. In 1972 Holm stated that tumors of the gastrointestinal tract were not suitable for ultrasound investigation.[1] Not only was gas seen to be an impediment to visualization of intra-abdominal organs, but unusual configurations of bowel and its content seemed likely to lead to inaccurate diagnosis. The splenic flexure and the stomach in particular were reported to produce pseudolesions of the kidney and the tail of the pancreas.[2, 3] Much of the attention therefore was centered around solutions to these diagnostic problems. In the upper abdomen, gastric pseudomasses were resolved by the use of gas in the form of citrocarbonate solution[4] or the rapid infusion of water with ultrasound visualization of the attendant microbubbles.[5, 6] In the lower abdomen and pelvis, pseudolesions were also encountered and were similarly resolved by the use of water, in the form of an enema, as a contrast medium.[7, 8] If this were to be the limit of the role of ultrasound in the gastrointestinal tract, then indeed the chapter's title should remain as suggested. However, several factors have contributed to an increasing role for ultrasound in the evaluation of bowel. Technical advances have probably made the greatest contribution. The advent of "gray scale" has been followed by even greater resolution. Real-time scanning with high resolution equipment has permitted continuous monitoring and visualization of peristalsis and movement of bowel contents between loops. Finally, endoscopic scanning and endosonography have provided greatly increased resolution of the mucosa and subsequent layers of the gut to allow better visualization of anatomical detail and of bowel pathology. The role of Doppler ultrasound in the evaluation of lesions of the gastrointestinal tract has not yet been fully investigated, although preoperatively it has contributed to our understanding of the reasons for failure of certain operative techniques.

Coinciding with the technological developments that have occurred in this area, and at least in part as a result of these developments, there is now a greater understanding of the sonographic anatomy of bowel and the contribution of bowel contents to different sonographic patterns.

APPEARANCES OF NORMAL BOWEL

Although bowel is anatomically subdivided into different sections, the basic structure throughout is that of a hollow tube. Sonographic appearances, therefore, are not solely dependent on the structure of the tube but also upon its contents and its degree of distention. There are anatomical differences, both in terms of shape and bowel wall configuration. These sometimes serve to identify specific bowel loops, but essentially appearances depend upon whether the bowel is collapsed or distended and if distended, whether filled with gas, fluid or both. These patterns are described as the mucus pattern, gas pattern or fluid pattern.[9]

The Mucous Pattern

The mucous pattern describes the appearance of the bowel in its collapsed state. The ultrasound appearance is described as a target consisting of a hyperechoic core of mucus and trapped gas surrounded by an hypoechoic halo of bowel wall (Fig. 6.1). It is possible, with high resolution equipment, to recognize that there are different layers of the bowel wall corresponding to its histologic features; there is an inner echogenic layer representing the mucosa, an echo poor muscularis mucosa and an echogenic submucosa, an echo poor muscularis propria, and an echogenic serosal layer. Although these appearances are better seen using endoscopic equipment, they may be recognized on transabdominal scanning, particularly during examination of the stomach[10, 11] (Fig. 6.2).

The target pattern is most commonly recognized at the esophagogastric junction, the pyloric antrum, and in the transverse colon (Fig. 6.3). While this pattern is characteristic of collapsed bowel, slight variations exist. These variations depend upon the degree of bowel collapse and the presence or absence of small amounts of trapped gas and fluid (Fig. 6.4A and 6.4B).

Fluid Pattern

Fluid distention in the normal bowel produces an appearance which is dependent upon whether the bowel is imaged along its long axis (a tubular pattern) or short axis (circular or cystic pattern) (Fig. 6.5). Different bowel segments are often recognized by their relative position within the abdomen. Thus the stomach is recognized by its continuity with the esophagogastric junction and its position in relation to the pancreas and other upper abdominal structures (Fig. 6.6). Similarly, the course of the ascending and descending colon,

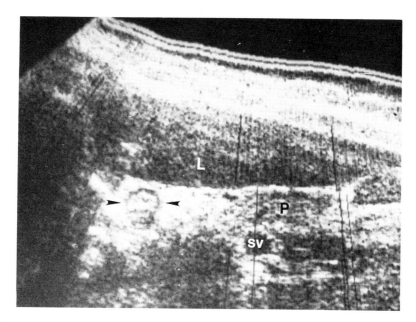

FIG. 6.1. Longitudinal scan just to the left of the aorta demonstrating the typical target appearance of the esophagogastric junction (arrowheads), situated posterior to the left lobe of the liver, *L*, and cephalad to the body of the pancreas, *p*. The course of the splenic vein, *sv*, posterior to the pancreas, is demonstrated.

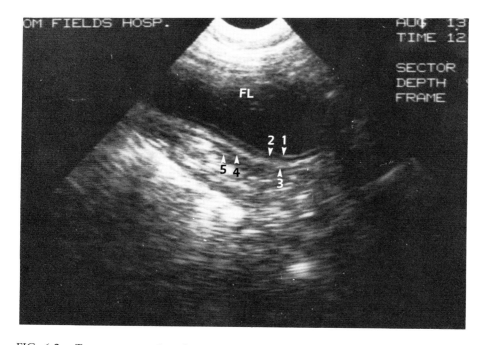

FIG. 6.2. Transverse section through the body of a fluid-filled stomach, *FL*, with some anterior reverberation within the fluid-containing stomach which obscures the anterior wall. However, on the posterior wall, the five layers of the gastric wall are identified. *1* = echogenic mucosa, *2* = echo poor muscularis mucosa, *3* = echogenic submucosa, *4* = echo poor muscularis propria, *5* = echogenic serosal layer.

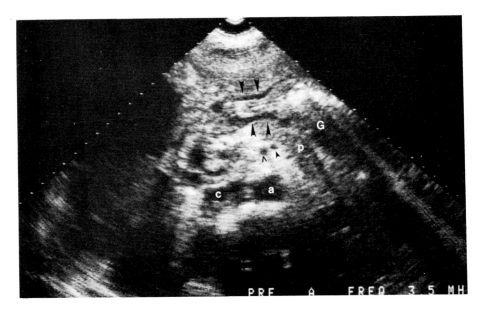

FIG. 6.3. Transverse scan of the upper abdomen demonstrating the long axis equivalent of the target appearance in the region of the pylorus of the stomach (large closed arrowheads). There is gas, *g*, in the more proximal portion of the stomach. (*a* = aorta, *c* = inferior vena cava, *p* = pancreas, small closed arrowhead = superior mesenteric artery, small open arrowhead = superior mesenteric vein.)

in particular, will frequently allow their accurate recognition. It is possible to differentiate bowel loops by the demonstration of specific anatomical features, particularly when the scan plane is aligned to the long axis of the bowel loop. In this way the first to third parts of the duodoenum can be identified by recognition of the characteristic C loop and its relationship with the pancreas[12] (Fig. 6.5). Other loops of bowel can be recognized by the particular structural features of the mucosa. Thus in the small bowel the valvulae conniventes produce what has been described as a "key-board" appearance or may be likened to a ladder (Fig. 6.7), whereas the ileum has smooth featureless walls, and the colon demonstrates haustral sacculations[13] (Fig. 6.8).

Gas Patterns

The significant acoustic impedance differences between gas and soft tissue produce marked reflection of sound at this interface together with a distal artifactual echographic appearance which is variable. These artifacts may be represented by a well defined acoustic shadow. These shadows contain low level reverberation echoes or closely spaced high level reverberation echoes (the so-called "ring down" artifact)[14, 15] (Fig. 6.9). Occasionally the "ring

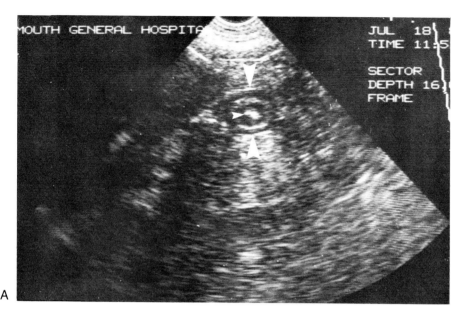

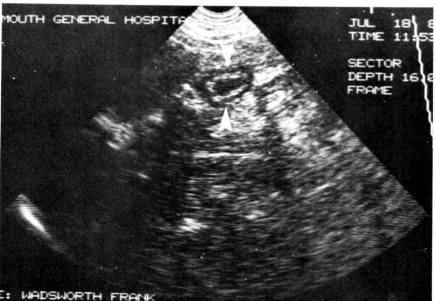

FIG. 6.4. Demonstration of the dynamic nature of bowel. (A) The target appearance is modified by bubbles of gas passing through the lumen, whereas in (B) the gas has been replaced by fluid.

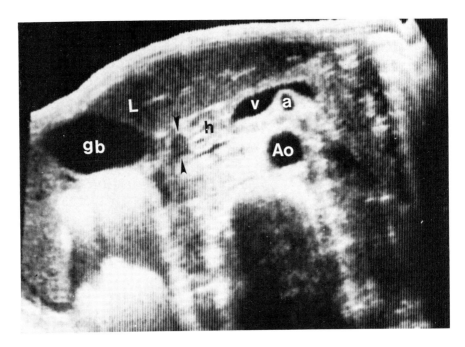

FIG. 6.5. The circular or cystic pattern of fluid-containing bowel seen "end on," identified in this case by the duodenum (arrowheads) situated to the right of the head of the pancreas, *h*. (*gb* = gallbladder, *L* = liver, *v* = splenic vein, *a* = superior mesenteric artery, *Ao* = aorta.)

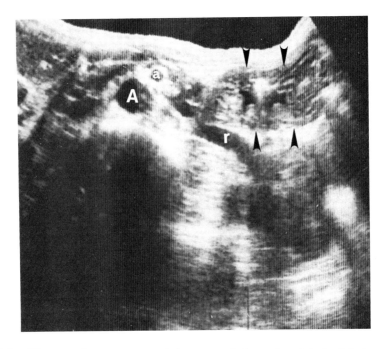

FIG. 6.6. Ultrasound appearance of the stomach (arrowheads). In this transverse scan of the upper abdomen the stomach contained small amounts of gas and fluid. The rugose nature of the gastric wall is also demonstrated. (*r* = left renal vein, *a* = superior mesentic artery, *A* = aorta.)

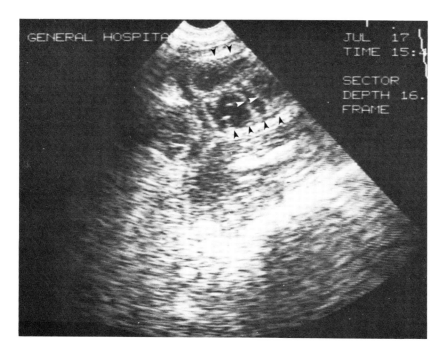

FIG. 6.7. Fluid-filled loops of small bowel may be frequently seen if the abdomen is examined after preparation for a pelvic ultrasound (i.e., ingestion of considerable volumes of fluid). In this image two loops of small bowel containing fluid are identified, (small black arrowheads) and in one of these the mucosal feature of jejunum, the valvulae conniventes (small white arrowheads) are demonstrated.

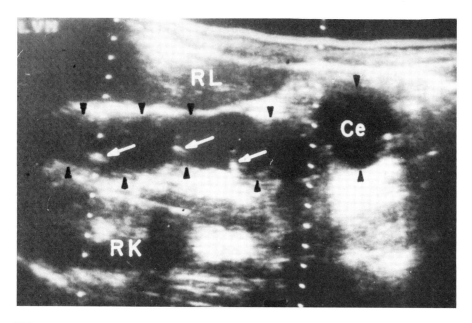

FIG. 6.8. Fluid-filled ascending colon (black arrowheads) in which the caecum, *ce* is clearly identified as well (arrows). (*RL* = right lobe of liver, *RK* = right kidney.)

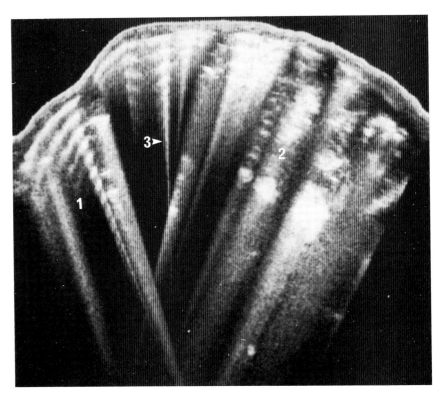

FIG. 6.9. Patient presented with acute small bowel obstruction. Although this is a patient with abnormal abdominal distention, this demonstrates all the characteristics of gas related artifact. *1* is an area of acoustic shadowing and immediately superficial to this there are closely spaced high level reverberation artifact. *2* is an area of low level reverberation artifact and *3* demonstrates an area of ring down artifact in the shape of a "comet tail."

down" artifact may demonstrate tapering. This has been described as a "comet tail" artifact.[16] This appearance is not specific for gas within the bowel, but is representative of gas within any location. It had been suggested that it would be possible to differentiate shadowing from a gas soft tissue interface and shadowing from a calculus soft tissue interface on the basis of the well defined shadow deriving from the latter, compared to the "dirty" distal acoustic shadowing deriving from gas.[17] However, although a clearly defined shadow is the rule in the presence of gallstones, reverberation occurs in a significant number of cases. Similarly, while some form of reverberation is demonstrated in most cases of bowel gas, clearly defined acoustic shadows are occasionally seen.[14]

None of these patterns represent a static appearance and evaluation of the bowel with real-time scanning will demonstrate peristalsis, the to and fro movement of intestinal contents termed "Brownian motion" by some authors,[18] and occasionally the mass movement of large bowel contents.

Colon Pseudotumor Pattern

While most of the features described for normal bowel can be said to be due to varying mixtures of fluid and gas, the appearances of the colon are sometimes atypical. Fluid, when present in the colon, may be echogenic because of the presence of suspended fecal material. Fecal masses, particularly in fecal impaction, may produce a highly reflective mass on sonography with distal acoustic shadowing.[19, 20] Where there is doubt about the nature of any such pseudomass, a plain abdominal radiograph will frequently demonstrate a "soap-bubble" appearance of a fecaloma or fluid levels in a distended, fluid filled, large bowel.[21] Where doubt remains it is possible to perform a water enema under real-time monitoring, which allows the differentiation of intraluminal, mural, and extraintestinal masses.[7, 8]

BOWEL WALL THICKNESS

It is possible to assess the thickness of bowel wall in vivo. This can be performed in the distended and nondistended state, regardless of the contents of the bowel. Usually the anterior bowel wall thickness is measured because of the possibility of pseudothickening that may be produced by unequal distribution of fluid and gas (Fig. 6.10). In normal patients the maximum bowel wall thickness is 3 mm when distended and 5 mm when nondistended. Normal colonic thicknesses of up to 9 mm and gastric thickness of up to 7 mm have been recorded[22, 23] but are unusual. In this author's opinion a

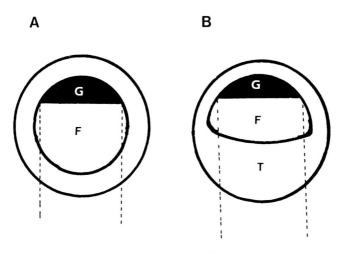

A   **B**

FIG. 6.10. Diagramatic representation of the effect of bowel contents on apparent bowel wall thickening. In (A) there is symmetrical bowel wall thickening, however the presence of gas, G, may produce a significant acoustic shadow which obscures the posterior bowel wall. Similarly the presence of a significant amount of fluid, F, which may be echo poor may produce a false impression of posterior asymmetric bowel wall thickening. In (B) asymmetrically thickened bowel may be obscured by the acoustic shadowing derived from gas, G.

bowel wall thickness of greater than 5 mm that does not change, either with peristalsis or with direct compression by the transducer, represents an indication for contrast radiology.

BOWEL MOTILITY

The study, by real-time ultrasound, of persitaltic movement of the gut is important in the recognition of bowel loops and also in the demonstration of abnormality. Bowel affected by inflammatory or neoplastic processes does not demonstrate the same motility as does normal bowel.

In the stomach it is possible to use ultrasound to quantify motility. Gastric contractions occurring every 20 seconds can be observed following the administration of a test meal.[24, 25] Gastric contractions do not appear to be related to antroduodenal flow but instead appear to be related to the mixing of gastric content. Trans-pyloric fluid movement occurs during relaxation of the pylorus and occurs in brief episodes lasting less than 4 seconds, followed by episodes of up to 5 seconds of retrograde flow.[26] This to and fro motion is also observed elsewhere in the gut. It is also possible, using ultrasound, to measure gastric emptying time and rate, by sequential measurement of antral volume following a test meal. Although such methods have been suggested to evaluate abnormal gastric emptying, a suitable application for these methods has yet to be described.[27, 28]

PATTERNS OF ABNORMAL BOWEL

Observation of the abnormal bowel will show variations upon the normal pattern. Since the appearances of abnormal bowel remain dependent upon their contents, there may be abnormal distention or distribution of gas distended bowel, abnormal dilatation of fluid filled bowel, or abnormal thickness of bowel wall altering the mucous pattern. Patterns of bowel abnormality are therefore first analyzed by utilizing the same descriptive patterns as are used for normal bowel and by identifying variation from the normal mucus, gas, or fluid patterns.

The Mucous Pattern

Alterations in bowel wall thickness should be detectable on ultrasound. The degree of bowel wall thickening will depend upon the degree of infiltration of the bowel wall by abnormal tissue. It was in the demonstration of the abnormal mucous pattern of bowel that the first reports of the diagnostic utility of ultrasound in the gastrointestinal tract were made. Although the first description of ultrasound demonstration of gastric neoplasm indicated that the characteristic pattern was that of a solid mass,[29] subsequent publications have indicated that the pattern of bowel involvement by any process which produces thickening is characteristic (Fig. 6.11). This pattern has been

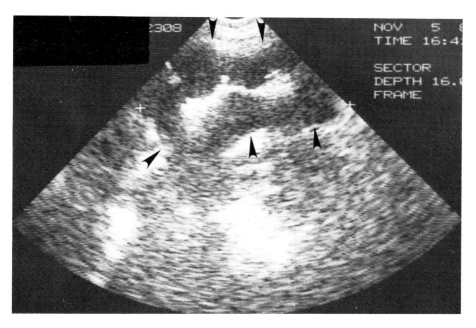

FIG. 6.11. Pseudokidney appearance of a carcinoma of the ascending colon (arrowheads). The characteristic echogenic core likened to the collecting system of the kidney and the echo poor thickened bowel wall likened to the renal parenchyma is clearly apparent.

variously described as the "target," "bulls-eye," "pseudokidney," "cockade," or "ring sign."[30–36] While being specific for an abnormality of bowel, this pattern is not specific for any particular bowel pathology and may be seen in both inflammatory and neoplastic processes within the bowel. A list of the reported causes of the pseudokidney sign is shown in Table 6.1. The site of involved bowel must be inferred by the relative position of the lesion in the abdomen. Thus a pseudokidney demonstrated in the right upper quadrant is likely to be pathology involving the hepatic flexure: in the epigastrium, the stomach; and in the pelvis, the sigmoid colon. Certain sites allow more exact delineation, particularly after the administration of fluid. For example, oral administration of fluid indicates the confirmation of a gastric or duodenal mass,[37] and administration of fluid via the rectum indicates the location of a lesion in the rectum and sigmoid colon.[7, 8]

It was thought in the first instance that it would be possible to differentiate certain groups of pathology one from the other, and in early work some authors indicated that this would be possible on the basis of the degree of thickening of the gastrointestinal wall. However, this suggestion was clearly not tenable, as one group reported that the thickening was greatest in tumors,[30] whereas another paper suggested that inflammatory thickening in infarction was more marked than in neoplasia.[34] Many different pathologies

TABLE 6.1. Lesions producing "atypical target" or pseudokidney appearance

Tumours
Adenocarcinoma
Lymphoma
Leiomyosarcoma
Carcinoid
Inflammatory Disease
Crohn's disease
Diverticular disease
Gastritis (including caustic)
Chronic granulomatous disease of childhood
Appendicitis
Tuberculosis
Peptic ulcer
Pancreatitis
Other
Infantile hypertrophic pyloric stenosis
Intussusception
Ischaemia
Intramural haemorrhage
Lymphangiectasia
Menetriers disease
Amyloidosis
Whipples disease
Radiation enteritis

can produce varying degrees of bowel wall thickening. These cannot be distinguished on the basis of either the thickness or on the degree of symmetry of thickening since both inflammatory (Crohn's disease) and neoplastic (lymphoma and certain sarcomata) can produce asymmetric thickening of the bowel wall. As a general rule however, inflammatory processes tend to involve longer segments of bowel than neoplastic processes (Figs. 6.11, 6.12). There are clearly exceptions to this: an intussusception, for instance, involves only a short segment of thickened bowel, and intestinal lymphoma may involve large segments. This author has demonstrated two adjacent carcinomas mimicking diverticular disease in the sigmoid colon (Figs. 6.13, 6.14).

Most workers would indicate that it is not possible to differentiate inflammatory from malignant pathology. However, certain recent work suggests that it is possible to demonstrate, with high resolution, high frequency ultrasound equipment, alternating layers of the mucosa, sub-mucosa, muscularis, and serosa via transabdominal scanning in the small and large bowel as

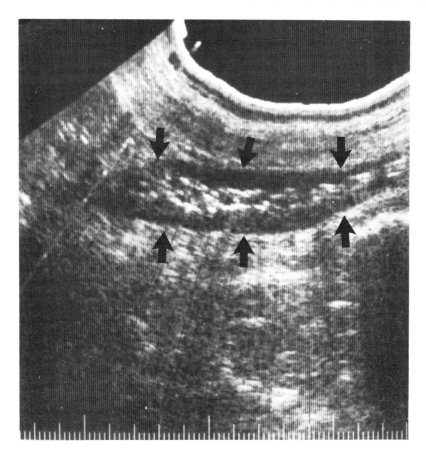

FIG. 6.12.   Involvement of long segment of bowel in inflammatory bowel disease (Crohn's disease, arrows) often allows the distinction between inflammatory and neoplastic involvement.

well as the stomach. These workers suggest that these layers are retained in inflammatory thickening but not retained in tumor. They also intimate that asymmetry of bowel wall thickening indicates the presence of tumor,[38] although this is not the experience of this author.

While these are nonspecific signs permitting the distinction between the many different causes of the "target appearance," some are sufficiently characteristic either in site, clinical context, or sonographic appearance to allow a confident diagnosis to be made.

INFANTILE HYPERTROPHIC PYLORIC STENOSIS

Ultrasound demonstration of thickening of the pyloric wall was first reported by Teele and Smith in 1977[39] (Fig. 6.15). Subsequently many authors have introduced measurements said to be specific for the condition. These are

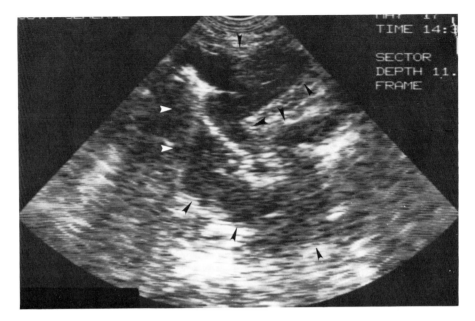

FIG. 6.13. Long irregular loop of bowel wall thickening is normally characteristic of inflammatory disease such as diverticular disease (arrowheads), but in this case secondary to two adjacent carcinomas.

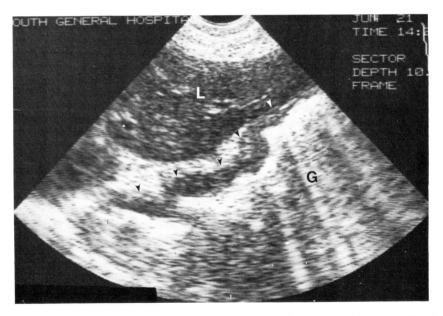

FIG. 6.14. Long segment of thickened intestine in the upper abdomen with the thickened intestinal wall identified by the arrowheads and the lumen containing considerable gas, *g*, suggesting an inflammatory process but representing instead linitis plastica of the stomach, an infiltrative neoplastic process. (*L* = liver.)

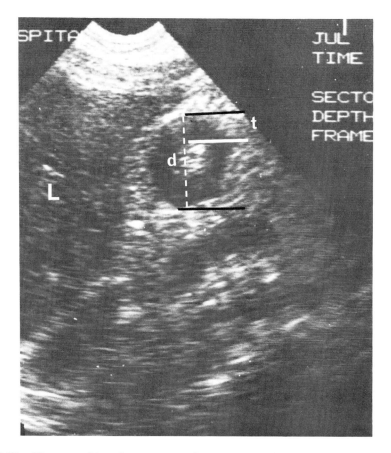

FIG. 6.15.   Hypertrophic pyloric stenosis demonstrating the thickened pyloric antrum and two of the measurements used to assess this condition: the thickness of the pyloric wall, *t*, and the diameter of the pylorus, *d*. (*L* = liver.)

the transverse diameter of the pylorus, the maximum thickness of the pyloric wall, and the length of the pyloric canal. Each of these measurements is generally larger in the child with pyloric stenosis than in the normal child, however, there is considerable overlap, particularly of the transverse diameter of the pylorus and of the wall thickness, although the length of the pylorus appears to be more specific[41-44] (Table 6.2). It is not surprising that there should be this overlap, since the dimensions of the pylorus increase with increasing age of the infant.[45] While the length of the pyloric canal appears to be the most sensitive and specific of the measurement parameters, the diagnosis should be based on a consideration of all these measurements together. Other sonographic signs, such as pre-pyloric hypertrophy and shouldering, and ultrasound equivalents of the "beak and tit" signs described in the study of the condition with barium meal should also be considered.[40]

TABLE 6.2. Pyloric dimensions in infantile hypertrophic pyloric stenosis (composite chart)

	Normals	IHPS
Pyloric transverse diameter	9.2 (6–15)	13.6 (9–19)
Wall thickness	1.7 (1–3.5)	3.75 (3–8)
Length	9.1 (5–16)	22.1 (16–28)

Further, the absence of demonstrable passage of gastric contents through the pylorus and increased peristalsis may also be demonstrated.[40]

It is possible to evaluate the pylorus postoperatively. When this is performed it can be demonstrated that all three measurement parameters return to normal values following the Rammstedt procedure.[46]

INTUSSUSCEPTION

Originally the appearances described for an intussusception were similar to those of other bowel associated target lesions, although interestingly were endowed with a different descriptive term, that of the "doughnut sign"[47, 48] (Fig. 6.16). Subsequently a further sign has been introduced which is produced by scanning the lesion in long axis to the loop of bowel. This sign, the "hay-fork" or "trident" sign, is seen to represent intussusceptum and

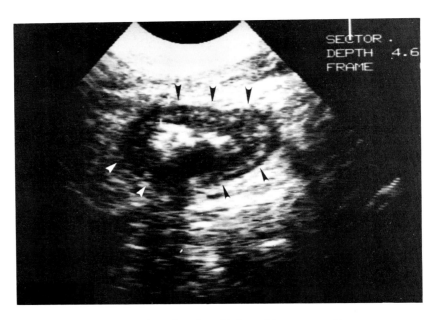

FIG. 6.16. The "doughnut" sign of intussusception.

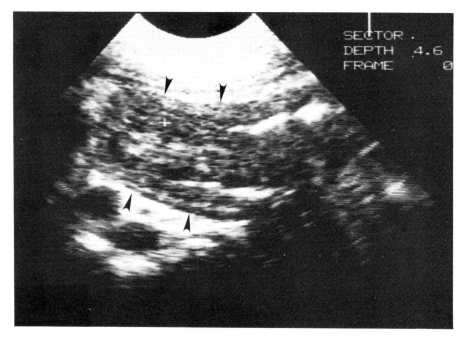

FIG. 6.17. The "hayfork" or "trident" sign of intussusception in its long axis with the intussusceptum and intussuscipiens.

intussuscipiens.[49–51] (Fig. 6.17). It has been suggested that it might be possible to predict those patients in whom hydrostatic reduction is likely to fail by the presence of marked wall thickening and almost complete obliteration of the central lumen.[52] Furthermore it is also possible to achieve reduction of an intussusception using ultrasound during reduction with water or saline, rather than utilizing contrast radiology.[53]

INFLAMMATORY DISEASE OF THE GUT

The ultrasonographic appearances seen in inflammatory bowel diseases depend upon the nature of the pathological involvement, the extent to which bowel is involved, and the presence or absence of complications. Unless the primary inflammatory pathology produces thickening of the bowel wall, ultrasound is unlikely to demonstrate significant abnormality in the absence of complications. Thus a condition that produces superficial ulceration without bowel wall thickening, such as ulcerative colitis, does not produce a demonstrable abnormality on ultrasound examination. Crohn's disease, with its transmural bowel involvement, will produce significant bowel wall thickening in the acute phase.[54] Thus, while there are many pathologies which may produce ulceration within the bowel, only those which involve the bowel transmurally will be detectable by ultrasound. These include Crohn's disease, diverticular disease, chronic granulomatous disease of childhood, and Ménétrier's disease. Bowel wall thickening demonstrated by ultrasound has also been reported in ileal tuberculosis,[55] and in antibiotic-associated colitis.

As a general rule, inflammatory bowel wall thickening may be symmetric or asymmetric, thick or thin, but usually involves a long segment of affected bowel.

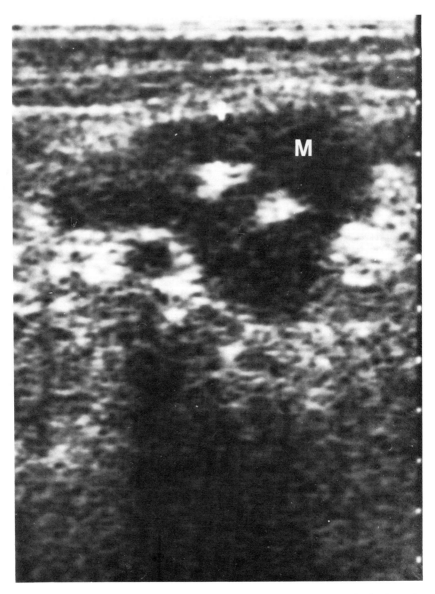

FIG. 6.18. Conglomerate mass, *M*, of matted loops of bowel with thickened wall in Crohn's disease.

Crohn's Disease

The sonographic findings in Crohn's disease are variable. They include the pseudokidney sign secondary to bowel wall thickening; a conglomerate mass which consists of irregular sonodense and sonolucent areas representing matted, thickened bowel (Fig. 6.18); and fatty conglomerations when the mesentery is included in the mass.[56] In addition, complications of the Crohn's inflammation such as abscess formation (Fig. 6.19) and bowel obstruction may be demonstrated by the presence of a fluid-filled mass, dilated fluid-filled loops, or an abnormal gas pattern.[54, 57–59] Occasionally it is possible to demonstrate fistulous tracts, although this requires great attention to detail during scan technique.[60]

The primary signs of Crohn's disease are, however, those of bowel wall thickening and conglomerate tumor formation. It is possible to quantify the degree of bowel wall thickening during active disease and to demonstrate a reduction in thickness with treatment.[54] The diagnostic accuracy of abdominal ultrasound in Crohn's disease suggests a sensitivity of 84 percent and a specificity of 83 percent.[61]

Ultrasound has been reported in the diagnosis of Crohn's disease in children but there are no specific features in this group.[62]

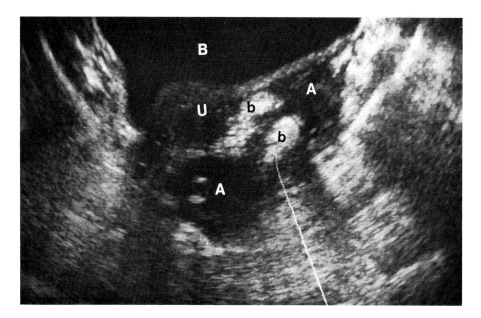

FIG. 6.19.   Pelvic abscess, *A* in association with Crohn's disease of the pelvic small bowel, *b*. (*B* = bladder, *U* = uterus.)

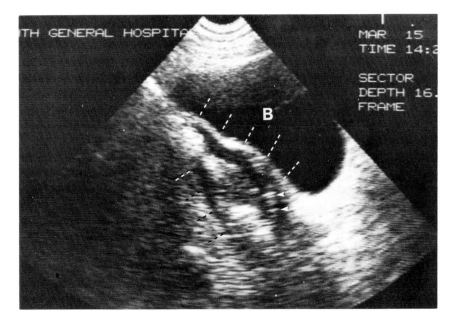

FIG. 6.20.   Diverticular disease of the sigmoid colon producing irregular bowel wall thickening but with some gas presumably within diverticula within the thickened bowel wall (arrowheads). (*B* = bladder.)

Diverticular Disease

Diverticular disease is recognized largely by its involvement of the distal descending and sigmoid colon. In acute diverticulitis there is thickening of the bowel wall and complications, such as abscess formation, may develop. The degree of bowel wall thickening may be followed during resolution with ultrasound and may prove to be an indicator as to the timing of the reintroduction of oral feeding. (Dubbins unpublished work). It is occasionally possible to see air-containing diverticula within the thickened bowel wall[63] (Fig. 6.20).

Ménétrier's Disease

In this condition gastric thickening is marked and the hypertrophied gastric rugae are demonstrated. There may be deformity of the exogastric component and rarely mesenteric lipomatosis.[64]

Necrotizing Enterocolitis of Infancy

There is little published work on the use of ultrasound in this condition but a short report suggests that the demonstration of the pseudokidney sign indicates the presence of gangrenous bowel and thus represents an indication for surgical intervention.[65]

Appendicitis

Although inflammatory involvement of the appendix again produces thickening of the wall of the appendix in common with other bowel involvement, its peculiar nature, and common occurrence merit separate consideration. Recent studies have indicated that it is possible to demonstrate an ultrasonic abnormality in a high proportion of patients with acute appendicitis. This is described as an echo poor or echo free lesion with a rounded ovoid or curved configuration representing thickened appendiceal walls with a dilated echo free appendiceal lumen separated by echogenic mucosa. This finding was best achieved using graded compression in the right iliac fossa (Fig. 6.21). Occasionally it is possible to see an appendicolith and other associated features such as dilated loops of bowel or free fluid in the peritoneum. The accuracy of this technique varies[66-68] but may be as high as 89 percent, which is clearly higher than for clinical examination and better than for plain radiology. However, the logistics of providing an acute ultrasound service of the technical expertise with the frequency required of this common condition have been called into doubt.[69]

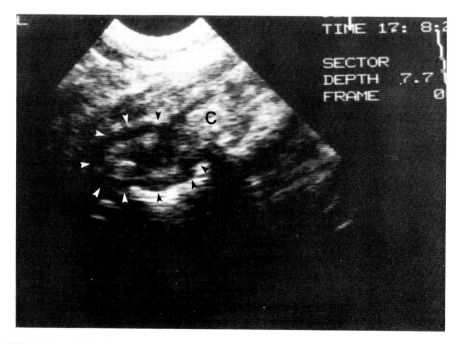

FIG. 6.21.   Markedly thickened appendix in patient with acute appendicitis (arrowheads). (C = caecum.)

Peptic Ulcer

If ultrasound has a role in the diagnosis of peptic ulcer, it has usually been described in the identification of complications. Perihepatic fluid collections, inflammatory involvement of the gallbladder fossa, ulcer penetration into the liver and the pancreas have been described.[70] More recently it seems possible to diagnose even small perforations by the detection of prehepatic air in the supine patient. This demonstration does not require an erect film of the patient and thus does not require patient movement.[71] There have been several case reports of demonstration of the ulcer crater itself, either as a cystic or gas-containing space or as a modified target lesion. However, these features are only seen in giant peptic ulcers[72, 73] (Fig. 6.22).

NEOPLASTIC DISEASE OF THE GASTROINTESTINAL TRACT

Many of the original articles describing bowel wall involvement in intestinal disease considered the detection of bowel cancer.[29–36] Although sonography is not suggested as an alternative to orthodox contrast radiology in the evaluation of bowel neoplasia, the detection rate for certain neoplasms is unexpect-

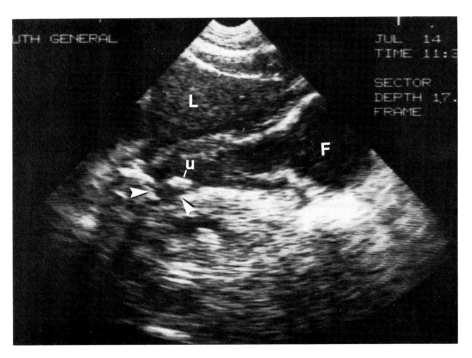

FIG. 6.22.   Giant peptic ulcer (arrowheads) in the region of the pyloric antrum of a fluid filled stomach, *F*. *"u"* identifies the mouth of the ulcer covered by echogenic material which could represent either mucus or blood. (*L* = liver.)

edly high in those patients with known gastric cancer, 97 percent being detected in one report.[74] Even when used as a primary imaging modality in the investigation of upper abdominal symptomatology, 72 percent of gastric cancers were diagnosed. The ability to recognize a gastric carcinoma depends largely on its position. It is possible to see anterior and posterior walls of the gastric antrum in 86 percent of normal patients, while this is possible for the gastric body in only 9 percent.[75] However, the role of ultrasound may be greater in staging, particularly gastric cancer. Not only may tumor be visualized and lymph node and hepatic metastases documented (Fig. 6.23), but local invasion may also be detected[76–78] (Fig. 6.24). Further, with new high resolution equipment it may be possible to identify the degree of involvement of the various intestinal layers by tumor without the need for recourse to endoscopic ultrasound.[11]

Although as a general rule ultrasound features of neoplastic lesions of the intestinal tract are those of the pseudokidney sign, certain tumors demonstrate characteristic patterns. Of these, involvement by lymphoma is the most common, but leimyosarcoma, being a predominantly exophytic lesion, demonstrates a pattern so characteristic that it may almost be pathognomic. The features are those of an eccentric bowel associated mass consisting of a mixture of solid and cystic areas representing the marked necrosis that occurs within this lesion[79] (Fig. 6.25).

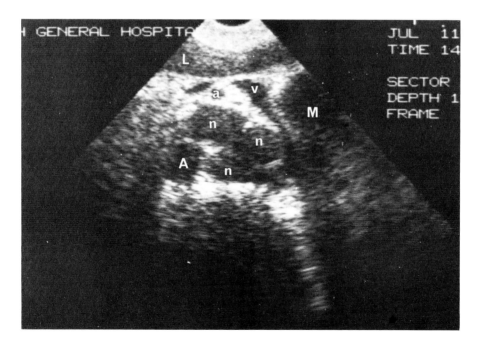

FIG. 6.23.   Scan of the upper abdomen demonstrating nodal masses, *n*, posterior to the superior mesenteric artery, *a*, and splenic vein, *v*. The aorta, *A*, is situated posteriorly to this. The gastric mass from which these nodal metastases arose is seen adjacent to this, *M*. (*L* = liver.)

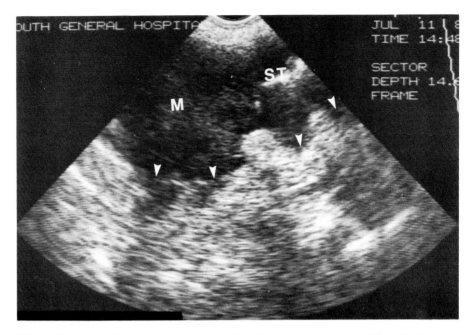

FIG. 6.24. Large irregular mass, *M*, arising from the stomach, *ST*, with irregular thickening of the gastric wall and extension of tumor through the serosa (arrowheads).

Intestinal Lymphoma

In this condition bowel wall thickening is the usual finding. In many cases this is indistinguishable from bowel wall thickening from other causes.[29-36] However, in gastric lymphoma the ultrasound pattern appears to be characteristic, recently described as a "spoke wheel" pattern of bowel wall thickening in many cases.[80] Although this feature had not been described previously in the literature, similar appearances had frequently been observed.[81, 82]

PSEUDO PSEUDOKIDNEY SIGN

The pseudokidney sign is taken as evidence of bowel wall thickening. However, the appearance may be seen in normal bowel, with unusual configuration and in other anatomic variations as well as certain pathological conditions and termed the pseudo pseudokidney sign (Table 6.3). This is particularly true in the colon where bowel wall thicknesses of up to 9 mm have been reported. Similarly, over-lapping loops of fluid-filled bowel may produce a confusing appearance suggestive of abnormal bowel. Similar patterns have been described in ovarian dermoids, mesenteric lymphoma ("sandwich sign"), and excess mesenteric fat. The most important of the bowel pathology mimics however, is the kidney itself. This should not constitute a problem when the kidney is in normal position, but in renal ectopia the kidney may

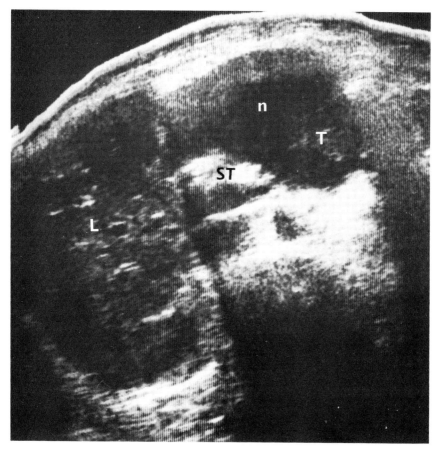

FIG. 6.25. Transverse scan through the upper abdomen demonstrating a tumor mass, *T*, arising from the stomach, *ST* with a large area of necrosis, *n*. This appearance is characteristic of a leiomyosarcoma. (*L* = liver.)

TABLE 6.3. Causes of pseudo pseudokidney

Normal kidney is unusual position
Multiple loops of fluid filled bowel
Dermoid
Normal colon
Gas in pancreatic head
Mesenteric lymphadenopathy
Mesenteric fat
Gallstones in thick walled gallbladder

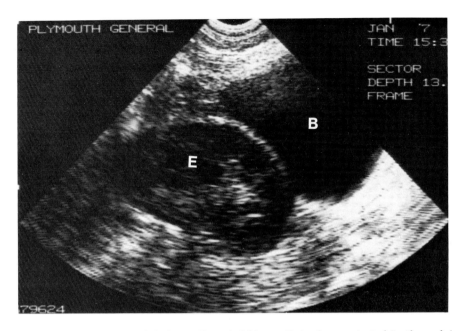

FIG. 6.26.   Pseudo pseudokidney. Ectopic kidney, *E*, is demonstrated in the pelvis adjacent to the bladder, *B*.

have a somewhat unusual configuration. In this condition it may be difficult to differentiate the kidney from bowel pathology unless the sonographer is aware of the need to evaluate both renal fossae (Fig. 6.26).

BIOPSY TECHNIQUE

The advent of fine needle aspiration biopsy guided by real-time ultrasound has allowed the sampling, at first, of cellular material and subsequently core biopsies from many different sites previously inaccessible to the transcutaneous approach. Although more recent work has suggested that it may be possible to differentiate, in some cases, benign from malignant lesions on the basis of ultrasound appearances alone, this suggestion is not yet widely accepted. Furthermore, cytological and histological analysis allows the differentiation of different cell types. Therefore, fine needle aspiration of bowel lesions of the pseudokidney type is of increasing importance, particularly in patients where confirmatory studies are either technically difficult or the findings nonspecific. Cytology allows the differentiation of adenocarcinoma from lymphoma and other lesions of the stomach, small, and large bowel.[83, 84]

ABNORMAL GAS AND FLUID PATTERNS

At first sight ultrasound has no role to play in the evaluation of intestinal obstruction and the consequent abnormality of content of bowel loops. The plain erect and supine radiograph of the abdomen, with the demonstration

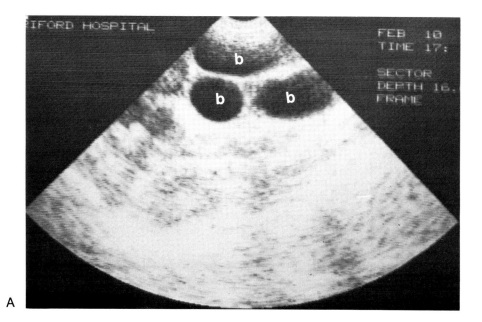

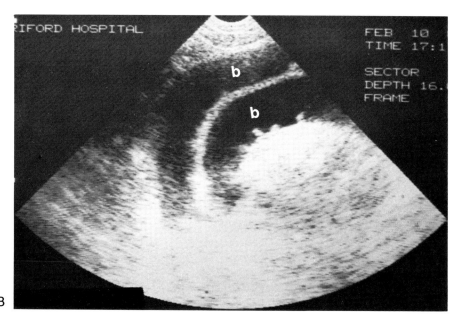

FIG. 6.27.   (A) demonstrates dilated fluid-filled loops of bowel in short axis, *b*. (B) fluid-filled loops of bowel, *b* in long axis. Somewhat effaced valvulae conniventes are shown in one of the loops.

of distended gas filled loops of bowel and air/fluid levels and the recognition of different anatomical features of involved bowel, will usually permit not only the diagnosis of obstruction, but also the level. However, several case reports stress that ultrasound may have a role in the evaluation of a closed obstructed loop as may occur in the afferent loop following gastrectomy,[85–87] or the internal or Richters hernia, or in intra-abdominal banding.[88] In these cases the obstructed loop may contain no gas and therefore will be invisible on the plain radiograph. The demonstration of fluid-filled loops indicates the retention of fluid within the bowel. The recognition of valvulae conniventes or haustra of the involved bowel may allow an assessment of the level of obstruction[9, 88] (Figs. 6.27 and 6.28). Absence of peristalsis within the affected loops is also a sign of an abnormality of intestinal transit, but the demonstration of fluid-filled bowel loops is not specific for obstruction and may be seen also in ileus of a paralytic nature. The major role, then, is in the evaluation of the gasless abdomen,[89] which is therefore radiographically obscure. Occasionally careful ultrasound evaluation may demonstrate the cause of the obstruction, for instance a strangulated inguinal hernia presenting as an inguinal pseudokidney.[90] However, such is the enthusiasm of some authors for the technique that one report indicates that in 48 cases of obstruction all were diagnosed by ultrasound, even when there was not a gasless abdomen on the plain radiograph of the abdomen. These workers used the decubitus position, placing the transducer in the most dependent portion.[91] In infants and children the distended gasless abdomen is considered a "fertile field for ultrasound."[92] Applying ultrasound in these cases revealed a variety of pathological entities, including small and large bowel obstruction, mesenteric cysts, and intestinal rupture including meconium peritonitis.

Although ultrasound will demonstrate distended fluid-filled loops of bowel, it must be remembered that not all fluid is without echoes. There are a number of reports indicating that bowel containing "echogenic fluid" may be confused with solid masses because of the heterogeneous nature of the contained fluid[19, 93–94] (Fig. 6.29). Furthermore, certain unusual mixtures within the gut may produce brightly reflective "masses" within the bowel lumen. This appears to be the case in malabsorption in infants where a suspension of milk, fluid, and air is thought to account for highly reflective contents within distended loops of bowel.[95]

ABNORMAL GAS PATTERNS

Rather less attention is paid to abnormal appearance or distribution of intraintestinal gas. For the most part the distribution of intestinal gas is considered only as an impediment to adequate ultrasound imaging, either of the bowel or of underlying organs. However, several authors have stressed the importance of bowel gas in evaluating the distribution and nature of ascitic fluid[96] (Fig. 6.30).

In cases of intestinal obstruction, distension of the abdomen by an excessive widespread distribution of bowel gas may be detected (Fig. 6.31). The configu-

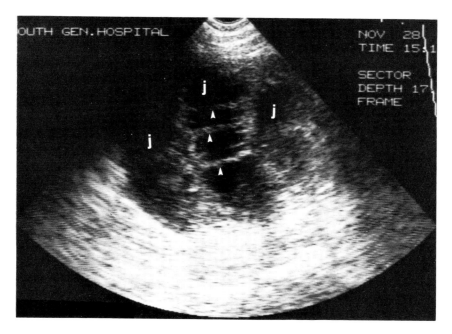

FIG. 6.28.   Dilated loops of small bowel in small bowel obstruction with the small bowel identified as jejunum, *j*, by the valvulae conniventes (arrowheads).

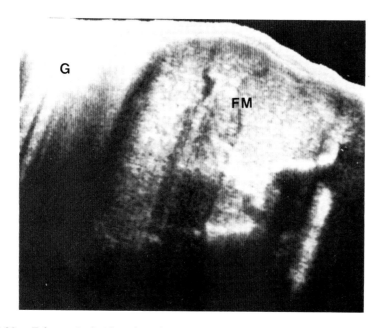

FIG. 6.29.   Echogenic fluid within distended bowel giving the appearance of a solid mass, *FM*. In this patient a carcinoma of the splenic flexure produced large bowel obstruction with retention of fluid fecal matter. (*G* = bowel gas.)

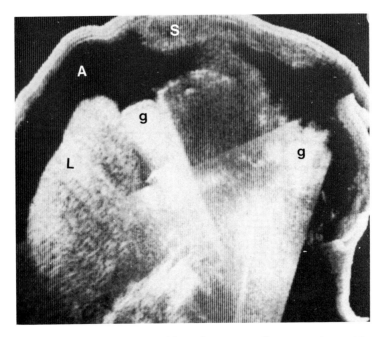

FIG. 6.30. Abnormal distribution of bowel gas in malignant ascites with tethering of bowel to the posterior abdominal wall, *g*. There are large plaque like serosal metastases, *S*. (*A* = ascitic fluid, *L* = liver.)

ration of bowel gas pattern and distribution may also be altered in certain malabsorption states in infants,[95] and this author has demonstrated an abnormal bowel gas pattern of unusual distribution in coeliac disease (Dubbins unpublished). In this situation multiple reverberant echoes are widely distributed within dilated small bowel loops (Fig. 6.32).

The pattern of bowel gas is a constantly changing one because of the movement of bowel contents by peristalsis. Qualitative analysis of intestinal motility depends on the demonstration of movement of gas microbubbles between bowel loops. Reduction or absence of motion of the microbubbles constitutes evidence of abnormal bowel motility.

A specific condition where evaluation of motion of gas microbubbles has a particular role is in the assessment of gastroesophageal reflux. Scanning the esophagogastric junction in long axis angled to the left of midline allows the demonstration of ascending microbubbles in the lower third of the esophagus. This technique may be used as a screening tool prior to formal contrast barium studies.[97]

Herniae

The herniation of loops of bowel into abnormal sites represents a special form of bowel gas of unusual distribution. As early as 1975 the first case report of the ultrasound demonstratio ⎎ of a spigelian hernia was recorded

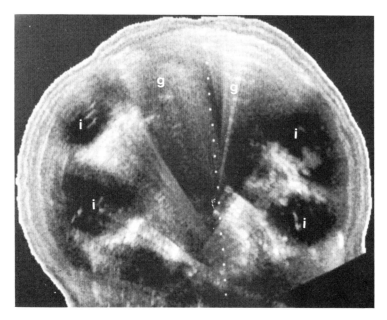

FIG. 6.31.   Small and large bowel obstruction with dilated loops of bowel, *i,* abdominal distention, and considerable amounts of bowel gas, *g.*

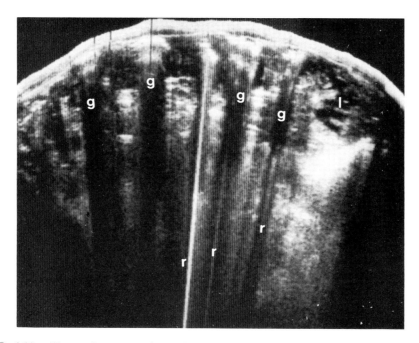

FIG. 6.32.   Unusual pattern of gas distribution, *g* with odd reverberation patterns, *r,* with some dilated loops of small bowel, *l,* seen in certain types of malabsorption, such as this patient with coeliac disease.

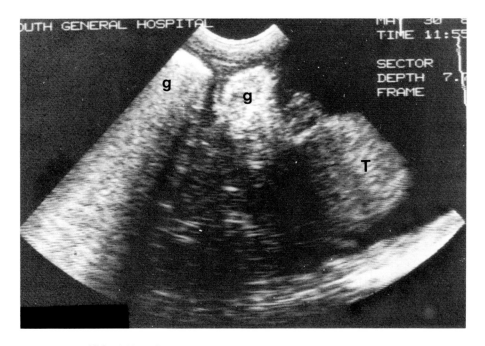

FIG. 6.33.   Gas containing scrotal hernia, *g*. (*T* = testis.)

by demonstration of the defect in the anterior abdominal wall and its fat and gas content.[98] Many other case reports have followed, and the value of ultrasound in the differentiation of this condition from other anterior abdominal wall swellings such as rectus sheath hematoma, etc. has been stressed.[99] It is also possible to diagnose herniae elsewhere and similarly to differentiate herniae from other pathology. Several workers suggest that ultrasound may allow a specific preoperative diagnosis in the evaluation of masses in the scrotum and in the inguinal region. The diagnosis of a hernia can be made on the ultrasound demonstration of hernial contents such as echogenic fat, fluid filled bowel loops, intestinal gas with shadowing, or on occasion, a pseudokidney appearance in an incarcerated hernia with an edematous bowel wall[90, 100–103] (Fig. 6.33).

NEW APPLICATIONS

Gastrointestinal ultrasound is no longer restricted to the interpretation of grey scale images produced by transabdominal insonation. The realization that ultrasound transducers could be used peroperatively, could be introduced into the body cavities, and used in conjunction with direct vision during formal endoscopy has resulted in fast expanding new fields of research and development for the role of ultrasound in the investigation of the gastrointestinal tract.

PEROPERATIVE ULTRASOUND

Much of the work concerning peroperative imaging has revolved around the demonstration of pancreatic tumors and the identification and location of calculus disease of the biliary and renal tract. The realization that high resolution ultrasound allows the demonstration of different mucosal and muscle layers of bowel has now led to the suggestion that peroperative staging of, for example, gastric cancer, is extremely accurate and allows the demonstration of depth of penetration and lateral wall extension of the gastric tumor.[104]

However, it is in the field of peroperative Doppler scanning in the assessment of intestinal viability that much attention has been focused. Early work had indicated that simple, continuous-wave Doppler flow meters could demonstrate patency of flow in small mesenteric vessels at the time of operation, and compromise of flow in experimental occlusion of mesenteric vessels could also be detected.[105] There are many situations, both pathological and iatrogenic, where the mesenteric circulation is at risk and the use of continuous wave Doppler scanning to predict intestinal viability has been shown to be of value in the assessment of blood flow following immobilization of the colon for esophageal bypass[106]; as an indication for reimplantation of the inferior mesenteric artery into the graft following aneurysmectomy, if temporary occlusion of the vessel produces diminished flow in the left colon[107]; in predicting ischemic stricture formation in patients undergoing resection of the small intestine or colon with primary anastomosis[108]; and in the determination of the extent of resection required in ischemic disease of the bowel.[109] In certain experimental work it appears that integrity of an anastomosis is assured if a Doppler signal is audible within 1 cm of the anastomosis, but if the last audible signal is greater than 2 cm from the anastomosis, a significant proportion will show evidence of stricture or anastomotic disruption.[110]

ENDOSONOGRAPHY

There are currently two different approaches to the introduction of ultrasound transducers into the lumen of the intestinal tract. The first, which may be described as endosonography, is the blind introduction of either a linear array or radial scanner into the rectum or esophagus. Although certain prototype blind esophageal scanners are under evaluation, there are no published works relating to this modality. However, the evaluation of the rectum by endosonography was first described by Wild and Reid in 1956, and an image demonstrating the muscular structure and mucosa of the colon was obtained with this early echo endoprobe[111] (Fig. 6.34). The introduction of high resolution, high frequency transducers to the evaluation of the rectal wall has markedly improved the accuracy of assessment of depth of invasion of tumor. It is possible to demonstrate whether tumor is confined to the muscularis or extends into the perirectal fat, although it remains difficult to determine

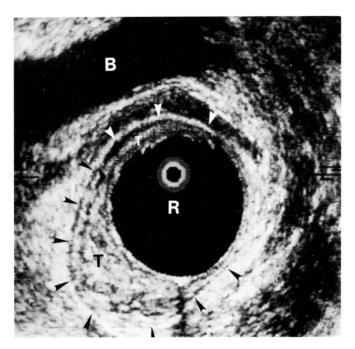

FIG. 6.34.   Transrectal ultrasound of rectal tumor, *T*. The radial transducer is within the rectum, *R*, and there is a large tumor mass involving the mucosal and submucosal layers. However, the echo poor muscularis propria and echogenic serosal layer (arrowheads) remain intact without evidence of tumor invasion. (*B* = bladder.) (Courtesy of Bruel & Kjaer U.K. Ltd., Harrow, Midox, England.)

stages T1 and T2, i.e., involvement of the mucosa and sub-mucosa versus the muscularis.[112] The ability to demonstrate the extent of the tumor and its degree of invasion can, however, have an influence on the choice of operative techniques, as well as determining the need for preoperative radiotherapy in those tumors which have extended beyond the muscularis propria[113] (Fig. 6-35). The accuracy of staging of rectal tumor varies between 72 percent and 86 percent[114, 115] and most of the errors are due to an overestimation of the depth of invasion, possibly due to coexisting inflammation.[116] A significant limitation of the technique however, is that, in those patients who present with a tumor producing marked stricturing of the colon, it is impossible to produce images of the tumor because of the failure to pass the instrument through the stricture.[117]

ENDOSCOPIC ULTRASOUND

Much of the evaluation of the applications of endoscopic ultrasound have been directed at organs immediately adjacent to the stomach, and for which the stomach provides a new acoustic window. The first report using a small A mode transducer in conjunction with a endoscope discussed the role of

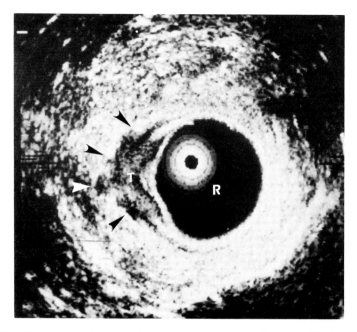

FIG. 6.35.   Transrectal ultrasound of recurrence of rectal tumor. *T*, the transrectal transducer, is identified within the rectum, R. There is an irregular tumor mass which has breached the five layers of the gut (arrowheads) with one area of tumor extension to the pelvic musculature (white arrowhead). (Courtesy of Bruel & Kjaer U.K. Ltd., Harrow, Midox, England.)

the technique in the context of the evaluation of masses deforming the gastric wall.[118] The introduction of small real-time linear array and radial scanners suggested the possibility of high resolution ultrasound evaluation of several of the upper abdominal organs.[119, 120] With the use of higher resolution transducers, it has become apparent that it is possible to characterize the mucosal and muscle layers of the upper intestinal wall, and thus assess the intramural and transmural infiltration of tumors in the esophagus, stomach, and duodenum, as well as detect extraesophageal and extragastric lymphadenopathy.[121–126] Indeed the accuracy of the assessment of the degree of vertical invasion by endoscopic ultrasound is reported to be between 83 percent in tumors limited to the mucosa and 100 percent when the degree of invasion has reached the serosa.[125]

It has also proved possible to introduce small Doppler crystals of both continuous wave and pulsed wave format to evaluate blood flow to the upper gastrointestinal tract. This has proved useful in the detection of blood vessels in close proximity to peptic ulcers, and therefore in predicting rebleeding rates;[126] in the assessment of proximity of vessels to the ampulla of Vater prior to papillotomy and evaluation of blood flow in esophageal varices before and after sclerosis.[127, 128]

CONCLUSION

Ultrasound evaluation of the gut is no longer restricted to an excuse for being unable to visualize other structures within the abdomen. An appreciation of the normal appearances of the gastrointestinal tract is vital to all those performing abdominal sonography. In certain pathologies such as idiopathic hypertrophic pyloric stenosis, intussusception, Crohn's disease, and even appendicitis, it provides an alternative method of diagnosis and management. In certain age groups, such as the very old, it may obviate the need for more invasive procedures in conditions such as tumors of the large bowel[76] and paradoxically almost, in certain cases of obscure intestinal obstruction.

The introduction of newer techniques, such as endosonography and endoscopic ultrasound and the application of transabdominal Doppler scanning in the evaluation of blood flow in gastric and mesenteric vessels may mean that the dream of being able to examine the entire mucosa and intestinal wall of the upper and lower gastrointestinal tracts, as well as determining the physiology and pathophysiology of blood supply simply with ultrasound, may become a reality.

REFERENCES

1. Holm HH, Rasmussen SN, Kristensen JK: Errors and pitfalls in ultrasonic scanning of the abdomen. Br J Radiol 45:835, 1972
2. Teele RL, Rosenfield AT, Freedman GS: The anatomic splenic flexure: An ultrasonic renal imposter. Am J Roentgenol 128:115, 1977
3. Berger M, Smith EH, Bartrum RJ, et al: False positive diagnoses of pancreatic tail lesions caused by colon. JCU 5:(5)343, 1977
4. Deeths TM, Kilcoyne RF: The use of gas as a contrast agent for abdominal ultrasound. JCU 3:(2)139, 1975
5. Yeh HC, Wolf BS: Ultrasonic contrast study to identify stomach tap water microbubbles. JCU 5:(3)170, 1977
6. Gooding GAW, Laing FC: Rapid water infusion: A technique in the ultrasonic discrimination of the gas-free stomach from a mass in the pancreatic tail. Gastrointest Radiol 4:139, 1979
7. Rubin CS, Kurtz AB, Goldberg BB: Water enema: A new ultrasonic technique in defining pelvic anatomy. JCU 6:28, 1978
8. Kurtz AB, Rubin CS, Kramer SL, Goldberg BB: Ultrasound evaluation of the posterior pelvic compartment. Radiology 132:677, 1979
9. Fleischer AC, Muhletaler CA, Everette JA: Sonographic patterns arising from normal and abnormal bowel. Radiol Clin North Am 18:(1)145, 1980
10. Matsue H: Ultrasonography of stomach: method and indication. J Medical Imagings 13:992, 1983
11. Nakagawa K, Nishiki M, Kawanishi H, et al: Ultrasonographic diagnosis of gastric carcinoma. Hiroshima J Med Sci 33:(4)739, 1984
12. Oliva L, Biggi E, Derchi LE, Cicio GR: Ultrasonic anatomy of the fluid-filled duodenum. JCU 9:245, 1981

13. Fleischer A, Dowling AD, Weinstein ML, Everette JA: Sonographic patterns of distended, fluid-filled bowel. Radiology 133:681, 1979

14. Suramo I, Paivansalo M, Vuoria P: Shadowing and reverberation artifacts in abdominal ultrasonography. Eur J Radiol 5:147, 1985

15. Avruch L, Cooperberg PL: The ring down artifact. J Ultrasound Med 4:21, 1985

16. Thickman D, Ziskin MC, Goldenberg NJ, Linder BE: Clinical manifestations of the comet tail artifact. J Ultrasound Med 2:225, 1983

17. Sommer FG, Taylor KJW: Differentiation of acoustic shadowing due to calculi and gas collections. Radiology 135:399, 1980

18. Weill F, Zeltner F, Rohmer P, et al: Les images gastriques et intestinales en ultrasonographie abdominale. J Radiol 60:(10) 579, 1979

19. Flanagan M, Dubbins PA: An unusual bowel pseudotumor, JCU 12:2926, 1984

20. Dubbins PA, Kurtz AB: Normal and abnormal bowel. p. 287. In Goldberg BB (ed): Abdominal Ultrasonography, 2nd Ed., John Wiley & Sons, New York, 1984

21. Derchi LE, Musante F, Biggi E, Cicio GR, Oliva L: Sonographic appearance of fecal masses. J Ultrasound Med 4:573, 1985

22. Fleischer AC, Muhletaler CA, Everette James A: Sonographic assessment of the bowel wall. AJR 136:887, 1981

23. Kuroiwa T, Hirata H, Yasumori K, Matsusaka T, Ninomiya K, Kawamura S: Ultrasonographic measurements of the normal gastric wall. Nippon Igaicu Hoshasen Gakkai 43:1273, 1983

24. Bateman DN, Leeman S, Metreweli C, Wilson K: A non-invasive technique for gastric motility measurement. Br J Radiol 50:526, 1977

25. Holt S, McDicken WN, Anderson T, Stewart IC, Heading RC: Dynamic imaging of the stomach by real-time ultrasound—a method for the study of gastric motility. Gut 21:596, 1980

26. King PM, Adam RD, Pryde A, McDicken WN, Heading RC: Relationships of human antroduodenal motility and transpyloric fluid movement: non-invasive observations with real-time ultrasound. Gut 25:1384, 1984

27. Bolondi L, Bortolotti M, Santi V, Calletti T, Gaiani S, Labo G: Measurement of gastric emptying time by real-time ultrasonography. Gastroenterology 89:752, 1985

28. Holt S, Cervantes J, Wilkinson A, Kirk Wallace JH: Measurement of gastric emptying rate in humans by real-time ultrasound. Gastro-enterology 90:918, 1986

29. Walls WJ: The evaluation of malignant gastric neoplasms by ultrasonic B-scanning. Radiology 118:159, 1976

30. Lutz HT, Petzoldt R: Ultrasonic patterns of space occupying lesions of the stomach and the intestine. Ultrasound Med Biol 2:129, 1976

31. Mascatello VJ, Carrera GF, Teele RL, Berger M, Holm HH, Smith EH: The ultrasonic demonstration of gastric lesions. JCU 5:383, 1977

32. Kremer H, Kellner E, Schierl W, Zollner N: Sonographische diagnosstik bei infiltrativen Magen-Darm-Erkrankungen. DMW 23:9, 1978

33. Bluth E, Merritt CRB, Sullivan MA: Ultrasonic evaluation of of the stomach, small bowel, and colon. Radiology 133:677, 1979

34. Morgan CL, Trought WS, Oddson TA, et al: Ultrasound patterns of disorders affecting the gastrointestinal tract. Radiology 135:129, 1980

35. Schwerk W, Braun B, Dombrowski H: Real-time ultrasound examination in the diagnosis of gastrointestinal tumors. JCU 7:425, 1979

36. Peterson LR, Cooperberg PL: Ultrasound demonstration of lesions of the gastrointestinal tract. Gastrointest Radiol 3:303, 1978

37. Derchi LE, Lerace T, De Pra L, et al: The sonographic appearance of duodenal lesions. J Ultrasound Med 5:269, 1986

38. DiCandio G, Mosca F, Campatalli A, et al: Sonographic detection of postsurgical recurrence of Crohn disease. AJR 146:523, 1986

39. Teele RL, Smith EH: Ultrasound in the diagnosis of idiopathic hypertrophic pyloric stenosis. N Engl J Med 296:1149, 1977

40. Graif M, Itzchak Y, Avigard I, et al: The pylorus in infancy: overall sonographic assessment. Pediatr Radiol, 14:14, 1984

41. Deeg KH, Zeilinger G, Bowing B, Brandl U: Sonographische Diagnose der hypertrophen pylorusstenose im kindesalter. Ultraschall 6:320, 1985

42. Stunden RJ, LeQuesne GW, Little KET: The improved ultrasound diagnosis of hypertrophic pyloric stenosis. Pediatr Radiol 16:200, 1986

43. Blumhagen JD, Noble HGS: Muscle thickness in hypertrophic pyloric stenosis. AJR 140:221, 1983

44. Strauss S, Itzchak Y, Manor A, et al: Sonography of hypertrophic pyloric stenosis. AJR 136:1057, 1981

45. dell'Agnola CA, Tomaselli V, Colombo C, Fagnani AM: Reliability of ultrasound for the diagnosis of hypertrophic pyloric stenosis. J Pediatr Gastroenterol Nutr 3:539, 1984

46. Sauerbrei EE, Paloschi GG: The ultrasonic features of hypertrophic pyloric stenosis, with emphasis on the postoperative appearance. Radiology 147:503, 1983

47. Sarti DA, Zablen MA: The ultrasonic findings in intussusception of the blind loop in a jejunoileal bypass for obesity. JCU 7:50, 1979

48. Burke LF, Clark E: Ileocolic intussusception—A case report. JCU 5:346, 1980

49. Montali G, Croce F, De Pra L, Solbiati L: Intussusception of the bowel: a new sonographic pattern. Br J Radiol 56:621, 1983

50. Alessi V, Salerno G, The "Hayfork" sign in the ultrasonic diagnosis of intussusception. Gastrointest Radiol 10:177, 1985

51. Bersani D, Wagner K, Lallemand M, Richert MP: Invagination intestinate aigue. J Radiol 66:739, 1985

52. Swischuk LE, Hayden CK, Boulden T: Intussusception: Indications for ultrasonography and an explanation of the doughnut and pseudokidney signs. Pediatr Radiol 15:388, 1985

53. Pracros JP, Tran-Minh VA, Wright C: Ultrasound diagnosis of intussusception (Letter) Lancet Vol 2. (8457) 733, 1985

54. Dubbins PA: Ultrasound demonstration of bowel wall thickness in inflammatory bowel disease. Clin Radiol 35:227, 1984

55. Bluth EI, McVay LV, Gathright JB: Ultrasonic Characteristics of Ileal Tuberculosis. Dis Colon Rectum 28:613, 1985

56. Holt S, Samuel E: Grey scale ultrasound in Crohn's disease. Gut 20:590, 1979

57. Sonnenberg A, Erckenbrecht J, Peter P, Neiderau C: Detection of Crohn's disease by ultrasound. Gastroenterology 83:430, 1982

58. Wellmann Von W, Gebel M, Freise J, Grote R: Sonographie in der diagnostik der ileitis terminalis Crohn, Frotschr Rontgenstr 133:146, 1980

59. Kaftori JK, Pery M, Kleinhaus U: Ultrasonography in Crohn's disease. Gastrointest Radiol 9:137, 1984

60. Jenss H, Klott KJ, Malchow H: Sonografie: Darstellung von fisteln und abszessen beim morbus Crohn. Leber Magen Darm 10:317, 1980

61. Cammarota T, Pera A, Bellando P, et al: L'esame ecotomografico nella diagnosi del morbo di Crohn. Radiol Med (Torino) 71:597, 1985

62. Dinkel E, Dittrich M, Peters H, Baumann W: Real-time ultrasound in Crohn's disease: characteristic features and clinical implications. Pediatr Radiol 16:8, 1981

63. Parulekar SG: Sonography of colonic diverticultis. J Ultrasound Med 4:659, 1985

64. Eisenscher A, Traverse G: Aspect echographique de la gastrite hypertrophique geante ou la maladie de Menetrier. J Radiol 61:527, 1980

65. Kodroff MB, Hartenberg MA, Goldschmidt RA: Ultrasonographic diagnosis of gangrenous bowel in neonatal necrotizing enterocolitis. Pediatr Radiol 14:168, 1984

66. Takada T, Yasuda H, Uchiyama K, Hasegawa H: Use of ultrasonography in the evaluation of acute appendicitis. Nippon Igaku Hoshasen Gakkai Zasshi 45:343, 1985

67. Karstrup S, Torp-Pederson S, Roikjaer O: Ultrasonic visualisation of the inflamed appendix. Br J Radiol 59:985, 1986

68. Puylaert JBC, Acute appendicitis: US evaluation using graded compression. Radiology 158:355, 1986

69. Dubbins PA: A sound approach to the diagnosis of acute appendicitis (editorial) Lancet 2 (8526):198, 1987

70. Madrazo BL, Hricak H, Sandler MA, Eyler WR: Sonographic findings in complicated peptic ulcer. Radiology 140:457, 1981

71. Seitz K, Reising KD: Sonographischer Nachweis freier Luft in der Bauchhohle. Ultraschall 3:4, 1982

72. Parulekar S, Lubert M: Ultrasound demonstration of giant duodenal ulcer. Gastrointest Radiol 8:29, 1983

73. Rosenburg ER, Morgan CL, Trought WS, Oddson TA: The ultrasonic recognition of a gastric ulcer. Br J Radiol 53:1014, 1980

74. Derchi LE, Biggi E, Neumaier CE, Cicio GR: Ultrasonographic appearances of gastric cancer. Br J Radiol 56:365, 1983

75. Rutgeerts L, Verbanck J: Sonographic detection of infiltrating gastric lesions. Acta Gastroenterol Belg XLVII:464, 1984

76. Owens AP, Banerjee B, Morewood DJW: Sonography as an aid to diagnosis of caecal carcinoma in the elderly. Clin Radiol 34:669, 1983

77. Derchi L, Biggi E, Rollandi GA, et al: Sonographic staging of gastric cancer. AJR 140:273, 1983

78. Simeone JF, Dembner AG, Mueller PR: Invasion of the pancreas by gastric carcinoma: ultrasonic appearance. JCU 8:501, 1980

79. Subramanyam BR, Balthazar EJ, Raghavendra BN, Madamba MR: Sonography of exophytic gastrointestinal leiomyosarcoma. Gastrointest Radiol 7:47, 1982

80. Derchi L, Banderali A, Chiara Bossi M, et al: The sonographic appearances of gastric lymphoma. J Ultrasound Med 3:251, 1984

81. Miller JH, Hindman BW, Lam AHK: Ultrasound in the evaluation of small bowel lymphoma in children. Radiology 135:409, 1980

82. Salem S, Hiltz CW: Ultrasonographic appearance of gastric lymphosarcoma. JCU 6:377, 1978

83. Ennis MG, MacErlean DP: Biopsy of bowel wall pathology under ultrasound control. Gastrointest Radiol 6:17, 1981

84. Solbiati L, Montali G, Croce F, et al: Fine needle aspiration biopsy of bowel lesions under ultrasound guidance; Indications and results. Gastrointest Radiol 11:172, 1986

85. Hauser JB, Stanley RJ, Geisse G: The ultrasound findings in an obstructed afferent loop. JCU 2:287, 1974

86. Feiss JS, Raskin MM, Wolfe J, et al: A case of afferent loop obstruction secondary to recurrent carcinoma of the stomach with ultrasound and C.T. scan findings. Am J Gastroenterol 68:77, 1977.

87. Berger LA: Chronic afferent loop obstruction diagnosed by ultrasound. Br J Radiol 53:810, 1980

88. Scheible W, Goldberger LE: Diagnosis of small bowel obstruction: The contribution of diagnostic ultrasound. AJR 133:3685, 1979

89. Bosiljevac JE, Harrison PB, Kouiri SH, Reeves BF: Intestinal obstruction: abdominal ultrasonography for diagnosis of difficult cases. J Kans Med Soc 207, 1981.

90. Avni EF, Brombart JC, Da Costa PM: L'examen echographique dans les occlusions intestinales. J Radiol 63:409, 1982

91. Meiser G, Meissner K: Sonographische Differentialdiagnose des darmverschlusses—Ergebnisse einer prospektiven untersuchung an 48 patienten. Ultraschall 6:39, 1985

92. Seibert JJ, Williamson SL, Golladay ES, et al: The distended gasless abdomen: A fertile field for ultrasound. J Ultrasound Med 5:301, 1986

93. Kurtz AB, Dubbins PA, Rubins CS: Echogenicity—analysis significance and masking. AJR 137:471, 1981

94. Soderlund V, Mortensson W, Nybonde T: Fluid filled structures simulating solid tumors at ultrasonography—a report on five cases. Pediatr Radiol 16:110, 1986

95. Avni EF, Gansbeke D, Rodesch P, et al: Sonographic demonstration of malabsorption in neonates. J Ultrasound Med 5:85, 1986

96. Edell SL, Geftel LUB: Ultrasonic differentiation of type of ascitic fluid. AJR 133:111, 1979

97. Naik DR, Moore DJ, Ultrasound diagnosis of gastroesophageal reflux. Arch Dis Child 59:366, 1984

98. Spangen L: Ultrasound as a diagnostic aid in ventral abdominal hernia. JCU 3:211, 1975

99. Fried AM, Meeker WR: Incarcerated Spigelian hernia: ultrasonic differential diagnosis. AJR 133:107, 1979

100. Subramanyan BR, Balthazar EJ, Rghavendra BN, Horii SC, Hilton S: Sonographic diagnosis of scrotal hernia. AJR 139:535, 1982

101. Deitch EA, Soncrant MC: The value of ultrasound in the diagnosis of nonpalpable femoral hernias. Arch Surg 116:185, 1981

102. Lineweaver W, Vlasak M, Muyshondt E: Ultrasonic examination of abdominal wall and groin masses. South med J 76:590, 1983

103. Deitch EA, Soncrant MC: Ultrasonic diagnosis of surgical disease of the inguinal-femoral region. Sur Gynecol Obstet 152:319, 1981

104. Machi J, Takeda J, Sigel B, Kakegawa T: Normal stomach wall and gastric cancer: evaluation with high resolution operation US. Radiology 159:85, 1986

105. Wright CB, Hobson RW: Prediction of intestinal viability using Doppler ultrasound technics. American J Surgery 129:642, 1975

106. Kurstin RD, Soltanzedeh H, Hobson RW, Wright CB: Ultrasonic blood flow assessment in colon esophageal bypass procedures. Arch Surg 112:270, 1977

107. Hobson RW, Wright CB, O'Donnell JA, et al: Determination of intestinal viability by Doppler ultrasound. Arch Surg 114:165, 1979

108. Cooperman M, Martin EW, Keith LM, Carey LC: Use of Doppler ultrasound in intestinal surgery. Am J Surg 138:856, 1979

109. Cooperman M, Martin EW, Carey LC: Evaluation of ischemic intestine by Doppler ultrasound. Am J Surg 139:73, 1980

110. Cooperman M, Pace WG, Martin EW, et al: Determination of viability of ischemic intestine by Doppler ultrasound. Surgery 83:705, 1978

111. Wild JJ, Foderick JW: The feasibility of echometric detection of cancer in the lower

gastrointestinal tract Part II. Am J Proctol Gastroenterol Colon Rectal Surg Vol 29:11, 1978

112. Hildebrandt U, Feifel G: Preoperative staging of rectal cancer by intrarectal ultrasound. Dis Colon Rectum 28:42, 1985

113. Pahlman L, Adalsteinsson B, Glimelius B, et al: Ultrasound in preoperative staging of rectal tumours. Acta Radiol (Diagn) 25:489, 1984

114. Alzin HH, Kohlberger E, Schwaiger R, Alloussi S: Valeur de l'echographie endorectale dans la chirurgie du rectum. Ann Radiol 26:334, 1983

115. Feifel G, Hildebrandt U, Dhom G: Die endorectale sonographie beim rectumcarcinom. Chirurg 56:398, 1985

116. Saitoh N, Okui K, Sarashina H, et al: Evaluation of echographic diagnosis of rectal cancer using intrarectal ultrasonic examination. Dis Colon Rectum 29:234, 1986

117. Dragsted J, Gammelgaard J: Endoluminal ultrasonic scanning in the evaluation of rectal cancer: a preliminary report of 13 cases. Gastrointest Radiol 8:367, 1983

118. Lutz H, Rosch W: Transgastroscopic ultrasonography. Endoscopy 8:203, 1976

119. Lux G, Heyder N, Lutz H, Demling L: Endoscopic ultrasonography—technique, orientation and diagnostic possibilities. Endoscopy 14:220, 1982

120. Hisanaga K, Hisanaga A, Nagata K, Ichie Y: High speed rotating scanner for transgastric sonography. AJR 135:627, 1980

121. Strohm WD, Classen M: Endoskopische Ultraschalluntersuchung des osophagus. Deutsche Medizinische Wochenschrift 20:783, 1985

122. Heyder Von H: Ultraschall-endoskopie—eine bereicherung der gastrointestinalen diagnostik. Fortschr Med 103:1044, 1985

123. Caletti G, Bolondi L, Labo G: Ultrasonic endoscopy—the gastrointestinal wall. Scand J Gastroenterol (Suppl) (94) 102:7:1984

124. Tio TL, Tytgat GN: Endoscopic ultrasonography in the assessment of intra and transmural infiltration of tumours in the oesophagus, stomach, and papilla of Vater and in the detection of extraoesophageal lesions. Endoscopy 16:2033, 1984

125. Yamanaka T, Yoshida Y, Ueno N, et al: Endoscopic ultrasonography in the diagnosis of the degree of vertical invasion of gastric cancer. Nippon Shokakibyo Gakkai Zassi 82:32, 1985

126. Beckly DB, Casebow MP: Prediction of rebleeding from peptic ulcer: experience with an endoscopic Doppler device. Gut 27:96, 1986

127. Martin RW, Gilbert DA, Silverstein FE, et al: An endoscopic Doppler probe for assessing intestinal vasculature. Ultrasound Med Biol 11:61, 1985

128. Silverstein FE, Deltlenre M, Tytgat G, et al: An endoscopic Doppler probe: preliminary clinical evaluation. Ultrasound Med Biol 11:347, 1985

7 Abdominal Fluid Collections: Percutaneous Aspiration and Drainage

MARTIN I. COHEN
GIOVANNA CASOLA
ERIC VANSONNENBERG

In recent years, both ultrasound and computed tomography (CT) have been used effectively for percutaneous aspiration and drainage of abdominal fluid collections. The safety and efficacy of these percutaneous procedures have made them the therapeutic method of choice. This chapter discusses the relative advantages and disadvantages of ultrasound compared with CT for the aspiration and drainage of abdominal fluid collections. We describe both the techniques for needle aspiration and catheter drainage, and the individualized management of specific fluid collections.

ADVANTAGES OF ULTRASOUND COMPARED TO CT

Ultrasound is a rapid and reliable method to search the abdomen for fluid collections. Ultrasound is especially accurate in the pelvis, liver, bile ducts, and perihepatic spaces. Following detection of an abscess, needle aspiration and catheter placement for definitive therapy are performed with ultrasound guidance, either in the ultrasound suite or at the patient's bedside.

One of the most significant advantages of ultrasound is its portable capability. This permits bedside imaging and intervention for critically ill patients who cannot be brought to ultrasound. Ultrasound has several other advantages compared to CT. The multiplanar imaging of ultrasound aids in differentiating subdiaphragmatic fluid collections from pleural effusions or empyema. The use of duplex Doppler scanning enables one to differentiate fluid collections from vascular structures such as pseudoaneurysms, for which inadvertent percutaneous drainage would be catastrophic. Ultrasound is the most appropriate imaging modality for pregnant patients and children in whom ionizing radiation from CT or fluoroscopy should be avoided. Finally, ultrasound is cheaper and more readily available than CT.

The major disadvantage of ultrasound is its limitation due to bowel gas. Bowel gas will not allow reliable exclusion of interloop abscesses or those juxtaposed to bowel. Bowel gas typically interferes with pancreatic imaging. This is especially true in toxic patients, in whom an ileus often is present. Due to the need for direct contact between the skin and transducer, open wounds, dressings, and drains also interfere with ultrasound imaging. Obesity is another factor which degrades ultrasound images.

Ultrasound has attractive benefits for percutaneous drainage. With real-time imaging, the trajectory of the needle tip can be followed directly into the fluid collection. Ultrasound-guided procedures usually can be performed in less time than that required for CT-guided procedures. Superficial abdominal wall collections and extremity abscesses are particularly amenable to ultrasound-guided aspiration and subsequent drainage. Ultrasound also is used extensively for percutaneous hepatic, biliary, renal, and gallbladder procedures. In these situations, avoidance of bowel loops is seldom a problem. Ultrasound is the guidance modality of choice for drainage of intra-abdominal fluid collections, and urinary and biliary tract drainage in pregnant patients and children. MRI may have a role in the management of fluid collections in pregnant women in whom ultrasound is inadequate.[1]

PATIENT PREPARATION

Following the discovery of an abdominal fluid collection by ultrasound, the patient is evaluated for percutaneous aspiration and drainage. Since the sonographic appearance of intra-abdominal fluid collections is nonspecific, needle aspiration is essential to ascertain the contents of the fluid collection. Noninfected collections including seromas, urinomas, bilomas, hematomas, and lymphoceles can all simulate the appearance of an abscess.

Prior to needle aspiration, informed consent is obtained, along with baseline hemoglobin and hematocrit levels, platelets, prothrombin time (PT), and partial thromboplastin time (PTT). Optimally, the PT should be within 3 seconds of control, the PTT less than 40 seconds, and platelets more than 50,000/cc prior to needle aspiration. Bleeding times are obtained only if there is a history of aspirin use, nonsteroidal antiflammatory medication, or renal failure. Coagulopathies are corrected by infusion of fresh-frozen plasma, platelets, and clotting factors. Patients are placed on clear liquids prior to the procedure, and an intravenous (IV) line is inserted. Intravenous sedation and analgesia are achieved with Versed or Valium, and fentanyl or Demerol respectively.

NEEDLE ASPIRATION AND DRAINAGE

Following diagnostic imaging, a site for the needle puncture is selected. The skin is marked using an indelible marker or pressure from a needle hub. The skin is prepped with Betadine and draped using sterile technique. Subsequently, 2 percent lidocaine is infused for local anesthesia and a skin nick is made with a #11 scalpel blade.

Determining a safe access route without transgression of bowel loops or other vital structures is essential for diagnostic needle aspiration and therapeutic catheter drainage. Traversing bowel loops may contaminate uninfected fluid collections or yield a false positive gram stain and culture. Ultrasound guidance is best suited for superficial fluid collections, percutaneous cholecystostomy, percutaneous nephrostomy, and fluid collections in the liver, retroperitoneum, and psoas muscles. There is minimal risk of inadvertent puncture of an overlying structure with ultrasound guidance in these locations.

The depth of puncture is determined from the diagnostic study, and the appropriate distance is marked on the shaft of the needle with sterile tape. A 22 gauge needle is used for all initial aspirations. Aspiration may be performed with or without a biopsy guide. The appropriate needle angulation is maintained as the needle is inserted into the fluid collection using real-time ultrasound guidance. Once the needle has entered the fluid, a few cc are aspirated, using extension tubing and a 20 cc syringe. If no fluid returns, the needle tip position is reassessed with ultrasound. If there is difficulty in localizing the needle, a number of techniques can be helpful. These include: (1) moving the stylet of the needle up and down: (2) moving the entire needle: (3) attempting to pass a 0.018-inch guidewire into the collection through the needle: or (4) injecting air or a small amount of sterile, nonbacteriostatic saline through the needle. Teflon-coated, roughened needles (Cook, Inc., Bloomington, Indiana) also improve needle visualization by ultrasound.[2]

If the needle tip is well-positioned and fluid cannot be aspirated, a larger gauge needle (20 or 18 g) is inserted using ultrasound guidance. If fluid is not aspirated at this time, biopsies of the lesion should be obtained using the needles already in position. Biopsies are obtained by connecting a 20 cc syringe directly to the hub of the needle and while suction is maintained on the syringe, the needle is moved up and down and rotated to obtain a core of tissue. Aspirated material is sent for cytology, chemistries, culture, and sensitivity. Infection within organized tissue or an unsuspected tumor may be diagnosed.

Usually fluid is recovered using the initial 22 g needle. Only a few cubic centimeters should be aspirated and sent for gram stain and culture. This ensures that the collection will remain as large as possible and therefore easier to insert a catheter into. If grossly purulent material is aspirated, broad spectrum antibiotics are administered by IV in anticipation of percutaneous catheter drainage. Occasionally, the gram stain will show polymorphonuclear leukocytes and no organisms, generally due to previous antibiotic therapy. Organisms without polymorphonuclear leukocytes indicate aspiraton of bowel contents or infection in an immunocompromised patient. Aspirated fluid also should be sent for chemical analysis including blood urea nitrogen (BUN), creatinine, amylase, bilirubin, and fat globule (lymphocele) levels to determine the origin of uncertain fluid collection.

CATHETER SELECTION

The character of the fluid aspirate is the most important determinant for catheter selection. Large bore 12 to 14 Fr double lumen catheters (i.e. vanSonnenberg Sump) (MediTech, Inc., Watertown, MA) are most effective for purulent collections. The collection must be large enough to accomodate all the catheter sideholes. Two or five hole standard sump systems are available. Sump catheters allow air to enter the collection so that the cavity wall does not collapse around the catheter and prevent drainage when suction is applied. Our preferred catheter is designed for trocar insertion, but also may be placed by Seldinger technique.[3]

Smaller, single lumen catheters in the 7 to 9 Fr range may be used for less viscous collections, such as bilomas, urinomas, and lymphoceles. Standard biliary and nephrostomy catheters are inserted using Seldinger technique. The Sacks catheter (Elecath, New Jersey) is designed for trocar insertion and is excellent for nonviscous collections. On occasion, small trocar catheters are placed directly for percutaneous nephrostomy.

CATHETER INSERTION

There are two basic methods of catheter insertion; trocar, and Seldinger. Following diagnostic aspiration and initiation of antibiotics, a deep incision is made through the skin and soft tissues adjacent to the previously inserted 22 g needle. Superficial tissues are spread using a hemostat to facilitate catheter placement. The catheter is mounted on the accompanying metal stiffening cannula through which a sharp 19 g stylet is inserted. The depth of insertion of the 22 g needle is measured and marked similarly on the drainage catheter. The previously introduced 22 g needle demonstrates a safe pathway for catheter insertion. The catheter is introduced into the collection in tandem with the 22 g needle to the appropriate depth. The inner stylet is removed and a small amount of fluid is aspirated to confirm that the catheter tip is within the collection. At this time, an .038-inch J-tipped guidewire is introduced and coiled into the cavity over which the catheter is advanced.[4] The guidewire prevents inadvertent perforation of the back wall of the collection or kinking by the catheter. This tandem trocar method is suitable for CT, ultrasound, or fluoroscopic guidance. It permits the procedure to be done using a single modality, rather than moving from one modality to another.

Seldinger technique usually is performed in conjunction with fluoroscopy.

The initial 22 g needle puncture is followed by tandem placement of a removable hub 22 g needle, or an 18 g needle, or a needle-sheath assembly.[5] The patient is moved from ultrasound or CT where initial detection and localization occurred. Fluid is aspirated from the needle or sheath prior to placement of an .038-inch guidewire into the fluid collection. Fluoroscopy is used for successive tract dilatation for the final catheter placement. The removable hub system permits coaxial insertion using only a fine needle puncture. This system is explained later in the section on Ultrasound Guided Nephrostomy.

Following catheter placement by either technique, the cavity is evacuated completely and irrigated with 15 to 20 cc aliquots of saline until the aspirated fluid is clear. Occasionally, upon completion of drainage of nonhemorrhagic collections, the aspirate will become blood-tinged. This most likely results from trauma to friable blood vessels in the cavity. Invariably this bleeding ceases spontaneously. Following saline irrigation, the catheter is secured and connected to suction.

Due to problems with skin infection and foreign body reactions to suture material, we no longer suture the catheter to the skin. Instead, using bonding cement, a stomahesive disc is glued to the skin. A Molnar disc secures the catheter by means of a plastic cinch. The Molnar disc is sutured to the elevated ring of the ostomy disc. If kept dry, this appliance will hold most catheters in place for 2 to 3 months.

PERCUTANEOUS ABSCESS AND FLUID DRAINAGE

Although the clinical presentation and sonographic appearance of a variety of intra-abdominal fluid collections are similar, approaches to catheter drainage and management may differ. For this reason, the approach to specific intra-abdominal fluid collections will be discussed.

Intra-abdominal abscesses are the most frequently drained fluid collections. The majority of patients present with fever, elevated WBC, and localizing signs. However, fever of unknown origin or an asymptomatic mass may be the presenting complaint. Intra-abdominal abscesses are most commonly postoperative, posttraumatic, or secondary to disease processes such as pancreatitis, Crohn's disease, diverticulitis, cholecysititis, appendicitis, or perforated peptic ulcer[6] (Fig. 7.1).

Regardless of the etiology, the drainage procedures follow similar guidelines. Ultrasound is most useful for drainage of upper abdominal, abdominal wall, or retroperitoneal and psoas abscesses, where interposed bowel loops rarely are a problem. Aspiration and drainage are performed as previously outlined in this chapter; generally a sump catheter is inserted to best evacuate the viscous contents of abscesses. Following evacuation of the abscess, the catheter is placed on low continuous suction. Irrigation is performed three to four times a day with 15 to 20 cc of sterile saline followed by a 5 cc flush into the drain and sump lumens to maintain patency.

A sinogram is performed at the time of initial drainage or within several days after drainage. Contrast is injected into the abscess cavity at sinography to check catheter position, size of the cavity, and to determine if any fistulas

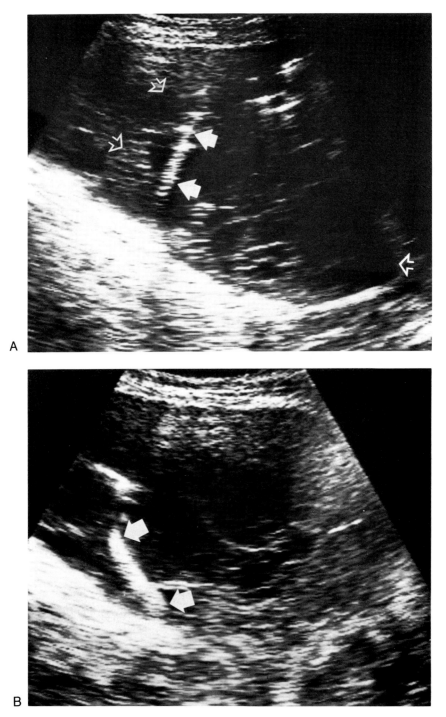

FIG. 7.1. Ultrasound-guided percutaneous abscess drainage: 70-year-old female with ovarian carcinoma 10 days post lysis of adhesions. WBC 37,000. (A) 22g needle (arrows) in 12 × 15 cm left upper quadrant abscess (open arrows). (B) 9 Fr catheter (arrows) in dependent portion of abscess. (*Figure continues.*)

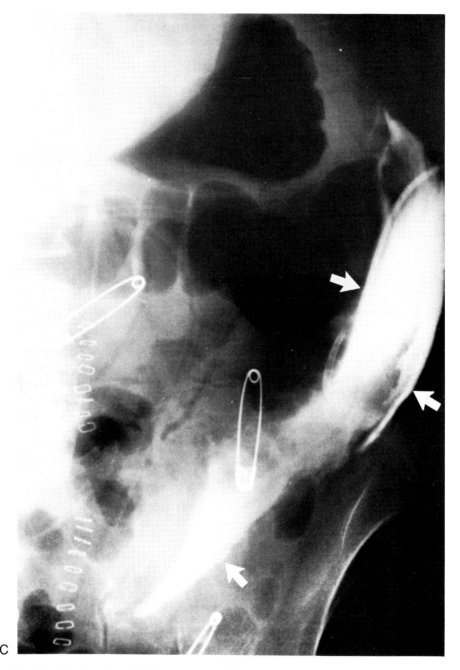

FIG. 7.1 (*Continued*). (C) Sinogram at 48 hours shows extensive abscess cavity in left paracolic gutter (arrows).

exist. Fistulas manifest clinically as high output drainage or a change in the character of the drainage. Frequently, the sinogram, several days after drainage, may detect a fistula that was not apparent at the time of initial sinography. Due to the possibility of inducing sepsis, care should be taken so that the abscess cavity is not overdistended by contrast injection. Abscesses are never injected with saline or contrast until they have been evacuated.

When the daily drainage drops below 10 cc a day and the patient's laboratory and clinical parameters no longer show evidence of toxicity, the catheter is withdrawn about 2 cm a day. This gradual catheter advancement allows the drainage tract to close without loculation of fluid within the tract or residual cavity. If there is a sudden increase in drainage, a sinogram should be repeated to determine if there is a connection to the bowel, pancreas, or the urinary or biliary tracts. If the patient remains septic after drainage, one must search for the presence of an undrained collection.

CATHETER CARE

During the course of catheter drainage, the most frequently encountered problem is a sudden decrease or absence of catheter output. Although this may be a favorable sign, a catheter-related problem must be considered. Dislodgement, kinking, clogging, and accidental stopcock closure are potential problems. Marking of the catheter with an indelible marker at the point of exit from the Molnar disc, tells if inadvertent catheter withdrawal has occurred (i.e., whether or not the catheter has pulled back). Kinking tends to occur at the point of fixation of the catheter to the Molnar disc. A kinked catheter can be temporarily splinted with plastic tubing or a portion of a tongue blade and tape. However, catheter exchange is necessary for long-term drainage. Larger (12 and 14 Fr) catheters are less likely to kink than small catheters. Inspissation of debris within the catheter lumen may entirely occlude the catheter, making irrigation difficult or impossible. Usually a 5 cc syringe filled with saline will generate enough pressure to clear the catheter. This should be followed by irrigation of the collection with 10 to 15 cc aliquots of sterile saline until the drainage clears. In the event that the lumen remains plugged, the patient should be transported to the fluoroscopy suite for catheter exchange. A variety of techniques, including exiting the guidewire out of a sidehole rather than the endhole, using the stiff end of the guidewire, placing a larger sheath over the occluded catheter, or placing a guidewire alongside the catheter tract, may be necessary for catheter exchange.[7]

SPECIFIC AREAS AND TYPES OF DRAINAGE

Amebic Abscess

Hepatic amebic abscess represents a subset of intra-abdominal abscesses where therapeutic considerations remain controversial. Medical therapy is effective in eradicating the parasites from the cyst. However, there are situations where percutaneous drainage is indicated. Most authors recommend percutaneous drainage of lesions that occur in the left lobe of the liver, and those throughout the liver in which impending rupture is feared. Additional indications include failure or intolerance of medical therapy and pregnancy.[8]

The initial needle aspiration is performed as outlined previously. In the majority of cases, trophozoites will not be aspirated. Biopsy of the cavity wall may yield these trophozoites.[8] Although the aspirate may have an "anchovy paste" appearance, it is commonly yellowish or hemorrhagic. In addition, amebic abscesses are not foul-smelling and gram stain demonstrates white blood cells without organisms. In a recent series,[8] we successfully treated 20 cases of hepatic amebic abscesses with an average of four days of percutaneous drainage. This is much more rapid than the typical course for intra-abdominal pyogenic abscesses. Early catheter removal is felt to decrease the incidence of bacterial superinfection of these collections and to expedite care. Most amebic abscesses may be drained successfully using ultrasound guidance.

Hematoma

Hematomas occur secondary to blunt or penetrating trauma, surgery, or a variety of bleeding disorders. The ultrasound appearance of hematoma ranges from hyperechoic to hypoechoic to cystic depending upon the age of the hematoma, and whether it is parenchymal or within the peritoneal cavity.[9] Septations frequently are identified within these collections, as are fluid/debris levels (Fig. 7.2). The role of percutaneous drainage in the treatment of hematomas has not been well established. Nevertheless, hematomas may cause pain, obstruct the urinary tract, or become infected; in these clinical situations, drainage often is necessary. Our experience with percutaneous drainage of hematomas has been variable. In some cases the hematoma is liquefied and catheter drainage is successful; in others, the hematoma is clot-filled and organized, and aspiration is difficult. In these cases, aggressive irrigation with saline and multiple catheters are helpful. If the patient is febrile and the collection is infected, a trial of percutaneous drainage should be attempted, even if the entire collection is not drained. Catheter drainage may help temporize the patient so that he or she is better suited for surgery. While instillation of streptokinase may be of benefit in helping to liquify hematomas,[10] the present clinical experience with this technique is limited.

Biloma

Bilomas most commonly present with upper abdominal distention or right upper quadrant discomfort in patients who have undergone recent gallbladder or hepatic surgery. Other causes include blunt trauma, percutaneous biliary drainage, or liver biopsy.[11] Bilomas tend to elicit an inflammatory reaction that confines these collections to the upper abdomen. Approximately

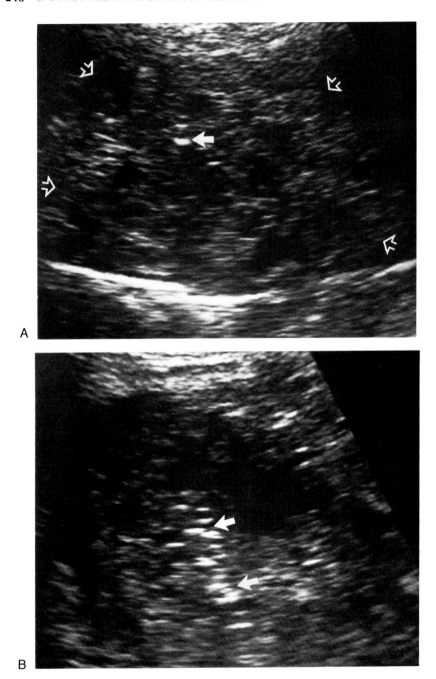

FIG. 7.2. Ultrasound-guided percutaneous hematoma aspiration and drainage: 35-year-old male, status post renal transplant removal, with lower abdominal hematoma. (A) 22 g needle (arrows) in complex fluid collection (open arrows) yielded nonclotting blood. Gram stain negative. (B) 8 Fr catheter (arrows) resulted in an additional 200 cc of nonclotting blood. (*Figure continues.*)

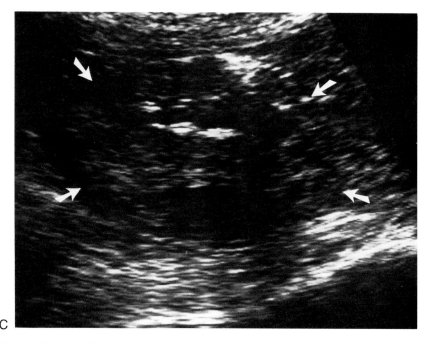

C

FIG. 7.2 (*Continued*). (C) Decreased size of collection (arrows), post aspiration. Due to noninfected contents, catheter was removed a day later.

two thirds occur in the right upper quadrant and one third in the left upper quadrant.[12] Once again, the ultrasound appearance of these fluid collections is nonspecific. A lattice of septations frequently is seen. Although small bilomas may be treated conservatively with serial ultrasound examinations to document regression, larger collections do require drainage (Fig. 7.3). Two radiologic series demonstrate the efficacy of percutaneous drainage in a total of 26 patients.[11, 12] The initial aspirate may be yellow, greenish, or frankly purulent if infected. Dipstick technique will immediately confirm the presence of bile. Single lumen or sump catheters are used, depending on the viscosity of the fluid.

In the absence of ongoing bile leakage, these collections resolve rapidly with percutaneous drainage. However, communication with major bile ducts or the gallbladder generally requires percutaneous biliary drainage to divert the flow of bile (Fig. 7.4). Surgical repair may be needed to conclude therapy.

Urinomas

Urinomas are collections of extravasated urine outside of the urinary tract. Causes are obstructive, including a calculus, surgical suture, or posterior urethral valves; alternatively, nonobstructive leakage secondary to surgery,

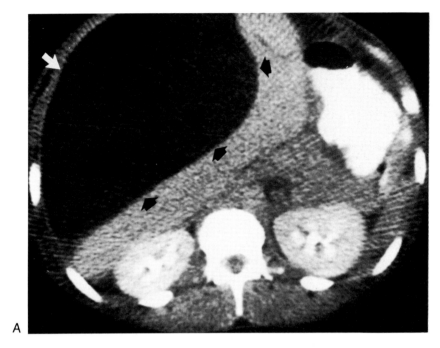

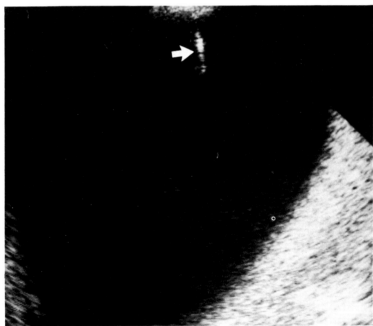

FIG. 7.3. Ultrasound-guided biloma drainage: 30-year-old male post surgery for gunshot wound to liver. Patient complained of increased abdominal girth. (A) CT scan through upper abdomen demonstrates huge right subdiaphragmatic fluid collection (arrows) displacing liver inferiorly and to the left. (B) Transverse ultrasound through upper abdomen shows 22 g needle (arrow) in anechoic biloma. (*Figure continues.*)

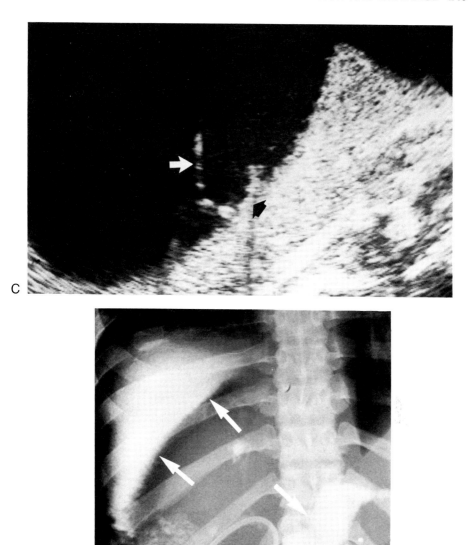

FIG. 7.3 (*Continued*). (C) Coil of catheter (arrows) within the biloma. (D) Sinogram shows contrast pooling in dependent portion of the huge biloma (arrows).

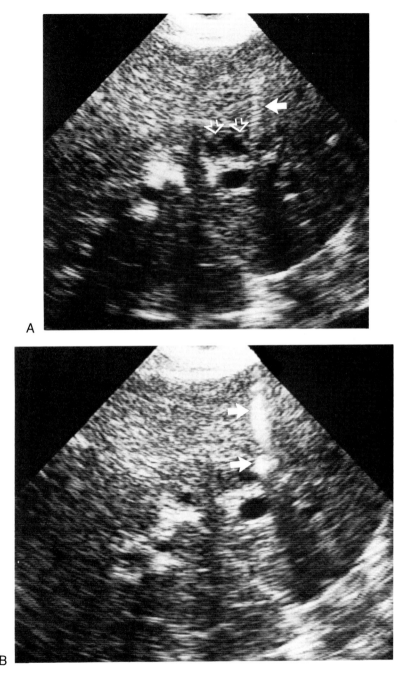

FIG. 7.4.   Ultrasound-guided drainage of bile ducts: 65-year-old male with sclerosing cholangitis and dilated left-sided bile ducts. (A) Transverse ultrasound through left lobe of liver shows 22 g needle (arrow) entering dilated left bile ducts (open arrows). (B) Dilator (arrows) entering duct. (*Figure continues.*)

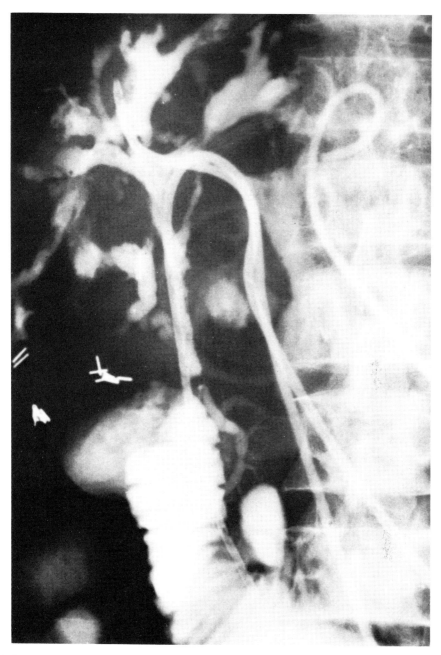

FIG. 7.4 (*Continued*). (C) Cholangiogram shows irregularly dilated bile ducts with three drainage catheters entering liver from left side.

instrumentation, or trauma may be causative. Urinomas are dynamic collections that will decrease in size or resolve completely if leakage of urine from the urinary tract ceases.[13] Percutaneous drainage is indicated with suspected infection, pain, or associated urinary tract obstruction. Diversion of the urinary flow by means of percutaneous nephrostomy or antegrade or retrograde stenting controls and decreases urine leakage. Additionally, placement of a catheter or stent allows healing of ureteral injuries. Stricture formation can be a result of surgical or catheter treatment in some patients. These are amenable to percutaneous balloon dilatation.

Due to the nonviscous nature of uninfected urinomas, medium bore 7 to 9 Fr single lumen catheters are adequate for drainage. However, with infection, these collections should be treated as abscesses, i.e., large bore sump catheters are indicated. Due to the retroperitoneal location of the majority of these collections, ultrasound guidance may be used for many cases (Fig. 7.5).

Pseudocysts

Pancreatic pseudocysts complicate 2 to 18 percent of cases of pancreatic inflammatory disease.[14] Most pseudocysts are due to alcoholic pancreatitis; other causes include idiopathic, biliary stone disease, trauma, postoperative, and tumor-related. Controversy exists as to whether pancreatic pseudocysts should be drained percutaneously or surgically. Pseudocysts that do not change in size over a period of 2 to 3 weeks and those that are greater than 4 cm in size are unlikely to resolve spontaneously. Percutaneous drainage should be attempted since these patients are at risk for complications (i.e., rupture, bleeding, infection). Additional indications for drainage include overt or suspected infection, severe pain, and biliary obstruction.[15] Although ultrasound frequently is used for initial detection, CT guidance is indicated for aspiration and catheter drainage in most patients. This is due to the better delineation of deep structures adjacent to the pancreas which must be avoided.

CT clearly defines the relationship of the pseudocyst to surrounding bowel loops. It also detects large varices which occasionally surround these collections. We no longer attempt single step needle aspiration for definitive drainage of these collections because the recurrence rate is high (about 70 percent).[15] Our current approach is diagnostic aspiration followed by catheter drainage. Following catheter drainage, a sinogram is performed to detect ductal communication and to assess cavity size. Ductal communication may not be appreciated during the initial sonogram but may be evident on follow-up studies. We have drained over 40 pancreatic pseudocysts with success in over 90 percent of cases. The average duration of drainage was 18 days and the range was 5 to 32 days. When the catheter drainage is less than 10 cc's a day, we clamp the catheter for 1 to 2 days and repeat an ultrasound or CT scan at this time. If no fluid has reaccumulated, the catheter is with-

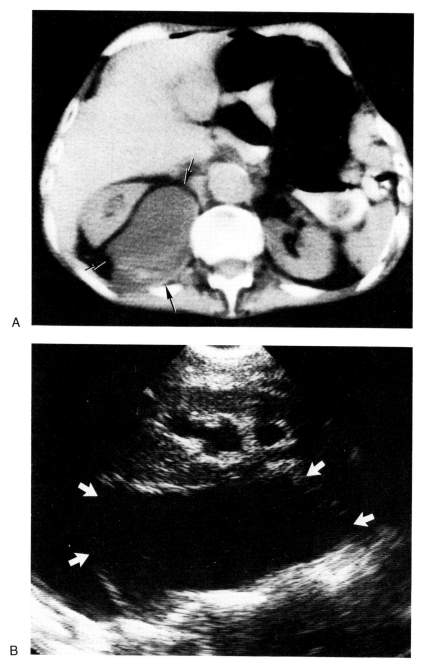

FIG. 7.5.   Ultrasound-guided urinoma drainage and percutaneous nephrostomy: 90-year-old male with bladder carcinoma. (A) Non-contrast CT shows right posterior pararenal urinoma secondary to obstruction at trigone. (B) Longitudinal ultrasound through right kidney shows grade 2 hydronephrosis and posterior fluid collection (arrows). (*Figure continues.*)

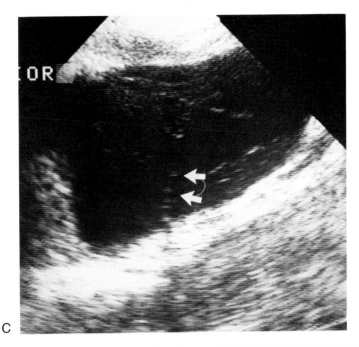

C

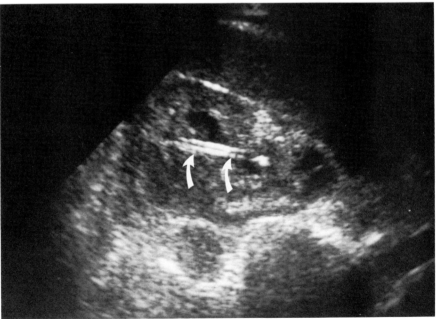

D

FIG. 7.5 (*Continued*).   (C) 22 g needle (arrow) in urinoma. (D) Longitudinal ultrasound through right kidney two weeks later shows complete resolution of urinoma. 10 Fr percutaneous nephrostomy in renal pelvis (arrows).

drawn. In the setting of a pancreatic fistula, protracted drainage may be necessary. Catheter drainage should be maintained until the fistula closes.

OTHER ULTRASOUND-GUIDED PROCEDURES

Ultrasound-Guided Percutaneous Nephrostomy

Percutaneous nephrostomy (PN) is a well established technique, first described by Casey and Goodwin in 1955.[16] Although optimally performed using both ultrasound and fluoroscopic guidance, PN can be performed using ultrasound or fluoroscopic guidance alone.

Ultrasound-guided PN is indicated for children and pregnant patients with urinary tract obstruction (Fig. 7.6). Ultrasound guidance also is helpful for the operator by eliminating or reducing radiation exposure. As such, it may be utilized in many patients who have moderate to severe hydronephrosis.

The technique of ultrasound-guided percutaneous nephrostomy involves placement of the patient in a prone-oblique position with the side of the obstructed kidney elevated 30 to 45 degrees. A preliminary ultrasound is performed in this position to determine the appropriate approach, preferably below the twelfth rib to avoid traversing the posterior pleura. Following antiseptic preparation of the flank, the skin is infiltrated with local anesthetic. A 22 g needle with a removable hub (Cook, Inc, Bloomington, Indiana) is introduced into the renal collecting system using real-time ultrasound guidance.[17] Following aspiration of urine, which is sent for culture, the hub of the 22 g needle is removed and the 18 g needle from the system is introduced to the same depth over the shaft of the 22 g needle, using a rotating motion. The 22 g needle is then removed and urine is again aspirated to confirm needle position. An .038-inch guidewire is introduced directly via the 18 g cannula and coiled in the renal pelvis. Subsequent dilatation with 6, 7, and 8 Fr dilators will allow placement of a 7.6 Fr pigtail catheter into the renal pelvis. Following aspiration of as much urine as is possible, the catheter is placed to gravity drainage.

Alternatively, trocar technique may be used in moderately to severely dilated collecting systems. Following aspiration of urine for confirmation of the position of the 22 g needle, the nephrostomy catheter is introduced directly, using a Sacks catheter in tandem with the fine needle.

PERCUTANEOUS CHOLECYSTOSTOMY

Ultrasound guidance is important for percutaneous aspiration and drainage of the gallbladder.[18, 19] The indications for percutaneous cholecystostomy include: acute cholecystitis, gallbladder empyema, stone dissolution, cholangiography, and bile duct and gallbladder drainage. It is uncertain whether punctures should always be through the bare area of the gallbladder. We use Seldinger technique with the removable hub, single large guidewire system[27] (Fig. 7.7).

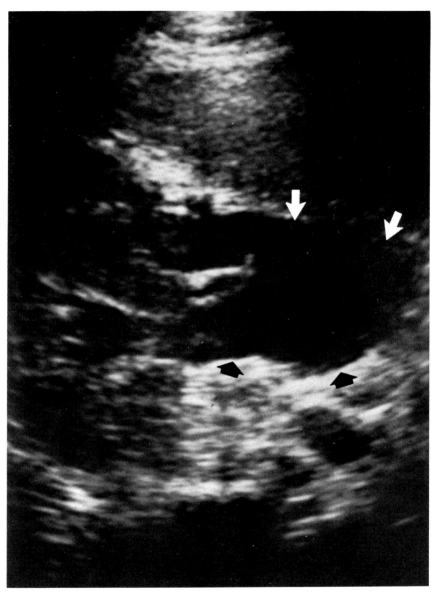

A

FIG. 7.6.   Ultrasound-guided percutaneous nephrostomy in a pregnant female: 25-year-old female with history of renal stone disease, 19 week gestation, and grade 2 right hydronephrosis. (A) Transverse sonogram showing dilatation of the collecting system (arrows). (*Figure continues.*)

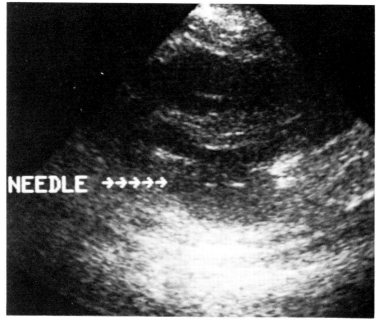

B

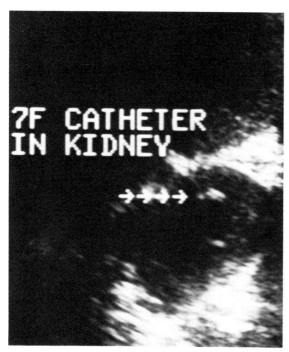

C

FIG. 7.6 (*Continued*). (B) 22 g needle in renal pelvis (longitudinal). (C) Coil of 7 Fr nephrostomy catheter in renal pelvis post procedure. Entire procedure was performed with ultrasound guidance.

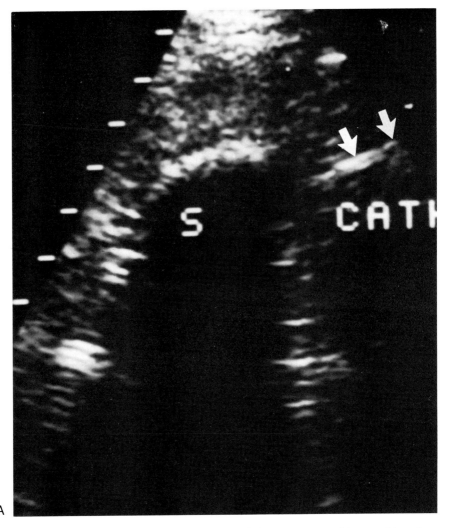

FIG. 7.7. Ultrasound-guided percutaneous cholecystostomy: 62-year-old male one week status post myocardial infarction presented with pain, fever, and leukocytosis secondary to hydropic gallbladder. (A) 7 Fr catheter (arrows) entering stone-filled gallbladder, s. *(Figure continues.)*

CONCLUSION

Ultrasound is an essential tool for the interventionalist. It has certain advantages over CT and fluoroscopy and clearly is preferrable in certain situations. A variety of procedures can be performed effectively using ultrasound, including puncture and drainage of virtually all organs in the abdomen. The easy accessibility, portable capability, and lack of radiation are distinctive benefits of ultrasound.

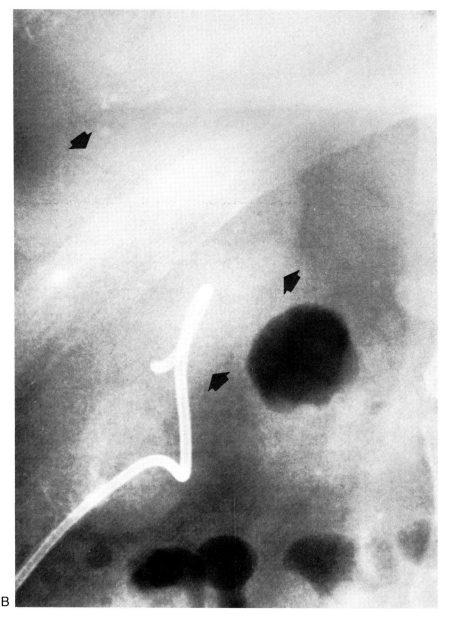

B

FIG. 7.7 (*Continued*). (B) Portable radiograph shows catheter in gallbladder (arrows) adjacent to air-filled duodenal bulb.

ACKNOWLEDGEMENT

Our thanks to Ms. Peggy Clark for preparation of the manuscript.

REFERENCES

1. vanSonnenberg E, Hajek P, Baker L, et al: Materials for MR-guided interventional procedures: laboratory and clinical experience. The Radiological Society of North America, 72nd Scientific Assembly and Meeting, Chicago, Illinois, November 30 to December 5, 1986

2. McGahan JP: Laboratory assessment of ultrasonic needle and catheter visualization. J Ultrasound Med 5:373, 1986

3. vanSonnenberg E, Mueller PR, Ferrucci JT Jr, et al: Sump catheter for percutaneous abscess and fluid drainage by trocar or seldinger technique. AJR 139:613, 1982

4. vanSonnenberg E, Polansky AD, Wittich GR, et al: The protective value of a guidewire with trocar puncture of fluid collections. AJR 145:831, 1985

5. vanSonnenberg E, Wittich GR, Schiffman HR, et al: Percutaneous drainage access: Simplified coaxial technique. Radiology 161:593, 1986

6. Olak J, Christou NV, Stein LA, et al: Operative versus percutaneous drainage of intra-abdominal abscesses. Arch Surg 121:141, 1986

7. Lee AS, vanSonnenberg E, Wittich GR, Casola G: Exchange of occluded catheters with transcatheter and pericatheter maneuvers. Radiology 163:273, 1987

8. vanSonnenberg E, Mueller PR, Schiffman HR, et al: Intrahepatic amebic abscesses: Indications for and results of percutaneous catheter drainage. Radiology 156:631 1985

9. vanSonnenberg E, Simeone JF, Mueller PR, et al: Sonographic appearance of hematoma in liver, spleen, and kidney: a clinical pathologic, and animal study. Radiol 147:507, 1983

10. Vogelzang RL, Tobin RS, Burstein S, et al: Transcatheter intracavitary fibrinolysis of infected extravascular hematomas. AJR 148:378, 1987

11. Vazquez JL, Thorsen MK, Dodds WJ, et al: Evaluation and treatment of intra-abdominal bilomas. AJR 144:933, 1985

12. Mueller PR, Ferrucci JT, Simeone JF, et al: Detection and drainage of bilomas: special considerations. AJR 140:714, 1983

13. Healy ME, Terg SS, Moss AA: Uriniferous pseudocyst: computed tomographic findings. AJR 153:757, 1984

14. Torres WE, Evert MB, Baumgartner BR, Bernardino ME: Percutaneous aspiration and drainage of pancreatic pseudocysts. AJR 147:1007, 1986

15. vanSonnenberg E, Wittich GR, Casola G, et al: Complicated pancreatic inflammatory disease: diagnostic and therapeutic role of interventional radiology. Radiology 155:335, 1985

16. Goodwin WE, Casey WC, Woolf W: Percutaneous trocar (needle) nephrostomy in hydronephrosis. JAMA 157:891, 1955

17. vanSonnenberg E, Lee AS, Wing VW, et al: Removable hub needle system for coaxial biopsy of small and difficult lesions. Radiology 152:226, 1984

18. McGahan JP, Walter JP: Diagnostic percutaneous aspiration of the gallbladder. Radiology 155:619, 1985

19. vanSonnenberg E, Wittich GR, Casola G, et al: Diagnostic and therapeutic percutaneous gallbladder procedures. Radiology 160:23, 1986

8 Gastrointestinal Duplex Doppler Ultrasound

KENNETH J. W. TAYLOR

Duplex Doppler ultrasound scanning has numerous applications in gastroenterology. Although many of these have already been described and are in clinical use, many others are only now becoming apparent. In attempting to review the practical applications of Doppler to the study of gastrointestinal physiology and pathology, it is helpful to consider the kinds of information which may be provided by this modality.

APPLICATIONS OF DOPPLER ULTRASOUND

Presence of Flow

This is the most simplistic and yet probably the most clinically valuable application for Doppler scanning. There are numerous clinical occasions on which it is important to know whether there has been arterial occlusion or venous thrombosis. The ability to obtain this information economically, noninvasively, and even portably in the intensive care unit is extraordinarily valuable.[1, 2]

Direction of Flow

Doppler is capable of demonstrating direction of flow. This may be helpful occasionally in demonstrating reversed flow in the portal vein or flow towards a patent shunt.

Flow Disturbance

Flow disturbance in the abdomen may occur as a result of atheroma, or aneurysmal dilatation producing turbulence. Atheroma or fibromuscular hyperplasia may produce a stenosis, resulting in a high velocity jet followed by distal turbulence. The recognition of these hemodynamic disturbances allows noninvasive diagnosis of the vascular abnormality.

Tissue Characterization

Tissue characterization is an intriguing area for current and future research and clinical application. Doppler is capable of characterizing tissue because of the specific perfusion patterns which are characteristic of some tissues or states of activity of the tissue. The vascular morphology and flow characteristics as demonstrated by angiography usually allow the nature of a structure to be recognized, as for example, cavernous transformation of the portal vein. In an analogous way, the demonstration of characteristic portal venous flow in a structure allows the same diagnosis to be made using noninvasive Doppler ultrasound.[3] In another example, hepatocellular carcinomas have a characteristic vascular appearance when demonstrated on angiography.[4] The same characteristics, namely arterioportal shunting, permit the noninvasive diagnosis of this malignancy by Doppler scanning.[5] A further example is the characteristic turbulent arterial flow occurring in pseudoaneurysms of the peripancreatic arteries.[6] It seems highly probable that functional tumors of the pancreas will give rise to typical flow characteristics similar to those now seen in functioning tumors of other organs.

Doppler Waveform Analysis

The Doppler time-velocity spectrum is related predominantly to the impedance of the receiving vasculature. This has found great application in the documentation of pathologic change, (e.g., in the rejecting renal transplant) or to indicate physiologic change (e.g., in the functioning ovary). In gastrointestinal (GI) applications, the technique can be used to evaluate physiologic changes such as the increased blood flow to the splanchnic circulation following a meal.[8, 9]

Measurement of Absolute Blood Flow

Many attempts have been made to measure flow in the normal portal vein and also in pathophysiologic disturbances associated with portal hypertension.[10] Although potentially of considerable value, few techniques described to date have been sufficiently accurate to be of clinical use. Nevertheless, the technique could be used to measure change in flow as a result of medication or surgery and may yet prove to be of considerable clinical interest.

   With such an overview in mind, the clinical applications of duplex Doppler scanning in GI disease can be reviewed. The technique and normal waveforms are first considered.

TECHNIQUE

A most important initial consideration is the acquisition of appropriate equipment. Many of the duplex Doppler machines were originally developed for use in cardiac applications. In the heart and great vessels, large volumes of blood are moving at high velocities giving rise to high amplitude and high Doppler shifted frequencies. Sensitivity of the Doppler equipment is therefore not an important issue. This holds true for equipment designed primarily for carotid work as well. However, the vessels with which we are concerned in the abdomen are often relatively small with a relatively low velocity and flow. Thus, a highly sensitive duplex Doppler device is mandatory. As a general rule, if the equipment is adequate for deep abdominal applications, it should be easily possible to detect parenchymal flow in numerous sites from invisible vessels within the liver and kidney.

A variety of types of scanners with different scanning geometry are available and are listed below.

Linear Array With an Off-Set Doppler Signal

A linear array has the advantage of simultaneous Doppler and image acquisition. It is one of the few commercially available machines in which the Doppler angle is optimal so that quantitation of flow is possible. Its major disadvantage is the relatively large size of the transducer and the difficulty in using this for an intercostal approach. Although it is adequate for lean individuals, obese patients and those with high livers require a sector scanner.

Sector Phased Array

Sector phased arrays also allow simultaneous imaging and Doppler acquisition. Unfortunately, many of these machines have a suboptimal image, especially in obese patients. It should be appreciated that simultaneous imaging and Doppler is not without a price as there is always some degradation of the image and/or the Doppler signal when there is time-sharing.

Mechanical Sector Scanner

Mechanical sector scanners have the disadvantage that imaging and Doppler acquisition are not simultaneous. With practice however, any such disadvantage may be easily overcome by experience. The quality of the Doppler signal is optimal and the image is good. The sector format also permits good access to the intercostal spaces. For these reasons, this is the instrumentation that has been utilized by the author.

For all adult abdominal work, a 3 MHz frequency is used both for imaging and for Doppler acquisition. The Food and Drug Administration (FDA) has shown concern that the output of Doppler devices has gradually increased and that some of them now have outputs approaching 1 W/cm.^{2} Concern is focused mainly on applications in obstetrics/gynecology. Nevertheless, it is clearly prudent to minimize the dosage in all patients and especially in those who might be pregnant.

Some of these machines start up at maximum power. Therefore, we routinely reduce the power output initially to 10 percent of maximum. The Doppler gain can then be increased until noise appears and then reduced to remove the noise. Once the vessel of interest is imaged, the Doppler cursor is aligned with the vessel, preferably at an angle between 30 and 60 degrees. In some vessels, such as the portal vein, this may not be possible, but it will still be easy to determine patency of the vessel even if the angle of attack is suboptimal. The optimal signal-to-noise ratio is usually attained with a sample volume of approximately 3 mm. Wall filters can be very high on machines designed for cardiac use (as high as 1600 Hz). For abdominal applications however, the lowest filter possible is used (50 to 100 Hz) since a high filter, as used in cardiac applications, can remove all evidence of flow from these low velocity abdominal vessels.

As each vessel of interest is investigated by placing the sample volume within the vessel lumen, we document both the image and the Doppler time-velocity spectrum. These are recorded as a horizontal pair of multiformat images so that the vessel of insonation and its waveform are documented together.

NORMAL WAVEFORMS

The normal waveforms are shown schematically in montages in Figures 8.1 and 8.2. The portal venous system demonstrates a very characteristic flow, which is found also in the splenic and superior mesenteric veins.[1] This consists of a low, rumbling flow with respiratory variation, at least in adults (Fig. 8.1E). This respiratory variation depends upon the changes in splanchnic outflow into the hepatic veins.[11] Increased resistance to flow occurs during inspiration in the hepatic bed due to the mechanical collapse of the intrahepatic vessels. This leads to decreased splanchnic flow on inspiration and increased splanchnic flow during expiration. The reduction or loss of this normal respiratory variation is a useful sign of portal hypertension, which will be discussed later.

The portal venous flow should be compared with the flow characteristics found in the inferior vena cava and hepatic veins (Figs. 8.1A and 8.1C). Here, complex waveforms are seen resulting from the combination of respiratory pressure changes on the low pressure systemic veins and the superimposed changes due to regurgitation from the right atrium during atrial systole. The resulting spectrum is a complex triphasic waveform.

The arterial waveforms show considerable diversity depending upon the size of the vessel and the impedance of the receiving vasculature (Fig. 8.2). The aortic waveform shows a clear window under the time-velocity spectrum

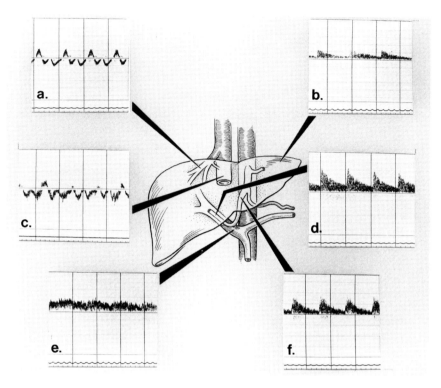

FIG. 8.1.   Montage to show waveforms in the perihepatic vasculature: (A) hepatic veins (B) parenchymal arterial flow (C) inferior vena cava waveform (D) main hepatic artery (E) portal vein (F) common hepatic artery. (Taylor KJW, Burns PN, Woodcock JP, Wells PNT: Blood flow in deep abdominal and pelvic vessels; ultrasonic pulsed-Doppler analysis. Radiology 154:487, 1985.)

(Fig. 8.2B). This implies the presence of a square wavefront (plug flow) indicating that all the red cells are moving at the same velocity at any one instant in time. Lower down in the aorta, a reversed component in diastole becomes apparent due to a reflected wave from the high impedance of the legs at rest. This maintains flow to the kidneys during diastole. Flow below the zero line, as, for example, in the left gastric artery (Fig. 8.2C), implies flow away from the transducer. The splenic artery is typically tortuous and this is reflected in the waveform, which is irregular and contains all frequencies from zero to the maximum (Fig. 8.2E). The very low flow in the gastroduodenal artery (Fig. 8.2F) should be compared with the very high velocities seen in most pancreatic tumors (see section on Doppler detection of neovascularity). The flow in the superior mesenteric artery (SMA) varies with sampling position and physiologic state. The waveform is more turbulent close to its origin (Fig. 8.2H) than more distally (Fig. 8.2G). Attempts to measure absolute blood flow in the SMA should be made more distally. The waveform also

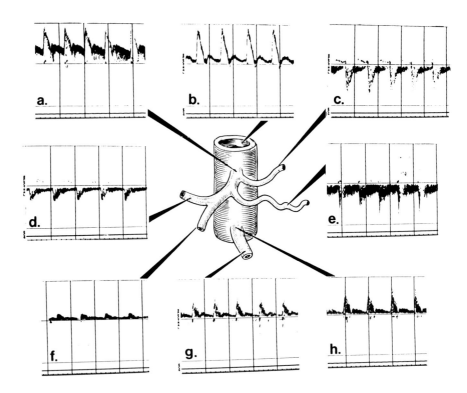

FIG. 8.2. Montage to show arterial waveforms in upper abdominal aortic branches. (A) celiac trunk (B) upper aorta (C) left gastric artery (D) main hepatic artery (E) splenic artery (F) gastroduodenal artery (G) distal superior mesenteric artery (H) proximal superior mesenteric artery. (Taylor KJW, Burns PN, Woodcock JP, Wells PNT: Blood flow in deep abdominal and pelvic vessels; ultrasonic pulsed-Doppler analysis. Radiology 154:487, 1985.)

varies with the physiologic state of the tissue. Thus, the relatively high impedance signal, (low diastolic flow), seen in the superior mesenteric artery after fasting, changes to a low impedance signal with rather marked diastolic flow after feeding. It is important to note that the hepatic artery and the divisions of the hepatic artery, down to the invisible arterial branches, should be easily detectable in numerous areas within the liver parenchyma (Fig. 8.1B). Thus, the diagnosis of hepatic arterial occlusion does not rely on the demonstration of the lack of flow in the main hepatic artery alone, but can be assessed from any area of the liver parenchyma.

ASSESSMENT OF ARTERIAL PERFUSION

Continuous wave (CW) Doppler scanning has been used successfully to detect viability of the gut intraoperatively.[12] When resection of the gut is necessary to excise a segment of gangrenous bowel, there may be difficulty in assessing the level at which the bowel becomes viable. By demonstrating the presence of arterial perfusion, Doppler indicates viability.

Doppler scanning may occasionally be useful in the recognition of mesenteric occlusion. However, while perfusion in the superior mesenteric artery (SMA) can be assessed in the vast majority of patients, the inferior mesenteric artery is less amenable to examination. However, the SMA is much more important in terms of the viability of the gut. Doppler scanning provides a potential method for assessing mesenteric ischemia. The normal response to a standard test meal has been documented (see section on quantitation of flow). The same test can be repeated on patients with recurrent, diffuse, abdominal pain and the adequacy of flow in the SMA thereby assessed.

Duplex Doppler scanning is invaluable for assessing the adequacy of the hepatic arterial anastamosis in recipients of liver orthografts[2] (Fig. 8.3). The overall incidence of arterial occlusion in liver transplants is 11 percent. Nevertheless, in children and in patients with difficult arterial anastamoses this incidence may be as high as 23 percent. The liver orthograft is deprived of any collateral blood supply, so that hepatic arterial occlusion is of very serious consequence. In adults it invariably leads to liver necrosis and death. It seems that some children may survive hepatic arterial occlusion, but a majority will require retransplantation.

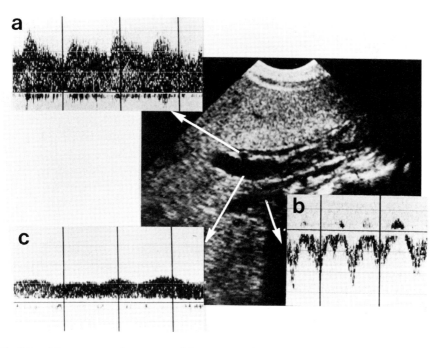

FIG. 8.3. Montage to show normal hepatic perfusion in liver orthograft. (A) right hepatic artery passing between the portal vein and the common duct (B) inferior vena cava (C) portal vein. (Taylor KJW, Morse SS, Weltin GG, et al: Liver transplant recipients; portable duplex US with correlative angiography. Radiology 159:357, 1986.)

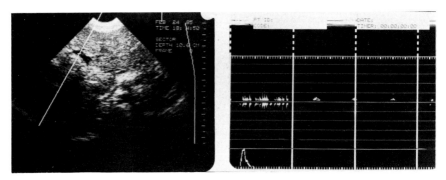

FIG. 8.4.   Acute hepatic arterial occlusion after liver transplantation. Timely diagnosis allowed successful reanastomosis. (Taylor KJW, Morse SS, Weltin GG, et al: Liver transplant recipients: portable duplex US with correlative angiography. Radiology 159:357, 1986.)

In our small series of patients with completed liver transplantation, hepatic arterial occlusion occurred on one occasion (Fig. 8.4). Such patients are invariably extraordinarily ill, and a portable evaluation in the intensive care unit is valuable. It should be stressed that hepatic arterial perfusion should be easily demonstrated in the main hepatic artery, in both left and right hepatic branches, and in numerous positions throughout the liver parenchyma.

In a large series of liver transplants reported from Pittsburgh, most of these patients did not have the benefit of Doppler scanning. One hundred-four angiograms were performed in 87 recipients of liver orthografts and 70 percent of these angiograms were abnormal.[13] Hepatic arterial occlusion occurred in 42 percent of 50 orthografts in children. Seventy-six percent of these children required retransplantation. Twelve percent of liver transplants in adults showed hepatic arterial occlusion and all required retransplantation. The experience of these authors demonstrates the need for repeated evaluation of arterial perfusion and our work shows that Doppler scanning can be used successfully, avoiding the need for repeated angiography.

EVALUATION OF PSEUDOANEURYSMS

Peripancreatic pseudoaneurysms are well documented complications of chronic pancreatitis, occurring particularly in alcoholics.[6] They occur as a result of arterial wall involvement in the autolytic process of the pancreatic phlegmon, and its organization to form a pseudocyst. Pseudoaneurysms may leak or rupture into the gut, producing repeated GI bleeding, or occasionally into the biliary system, producing hemobilia. The possibility of a leaking aneurysm should be considered in any patient with persistent anemia and evidence of GI bleeding during recovery from pancreatitis. These patients are difficult to diagnose because GI bleeding in alcoholics is frequently the result of bleeding from other sites, including esophageal varices, alcoholic

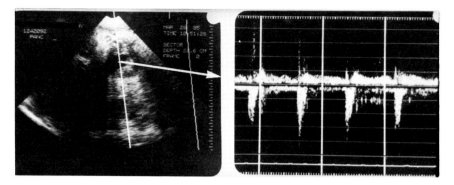

FIG. 8.5.   A complex pancreatic mass with a cystic center is seen. Doppler examination of this cystic area demonstrated turbulent arterial flow making the diagnosis of a pseudocyst of a peripancreatic artery. (Falkoff GE, Taylor KJW, Morse S: Hepatic artery pseudoaneurysm: diagnosis with real-time and pulsed Doppler ultrasound. Radiology 158:55, 1986.)

gastritis or peptic ulceration. This diagnosis is difficult to make; in one series reported in the literature, six of eleven patients had undergone bowel resection without preventing further episodes of GI bleeding.[14]

Figure 8.5 shows a pancreatic mass considered, in the light of the patient's clinical history, to be chronic pancreatitis. The center of this mass displays

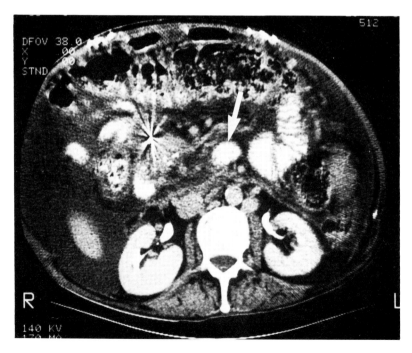

FIG. 8.6.   CT showing highly vascular center of pancreatic mass (arrow).

a fluid consistency which was initially assumed to be a pseudocyst. A Doppler examination of this fluid-filled center demonstrated a turbulent arterial flow. On the basis of the Doppler findings alone, the diagnosis of a pseudoaneurysm was made. This is a good example of tissue characterization and the unique information about perfusion which led to the realization of the true nature of this cystic mass. The diagnosis was confirmed by CT (Fig. 8.6). However, the definitive test here was angiography, which demonstrated a pseudoaneurysm derived from the replaced right hepatic artery and success-

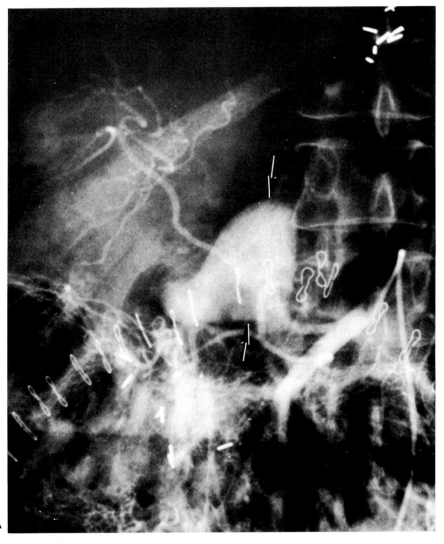

A

FIG. 8.7. (A) Angiogram demonstrating pseudoaneurysm arising from a replaced hepatic artery (arrows) (*Figure continues.*)

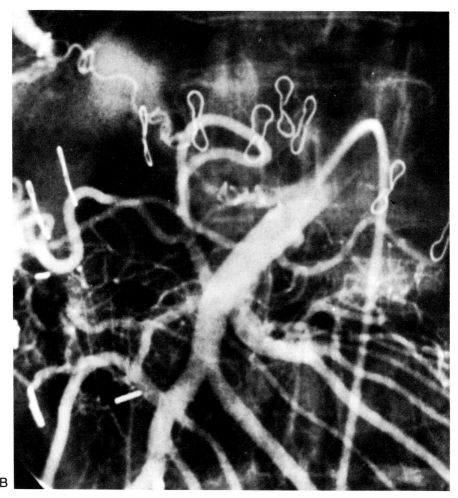

FIG. 8.7 *(Continued)*. (B) Angiogram showing successful embolization of pseudo-aneurysm. (Falkoff GE, Taylor KJW, Morse S: Hepatic artery pseudoaneurysm: diagnosis with real-time and pulsed Doppler ultrasound. Radiology 158:55, 1986.)

ful embolization was performed (Fig. 8.7). The patient has suffered no further episodes of GI bleeding.

PORTAL VEIN EVALUATION

Concern about the patency of the portal vein is a frequent clinical problem. In newborn special care units, especially in infants who have had umbilical catheters, the possibility of portal venous thrombosis is often raised, particularly in infants with ascites of unknown origin. It is extremely valuable in such infants to be able to exclude portal venous thrombosis, hepatic venous thrombosis, and caval thrombosis. Portal venous thrombosis is also common in cirrhotics who present with sudden decompensation of their cirrhosis and exacerbation of ascites.

Other patients with a propensity to portal venous thrombosis are recipients of liver transplants. In our series of twelve patients, we found two patients with portal venous thrombosis and two with portal vein stenosis.[2] Here, Doppler scanning can be most helpful, especially in acute venous thrombosis. Figure 8.8 demonstrates the left portal vein, which appears patent, and yet Doppler scanning correctly indicates the absence of flow. In a large series of liver transplants reported from Pittsburgh, portal vein thrombosis or stenosis was found in 13 percent of 87 patients.[13] Portal vein stenosis can be diagnosed by duplex Doppler ultrasound[2] (Fig. 8.9). The criteria for diagnosis are similar to those utilized for carotid artery stenosis. The waveform before the stenosis is normal. At the stenosis, there is a high velocity jet which subsequently gives rise to vortices and eddy currents. These spin off and give rise to a disrupted waveform and to flow in both directions. In our one surviving patient with portal vein stenosis, the condition has been stable over a two year period. Thus, although angiography was originally performed to confirm the diagnosis, subsequently duplex Doppler ultrasound scans alone have been performed to exclude progression.

A further entity which can be diagnosed by duplex technique is cavernous transformation of the portal vein[3] (Fig. 8.10). Portal venous thrombosis may occurr as a result of sepsis of the umbilical vein neonatally, intra-abdominal infection leading to pylephlebitis and thrombosis, and pancreatitis or any cause of hemo-concentration. It may be followed by the development of collateral vessels around the thrombosed portal vein. This was formerly

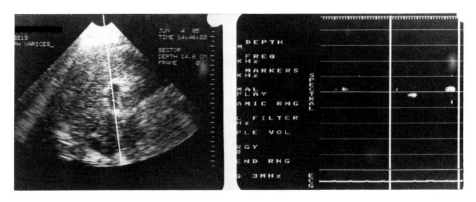

FIG. 8.8. Portal vein thrombosis. The left portal vein is seen at the porta hepatis and a Doppler cursor within it demonstrates only transmitted cardiac pulsation from movement of the whole liver. There is no evidence of normal portal venous flow. (Taylor KJW, Morse SS, Weltin GG, et al: Liver transplant recipients; portable duplex US with correlative angiography. Radiology 159:357, 1986.)

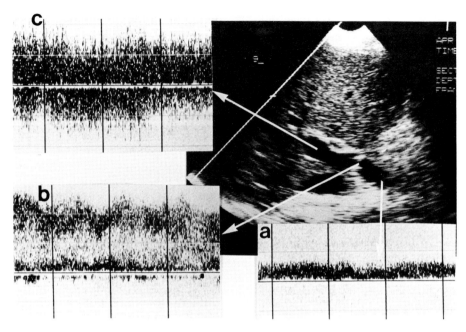

FIG. 8.9. Portal venous stenosis. A constriction is seen in the portal vein at the site of the anastomosis. (A) Flow before the stenosis is of normal low velocity, (B) flow at the stenosis shows a high velocity jet, (C) flow beyond the stenosis shows an irregular waveform with flow in both directions (above and below the zero line), consistent with eddy currents. (Taylor KJW, Morse SS, Weltin GG, et al: Liver transplant recipients; portable duplex US with correlative angiography. Radiology 159:357, 1986.)

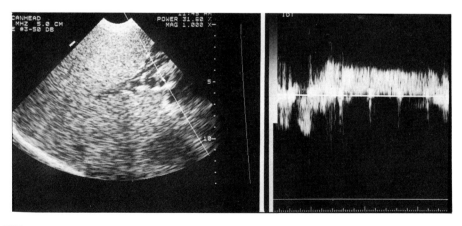

FIG. 8.10. Cavernous transformation of the portal vein. Longitudinal sections of the porta hepatis show multiple serpiginous channels replacing the normal portal vein. Doppler examination of these demonstrates portal venous flow.

thought to be a primary angiomatous malformation, but is now considered to be due to the formation of collateral vessels. It occurs in approximately one-third of patients after portal vein thrombosis. Others may open up portosystemic anastomoses, such as esophageal varices, which may be more life threatening. The classical appearance of cavernous transformation is the combination of serpiginous vessels and the thrombosed portal vein. Ultrasound imaging alone may suffice to suggest the diagnosis. However, the demonstration of portal venous flow within these vessels removes any uncertainty. In other patients, larger multicystic masses may be seen and the additional use of Doppler scanning, to allow tissue characterization of the nature of the mass, is essential.

The observation of air in the portal vein is virtually always of serious prognostic significance and indicates the need for laparotomy.[15] We observed this in one patient with a liver transplant in whom surgery revealed a large mesenteric abscess with bowel necrosis.[2] It has been most frequently documented, however, in patients with necrotizing enterocolitis (NEC) (Fig. 8.11). In this condition, it appears that the presence of air in the portal vein may result in an earlier diagnosis of NEC than the presence of intestinal pneumatosis, which is a later manifestation. The amplitude of the Doppler shifted signal from blood within the portal vein is relatively small. The huge impedance mismatch between blood and air implies that a much larger amplitude signal is obtained from bubbles of air within the portal vein. In theory, one would expect Doppler to be more sensitive than imaging for the detection of microbubbles, but this is yet to be proven. Certainly, Doppler signals from air in the portal vein are of large amplitude, which overwhelm the electrical circuits and produce the spikes noted in Figure 8.11.

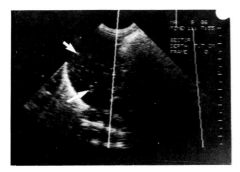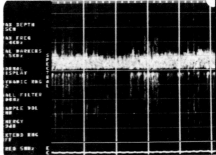

FIG. 8.11. Necrotising enterocolitis (NEC). Scans of the liver demonstrate multiple high level echoes through the liver parenchyma consistent with air in the portal venous radicles (arrowed). Examination of the Doppler spectrum in the portal vein demonstrates multiple high amplitude spikes due to air bubbles passing up the portal vein. (Taylor KJW, Burns PN, Wells PNT (eds): Doppler Ultrasound in Diagnostic Imaging. Raven Press, New York, 1987.)

PORTAL HYPERTENSION

The sonographic findings in portal hypertension (Table 8.1) allow for a presumptive diagnosis based upon ultrasonic imaging alone.[16] The portal vein shows a very low velocity flow. Some of these findings, such as a large patent para-umbilical vein, allow for a definitive diagnosis.[17–19] However, most of these signs are relative and must be assessed together. Furthermore, the Doppler scanning demonstration of typical hypertensive portal venous flow in varices adds certainty to the diagnosis. Portal hypertension is most frequently due to cirrhosis and obstruction of the portal venous radicals by fibrosis and the disorganized architecture of regenerating nodules. Less frequently, it may result from portal venous thrombosis or other causes of portal venous obstruction. The end result of any of these conditions is an increased pressure in the splanchnic venous system and the formation of spontaneous porto-systemic anastomoses (Fig. 8.12). These are conventionally described in four anatomic sites, although it should be appreciated that spontaneous porto-systemic anastamoses may occur at any anatomic site where the portal and systemic veins are in close proximity. Thus, in addition to the well described sites, one should add the retroperitoneum and the body wall. Here spontaneous shunting can occur between the portal system and the systemic veins such as the renal veins or lumbar veins. The four groups of collateral vessels conventionally described are mentioned below.

TABLE 8.1. Sonographic findings in portal hypertension

Dilated portal vein

Dilated splenic and superior mesenteric veins (SMV)

Patent paraumbilical vein

Varices

Splenomegaly with dilated splenic radicles

Diminished response to respiration in splenic vein
  and SMV

Dilated hepatic and splenic arteries

Ascites

Small liver with irregular surface or large liver
  with abnormal texture

(Reprinted with permission from DiCandio G, Campatelli A, Mosca F, et al: Ultrasound detection of unusual spontaneous portosystemic shunts associated with uncomplicated portal hypertension. J Ultrasound Med 4:297. Copyright 1985 by the American Institute of Ultrasound in Medicine.)

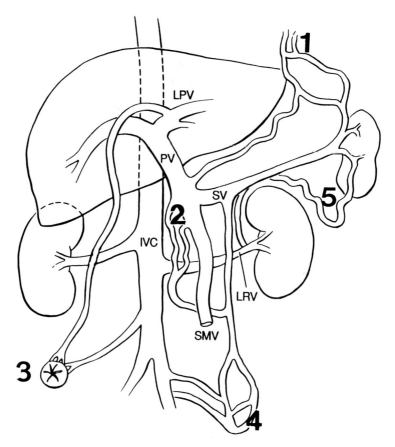

FIG. 8.12. Schema to show sites of spontaneous portosystemic anastomoses. (1) Clinically, the most important site is the lower esophageal region. Varices are derived from between the esophageal branches of the left gastric vein and the esophageal branches of the azygos and hemiazygos veins. (2) Numerous retroperitoneal anastomoses may develop between the mesenteric veins and the veins of the body wall such as the lumbar veins. (3) A patent paraumbilical vein may form a large communication between the left portal vein, *LPV*, and the veins of the anterior abdominal wall such as the epigastric veins around the umbilicus. (4) Hemorrhoidal anastomoses may form between the superior, middle and inferior rectal veins. (5) Spontaneous spleno-renal shunts may also develop. (*IVC* = inferior vena cava, *PV* = portal vein, *SV* = splenic vein, *SMV* = superior mesenteric vein, *LRV* = left renal vein.) (Taylor KJW, Burns PN, Wells PNT (eds): Doppler Ultrasound in Diagnostic Imaging. Raven Press, New York, 1987.)

Gastroesophageal Region

Lower esophageal varices occur where the esophageal branches of the left gastric vein (coronary vein) form anastomoses with branches of the azygos and hemiazygos veins in the submucosa of the lower esophagus.[19] The resulting esophageal varices may rupture and are the most frequent cause of death in patients with portal hypertension.

Para-umbilical Vein

This appears as a continuation of the left portal vein and extends down the anterior abdominal wall to the umbilicus. Here, anastomoses, known as the caput medusa, occur with the epigastric veins, and varices may become visible around the umbilicus.

The para-umbilical vein can be seen clearly in many patients and the direction of flow established by concommitant pulsed Doppler scanning (Fig. 8.13). It should be noted that a small vessel extending through the ligament teres down the anterior abdominal wall to the umbilicus may occur in normal patients. Saddekni et al. reviewed 12 patients with a vessel in the ligament teres.[20] In ten patients, the vein exceeded 3 mm in diameter. All of these had liver disease, six with esophageal varices. Three of ten normal controls also had a patent vessel but this was less than 3 mm in diameter. However, it appears that the observation of a para-umbilical vein exceeding 3 mm in diameter is highly suggestive of portal hypertension.

Hemorrhoidal Anastomoses

These anastomoses are between the superior and middle hemorrhoidal veins. They derive from the inferior mesenteric vein and the inferior hemorrhoidal vein and drain into the internal iliac vein. This is a rare cause for hemorrhoids.

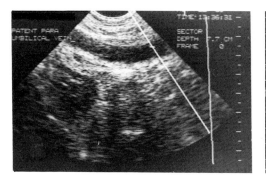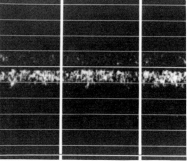

FIG. 8.13. Patent paraumbilical vein. A large vessel measuring approximately 8 mm is seen passing down the anterior abdominal wall. A Doppler cursor within this demonstrates continuous portal venous flow typical of the portal hypertensive state. (Taylor KJW, Burns PN, Wells PNT (eds): Doppler Ultrasound in Diagnostic Imaging. Raven Press, New York, 1987.)

Retroperitoneal Anastomoses

Doppler aids in the diagnosis of varices by allowing reliable recognition of the nature of these small vessels. Vessels may be seen in the lesser omentum and thicken it. This has been described as a sign of portal hypertension in children.[21] Numerous small vessels are frequently seen around the pancreas in patients with portal hypertension. Again, Doppler is helpful in determining whether or not these vessels are varices. (Fig. 8.14).

Respiratory Variation

Bolondi et al. reported that the normal portal venous branches of the superior mesenteric vein and the splenic vein exhibited diminished respiratory variation in portal hypertension.[11] Normal respiratory variation is due to collapse of the intrahepatic vessels on inspiration. In the hypertensive portal venous system, this respiratory variation may be entirely lost. Bolondi et al. reported a sensitivity of 80 percent and a specificity of 100 percent for this sign of portal hypertension.[11]

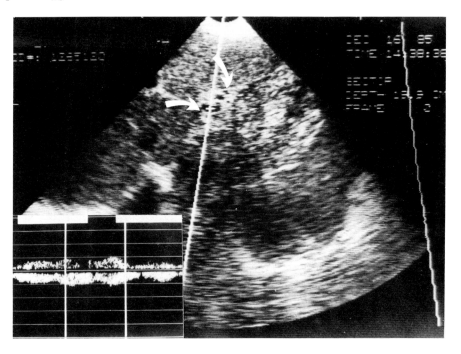

FIG. 8.14. Transverse section of the liver demonstrating the lesser omentum (arrows) with multiple small anechoic channels within it. Doppler demonstrates that these are portal venous radicles, thereby identifying these channels as varices. (Taylor KJW, Burns PN, Wells PNT (eds): Doppler Ultrasound in Diagnostic Imaging. Raven Press, New York, 1987.)

EVALUATION OF PORTOSYSTEMIC SHUNTS

Surgical portosystemic shunts are created to decompress the hypertensive portal venous system, and thereby decrease the flow through life-threatening esophageal varices which are spontaneous portosystemic shunts. These major surgical procedures are tending to be used less due to the increasing success of sclerotherapy.

Methods currently available for assessing the patency of shunts include duplex sonography, dynamic computerized tomography, magnetic resonance imaging and angiography. The success of duplex scanning depends much upon the body habitus of the patient, the type of shunt, and the experience of the operator. Obese patients with extensive postoperative scarring certainly challenge the sonographer. The most valuable technique for visualizing these shunts is firm pressure on the gas-filled intestine, which deflects intestinal gas from the ultrasound beam path. The sonographer must be completely aware of the type of shunt that has been effected so that the relevant anatomy is immediately appreciated.

The types of shunts that are performed include an end-to-side portocaval shunt, a side-to-side portocaval shunt, a proximal splenorenal, a distal splenorenal, and a mesocaval shunt. The portocaval shunts are usually easily visualized by duplex techniques, using either the liver or the gallbladder as an acoustic window (Fig. 8.15). Splenorenal shunts may be difficult in obese patients or if the spleen has been removed during the procedure. Nevertheless, most of these can be visualized after firm pressure on the abdomen to displace air within the gut, and providing that the examiner knows the anatomy of the anastomosis, since the surrounding landmarks may not be optimally imaged (Fig. 8.16). Mesocaval shunts are rarely performed at our institution.

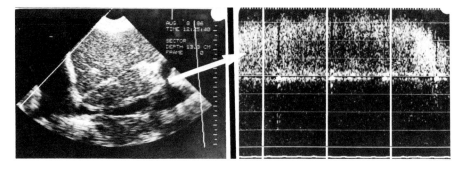

FIG. 8.15. Patent end-to-side portocaval shunt. This parasagittal section shows the end of the portal vein anastomosed to the inferior vena cava. The inferior vena cava at this site shows an enlargement, a so-called pseudoaneurysm, due to the commingling of flow. Doppler examination at the ostium demonstrates high velocity flow through the shunt. (Taylor KJW, Burns PN, Wells PNT (eds): Doppler Ultrasound in Diagnostic Imaging. Raven Press, New York, 1987.)

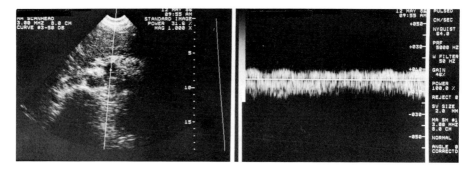

FIG. 8.16. Patent splenorenal shunt. A large communication is seen between the splenic and left renal veins situated just to the left of the SMA. A Doppler cursor in this region shows patency of the shunt. (Taylor KJW, Burns PN, Wells PNT (eds): Doppler Ultrasound in Diagnostic Imaging. Raven Press, New York, 1987.)

DETECTION OF OTHER VENOUS THROMBOSES

The reliable exclusion of venous thrombosis by a noninvasive means in many other deep veins is useful and often precludes the need for other studies. Figure 8.17 shows a patient with a thrombosis of the superior mesenteric vein. In patients with deep vein thrombosis of the femoral veins (Fig. 8.18A), the patency of the iliac veins can be established by duplex scanning (Fig. 8.18B). The possibility of caval thrombosis is raised in patients presenting with ascites of unknown origin or in patients with bilateral pedal edema. It is extremely useful to be able to demonstrate normal caval flow in such patients or to be able to localize the extent of thrombosis (Fig. 8.19).

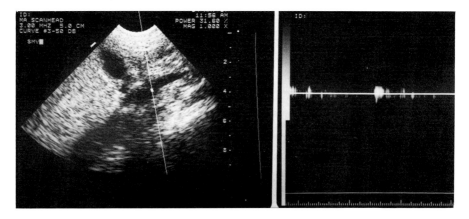

FIG. 8.17. Superior mesenteric venous thrombosis. This alcoholic patient presented with chronic pancreatitis and splenic vein thrombosis. The longitudinal section shows the SMV with no evidence of flow on the Doppler examination.

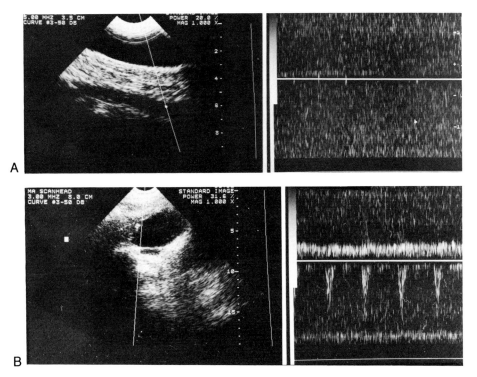

FIG. 8.18.   Deep venous thrombosis. (A) The femoral vein appears distended and pressure on it during real-time examination failed to obliterate the lumen, thereby suggesting thrombosis. Thrombosis was confirmed by the absence of flow on Doppler examination. (B) Examination of the iliac vessels in the same patient shows normal arterial and venous spectra. (Taylor KJW, Burns PN, Wells PNT (eds): Doppler Ultrasound in Diagnostic Imaging. Raven Press, New York, 1987.)

QUANTITATION OF FLOW

The estimation of flow using Doppler techniques is superficially simple. Flow is the product of the area of the vessel and the mean velocity of blood flowing within it.[10] The first moment of the Doppler shift frequency should provide an estimate of the centroid mean velocity. Ohnishi et al. stated quite incorrectly that the mean velocity cannot be estimated by Doppler and utilized the maximum velocity which is then reduced by an empirical factor to provide the mean velocity. For this to be valid, it must be assumed that the flow profile does not change under physiologic and pathologic conditions, and such an assumption is unwarranted. The normal portal vein is oval in cross-section, whereas the hypertensive portal vein is more circular. This change in shape in itself leads to profound changes in the blood flow profile. Then there are the respiratory variations in the portal venous velocity. These have been ignored by some investigators with estimations made only during inspi-

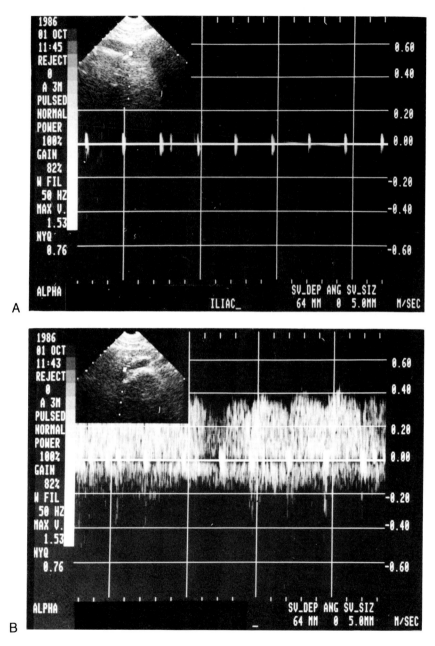

FIG. 8.19.   Caval thrombosis (A) A Doppler cursor in the lower inferior vena cava shows absence of normal flow indicating thrombosis. (B) There is brisk inflow into the cava at the level of the renal veins, showing that these are patent and that the cava is also patent above this level. (Taylor KJW, Burns PN, Wells PNT (eds): Doppler Ultrasound in Diagnostic Imaging. Raven Press, New York, 1987.)

ration. Even the area of a vessel is not necessarily easy to establish with accuracy. For example, the portal venous area varies with respiratory activity, whereas most arteries demonstrate a significant increase in area during systole. Finally, there are the difficulties associated with the angle of attack. For reasonably accurate determination of velocity, it is desirable that this angle be between 30 and 60 degrees. Angles exceeding 70 degrees involve the possibility of a substantial error. Linear scanners with an off-set Doppler transducer offer the possibility of a good angle, but the configuration of the transducer may be unusable on many obese abdomens. Using the mechanical sector scanners with an axial Doppler, the angle between the portal vein and the ultrasound beam is often in excess of 70 degrees.

The accuracy of estimates of flow is difficult to assess. Comparison with an in vitro measurement may show good correlation but the in vivo conditions are much more variable. Unfortunately, it is difficult, both in normals and in abnormals, to measure in vivo portal venous flow by Doppler scanning simultaneously with another method to obtain a good estimate of the accuracy of the estimation.

There is a further important point which may limit the utility of any technique for the measurement of portal venous flow. It is the amount of blood which bypasses the portal vein through esophageal varices which is most threatening to the patient's life. Thus, the flow through the portal vein is of limited interest. However, these considerations should not negate the use of the technique for comparative purposes. Even where inaccuracy exists in the estimation, it might be quite useful to compare flow estimates before and after therapy as, for example, when the patient is given propanolol.

Gill has demonstrated that portal venous flow can be accurately measured. He has achieved this by the use of specialized equipment, namely the Octoson.[22] In this equipment, any one of several transducers can be selected to obtain the Doppler data. The operator is able to select the transducer which is at the optimal angle (30 to 60°) in relation to the portal vein. Using such specialized equipment, Gill has achieved a systematic error of only six percent.

Quantitative measurements have also been made of waveform characteristics and absolute blood flow in the superior mesenteric artery.[8, 9, 23] Qamar, et al. quantitated time-velocity waveforms in 82 normal individuals using the pulsatility index (PI). In the fasting state, a high pulsatility of 3.5 ± 0.11 indicated vasoconstriction in the splanchnic circulation. In fifteen patients re-examined after a meal, the PI had decreased by 46 percent and this vasodilatation persisted for two hours. These authors also estimated absolute blood flow using the duplex technique to measure the luminal area and the mean velocity. At rest the blood flow in the SMA was 570 ml per minute and it doubled after a solid meal. Exercise reduced both the resting and the post-prandial increase in flow in the SMA. Aldoori, et al. also looked at flow in patients with the dumping syndrome following gastric surgery.[23] In these patients, the flow also doubled within five minutes of a standard meal, but the increased flow persisted to a greater extent than in the controls.

This led the authors to suggest that an abnormal distribution of splanchnic blood flow may contribute to the symptoms of the dumping syndrome. These examples show how duplex technology can be used to study both gastrointestinal physiology and pathophysiology.

DOPPLER DETECTION OF NEOVASCULARITY

Doppler detection of neovascularity has been reported in two large series of patients with carcinoma of the breast.[24, 25] In these experiments, continuous wave Doppler was used at a frequency of 9 to 10 MHz. The amplitude of the returned Doppler signal increases with the fourth power of the frequency so that reducing the frequency to 3 MHz for abdominal applications and the use of pulsed Doppler in addition reduces the sensitivity of the technique by a factor approaching 10^4 (i.e. 10,000). Despite these limitations, we have demonstrated Doppler signals in several tumors related to the GI tract.[5, 26] These have been found in recurrent tumor of the colon, (when accessible to the ultrasound beam) (Fig. 8.20) most pancreatic cancers, and in all hepatomas to date (Fig. 8.21).

We have investigated the Doppler signals in patients presenting with focal masses in the liver.[5] Of 72 patients, 15 proved to be hemangiomas by clinical follow-up. Seventeen proved to be hepatomas by biopsy and 40 were biopsy proven metastases. Of the hepatomas, two returned signals of 3 kHz and all the remaining tumors returned signals of 5 to 10 kHz. In contrast, the hemangiomas showed no evidence of abnormal flow. Of the metastases, approximately two-thirds demonstrated no signal and a third showed signals

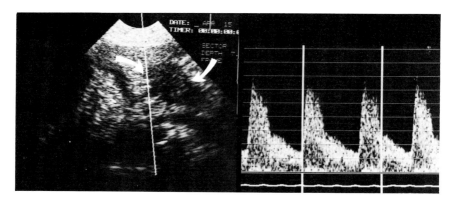

FIG. 8.20. Transverse section showing pancreas with an irregular mass contiguous with it (arrows). With the Doppler cursor situated at the periphery of this mass, an 6.5 kHz Doppler shift frequency was elicited. This corresponds to velocities in the region of 400 cm/s and is consistent with arteriovenous shunting around the growing edge of a tumor. Biopsy revealed recurrent tumor from a colonic carcinoma, adherent to the body of the pancreas.

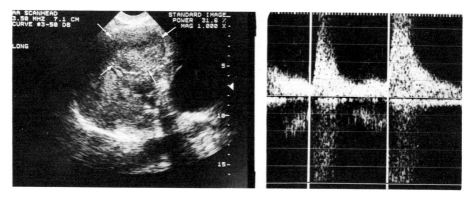

FIG. 8.21.   This parasagittal section shows a focal mass (arrows) in the porta hepatis producing biliary obstruction and which returns very high velocity signals exceeding 8 kHz. Note that aliasing has occurred. In over one hundred liver tumors examined to date, such high velocities have been obtained only in hepatomas and probably result from arterioportal shunts.

up to a maximum of 4 kHz. This method then provides a complete differentiation between hepatomas and hemangiomas, both common causes for echogenic masses, particularly in cirrhotic patients. The cause for this major difference in vascularity is well documented in the pathologic and angiographic literature. In hemangiomas, there is slow flow of a small amount of blood into large cavernous spaces. Hence, the need for delayed CT scans and labeled red cell scans. These low velocities are filtered out by the wall filter. In contrast, a well recognized feature of hepatomas is arteriovenous or more specifically, arterioportal, shunting. This pressure gradient causes the static energy to be converted into kinetic energy, thereby giving rise to high velocity shunts. It is interesting to note that the vascular metastases were all echogenic, supporting the concept proposed by other authors that echogenicity was related to vascularity. This also suggests why the majority, approximately 95 percent of the hepatomas, are also echogenic.

These signals occur in many different tumor types and we have seen them in tumors of the kidney, pancreas, adrenal, and colon (Fig. 8.20). The detection of neovascularity may be quite useful, not only for diagnosis but also to investigate the effects of agents which modify this response. Continuous production of new vessels appears to be essential to the continued growth and spread of malignant tumors.

CONCLUSION

The addition of Doppler scanning to ultrasonic imaging of the abdomen is of great value in demonstrating the perfusion characteristics of organs and vessels. It is probably most useful in its most simplistic application, for the exclusion of arterial or venous occlusion. Nevertheless, new applications are becoming apparent, and the estimation of blood flow may be of considerable physiologic and pathophysiologic interest. Finally, the demonstration of neovascular flow in tumors may be quite helpful in patient management. This is especially true where a pancreatic cancer is concealed by surrounding pancreatitis and even multiple open biopsies at surgery may yield misleading results. Clearly, much more work needs to be performed. The addition of color flow imaging will simplify perception of flow, yet careful evaluation will be necessary to ensure that the sensitivity of the duplex technique is not sacrificed for the easier use of color. Duplex Doppler scanning remains heavily dependent upon operator skill, but in the coming era of an oversupply of physicians, this is most desirable.

ACKNOWLEDGEMENTS

I would like to thank Jill Scognamillo for secretarial assistance and Cheryl Wilcox for editing.

REFERENCES

1. Taylor KJW, Burns PN, Woodcock JP, Wells PNT: Blood flow in deep abdominal and pelvic vessels; Ultrasonic pulsed-Doppler analysis. Radiology 154:487, 1985
2. Taylor KJW, Morse SS, Weltin GG, et al: Liver transplant recipients; portable duplex US with correlative angiography. Radiology 159:357, 1986
3. Weltin G, Taylor KJW, Carter AR: Duplex Doppler: An aid in the diagnosis of cavernous transformation of the portal vein. AJR 44:999, 1984
4. Okuda K, Musha H, Yamasaki T, et al: Angiographic demonstration of intrahepatic arterioportal anastomoses in hepatocullular carcinoma. Radiology 122:53, 1977
5. Taylor KJW, Ramos I, Morse SS, et al: Focal liver masses: differential diagnosis with pulsed Doppler ultrasound; a useful predictor of hepatocellular carcinoma. Radiology 164:643, 1987.
6. Falkoff GE, Taylor KJW, Morse S: Hepatic artery pseudoaneurysm: diagnosis with real-time and pulsed Doppler ultrasound. Radiology 158:55, 1986
7. Taylor KJW, Burns PN: Duplex Doppler scanning in the pelvis and abdomen. Ultrasound Med Biol 11:643, 1985
8. Qamar MI, Read AE, Skidmore R, et al: Noninvasive assessment of the superior mesenteric artery blood flow in man. Gut 25:A546, 1984
9. Qamar MI, Read AE, Skidmore R, et al: Transcutaneous Doppler ultrasound measurement of superior mesenteric artery blood flow in man. Gut 27:100, 1986
10. Ohnishi K, Saito M, Koen H, et al: Pulsed Doppler flow as a criterion of portal venous velocity: comparison with cineangiographic measurements. Radiology 154:495, 1985
11. Bolondi L, Gandolfi L, Arienti, V, et al: Ultrasonography in the diagnosis of portal hypertension: diminished response of portal vessels to respiration. Radiology 142:167, 1985
12. Wright CB, Hobson RW: Prediction of intestinal viability using Doppler ultrasound techniques. Am J Surg 129:642, 1975
13. Wozney P, Zajko AB, Bron KM, et al: Vascular complications after liver transplantation: a 5 year experience. AJR 147:657, 1986
14. Bivens BA, Sachatello CR, Chuang VP, Brady P: Hemosuccus pancreatitis (hemoductal

pancreatitis): gastrointestinal hemorrhage due to rupture of splenic artery aneurysm into the pancreatic duct. Arch Surg 113:751, 1978

15. Traverso LW: Is hepatic portal venous gas an indicator for exploratory laparotomy? Arch Surg 16:936, 1981

16. Di Candio G, Campatelli A, Mosca F, et al: Ultrasound detection of unusual spontaneous portosystemic shunts associated with uncomplicated portal hypertension. J Ultrasound Med 4:297, 1978

17. Lafortune M, Constantin A, Breton G, et al: The recanalized umbilical vein in portal hypertension: A myth. AJR 144:549, 1985

18. Fakhry J, Gosink BB, Leopold GR: Recanalized umbilical vein due to portal vein occlusion: documentation by sonography. AJR 137:410, 1981

19. Aagaard J, Jensen LI, Sorensen TIA, et al: Recanalized umbilical vein in portal hypertension. AJR 139:1107, 1982

20. Saddekni S, Hutchinson DE, Cooperberg PL: The sonographically patent umbilical vein in portal hypertension. Radiology 145:441, 1982

21. Brunelle F, Alagille D, Pariente D, Chaumont P: An ultrasound study of portal hypertension in children. Ann Radiol (Paris) 24:121, 1981

22. Gill RW: Pulsed Doppler with B-mode imaging for quantitative blood flow measurement. Ultrasound Med Biol 5:223, 1979

23. Aldoori MI, Qamar MI, Read AE, Williamson RCN: Increased flow in the superior mesenteric artery in dumping syndrome. Br J Surg 72:389, 1985

24. Jellins J, Kossoff G, Boyd J, Reeve TS: The complementary role of Doppler to the B mode examination of the breast. J Ultrasound Med 10:29, 1983

25. Burns PN, Halliwell M, Webb AJ, et al: Ultrasonic Doppler studies of the breast. Ultrasound Med Biol 8:127, 1982

26. Taylor KJW, Ramos I, Carter D, et al: Correlation of Doppler US tumor signals with neovascular morphologic features. Radiology 166:57, 1988.

Index